The domestic cat:

the biology of its behaviour

Edited by

Dennis C. Turner

*Lecturer in Ethology and Wildlife Research
University of Zürich-Irchel, Switzerland*

and

Patrick Bateson, FRS

*Professor of Ethology, University of Cambridge
United Kingdom*

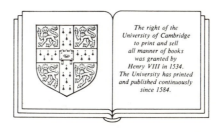

The right of the
University of Cambridge
to print and sell
all manner of books
was granted by
Henry VIII in 1534.
The University has printed
and published continuously
since 1584.

CAMBRIDGE UNIVERSITY PRESS
Cambridge
New York   Port Chester   Melbourne   Sydney

Published by the Press Syndicate of the University of Cambridge
The Pitt Building, Trumpington Street, Cambridge CB2 1RP
40 West 20th Street, New York, NY 10011, USA
10 Stamford Road, Oakleigh, Melbourne 3166, Australia

First published 1988
Reprinted 1989, 1990

Printed in Great Britain by the Bath Press

British Library cataloguing in publication data

Cats '86: the Behaviour and Ecology of the
Domestic Cat, conference : University of
Zürich-Irchel.
The Domestic Cat : the biology of its
behaviour.
1. Pets : Cats, behaviour
I. Title II. Turner, Dennis C. *1948–*   III. Bateson,
P.P.G. (Paul Patrick Gordon), *1938–*
636.8

Library of Congress cataloguing in publication data

The Domestic cat : the biology of its behaviour / edited by Dennis C.
Turner and Patrick Bateson.
    p.   cm.
Based on a symposium Cats '86, held at the University of Zürich-
Irchel, Switzerland, Sept. 1–3. 1986.
Bibliography: p.
Includes index.
1. Cats – Behavior. 2. Cats – Social aspects. I. Turner, Dennis
C., 1948– . II. Bateson, P. P. G. (Paul Patrick Gordon), 1938–
III. Cats '86 (1986 : University of Zürich-Irchel)
SF446.5.D65 1988
599.74'4280451 – dc 19   88–7346 CIP

ISBN 0 521 35447 1 hard covers
ISBN 0 521 35727 6 paperback

WD

Contents

List of contributors   vii
Preface and acknowledgements   ix

I Introduction
  1 Why the cat?   *Dennis C. Turner and Patrick Bateson*   3

II Development of young cats
  2 Behavioural development in the cat   *Paul Martin and Patrick Bateson*   9
  3 Factors influencing the mother–kitten relationship   *John M. Deag, Aubrey Manning and Candace E. Lawrence*   23
  4 Individuality in the domestic cat   *Michael Mendl and Robert Harcourt*   41

III Social life
  5 The tame and the wild – another Just-So Story?   *Paul Leyhausen*   57
  6 Cat society and the consequences of colony size   *G. Kerby and D. W. Macdonald*   67
  7 Spatial organisation and reproductive tactics in the domestic cat and other felids   *Olof Liberg and Mikael Sandell*   83
  8 The mating system of feral cats living in a group   *Eugenia Natoli and Emanuele De Vito*   99

IV Predatory behaviour
  9 Hunting behaviour of the domestic cat   *Dennis C. Turner and Othmar Meister*   111
  10 Diet of domestic cats and their impact on prey populations   *B. M. Fitzgerald*   123

V Cats and people
    11 The domestication and history of the cat   *James A. Serpell*   151
    12 The human–cat relationship   *Eileen B. Karsh and Dennis C. Turner*   159
    13 Practical aspects of research on cats   *Claudia Mertens and Rosemarie Schär*   179

VI Postscript
    14 Questions about cats   *Patrick Bateson and Dennis C. Turner*   193

    References   202
    Index   216

Contributors

Patrick Bateson, *Sub-Department of Animal Behaviour, University of Cambridge, Madingley, Cambridge CB3 8AA, UK*

John M. Deag, *Department of Zoology, University of Edinburgh, Kings Buildings, West Mains Road, Edinburgh EH9 3JT, Scotland, UK*

Emanuele De Vito, *Cattedra di Ecologia ed Etologia Animale, Dipartimento di Biologia Molecolare, Universitá di Roma, Via Lancisi no 29, 00100 Roma, Italy*

B. M. Fitzgerald, *Ecology Division, Department of Scientific and Industrial Research, Private Bag, Lower Hutt, New Zealand*

Robert Harcourt, *Sub-Department of Animal Behaviour, University of Cambridge, Madingley, Cambridge CB3 8AA, UK*

Eileen B. Karsh, *Department of Psychology, Temple University, Philadelphia, PA 19122, USA*

G. Kerby, *Department of Zoology, University of Oxford, South Parks Road, Oxford OX1 3PS, UK*

Candace E. Lawrence, *Department of Zoology, University of Edinburgh, Kings Buildings, West Mains Road, Edinburgh EH9 3JT, Scotland, UK*

Paul Leyhausen, *emer. Prof., Auf'm Driesch 22, D-5227 Windeck 1, West Germany*

Olof Liberg, *Institute of Zoology, University of Stockholm, S-106 91 Stockholm, Sweden*

D. W. Macdonald, *Department of Zoology, University of Oxford, South Parks Road, Oxford OX1 3PS, UK*

Aubrey Manning, *Department of Zoology, University of Edinburgh, Kings Buildings, West Mains Road, Edinburgh EH9 3JT, Scotland, UK*

Paul Martin, *Sub-Department of Animal Behaviour, University of Cambridge, Madingley, Cambridge CB3 8AA, UK*

Othmar Meister, *Ethology and Wildlife Research, Institute of Zoology, University of Zürich-Irchel, Winterthurerstrasse 190, CH-8057 Zürich, Switzerland*

Michael Mendl, *Department of Clinical Veterinary Medicine, University of Cambridge, Madingley Rd, Cambridge CB3 0ES, UK*

Claudia Mertens, *Ethology and Wildlife Research, Institute of Zoology, University of Zürich-Irchel, Winterthurerstrasse 190, CH-8057 Zürich, Switzerland*

Eugenia Natoli, *Dipartimento di Biologia Animale, Universitá di Catania, Via Androne no 81, 95124 Catania, Italy*

Mikael Sandell, *Department of Ecology, University of Lund, Ecology Building, S-223 62 Lund, Sweden*

Rosemarie Schär, Ethological Station Hasli, University of Berne, Wohlenstrasse 50a, CH-3032 Hinterkappelen, Switzerland

James A. Serpell, *Sub-Department of Animal Behaviour, University of Cambridge, Madingley, Cambridge CB3 8AA, UK*

Dennis C. Turner, *Ethology and Wildlife Research, Institute of Zoology, University of Zürich-Irchel, Winterthurerstrasse 190, CH-8057 Zürich, Switzerland*

Preface

This book arose from a symposium held at the Institute of Zoology, University of Zürich-Irchel in September 1986. The goals of that symposium were four-fold: (1) to bring together outstanding students of cat behaviour – both those researching the behaviour and ecology of free-ranging cats in the field and those observing the behaviour of captive cats in colonies – for the exchange of information and ideas; (2) to separate what is known about cat behaviour, i.e. can be substantiated by carefully collected data, from subjective impressions that still need verification; (3) to integrate what is known on a particular topic into a review (both spoken and written) and to present those reviews in a logical order so that the participant (and later, reader) gains as complete a picture of cat behaviour as possible; and (4) to inform both the professional and interested layman of the conference results during a public session and, later on, in book form.

Although emanating from a symposium, this volume is not simply a collection of conference proceedings. Most chapters are broad reviews of more general topics, including the authors' own research; each chapter has been subjected to an anonymous critical review before being included. The following persons reviewed one or more of the manuscripts, for which we are grateful: T. Althaus, P. Apps, T. Caro, L. Corbett, V. Dasser, J. Eisenberg, M. Fischbacher, O. Liberg, D. Macdonald, P. Messent, J. Rosenblatt, and of course, the editors themselves.

Constructive input during the symposium also came from the following researchers, who will be publishing their results later: K. Geering, U. Matter, J.-M. Pericard, J.-L. Renck and H. Rodel.

The symposium and this volume cover most, but not all aspects of domestic cat behaviour and ecology. Further research on cats is in progress and more may be stimulated by this volume; we therefore expect that much more will be discovered about the behaviour of cats in the future. We asked our authors to write their chapters in such a way that they serve as up-to-date reference sources for the zoologist and small animal veterinarian, but also be useful to the layman, particularly the cat-owner/breeder, interested in understanding the natural behaviour of these fascinating animals.

A number of persons were instrumental in organising the original symposium and/or preparing the manuscript for this book. All have our gratitude, but the following deserve special notice: M. Senn, Effems Beratung für Kleintierhaltung; I. Burrows, Waltham Centre for Pet Nutrition; H. Kummer, C. Ganz and K. Geering, Ethology and Wildlife Research, Univer-sity of Zürich; and Melissa Bateson, Cambridge, for preparing the illustrative line-drawings and cover design. Last but certainly not least, we thank our authors for their cooperation, patience and contributions.

Dennis C. Turner
Patrick Bateson
Zürich and Cambridge
June 1987

I

Introduction

1

Why the cat?

Dennis C. Turner and Patrick Bateson

The cat is a much loved and well-known animal. In Western countries it is becoming the most popular pet. On farms its value as a rodent catcher has been appreciated for years. Loved and familiar though it is, the cat remains an enigma. He is friendly to people and yet, in Rudyard Kipling's phrase, 'walks by himself', readily accepting the comforts of the human home and yet behaving as though his independence were total. Perhaps these paradoxical qualities cause some mistrust and even hatred. Certainly the cat, more than any other domestic animal has been as much persecuted as it has been appreciated. It is surrounded by fables and myths. Even many of the people who love cats are inclined to treat them as mysterious. However, in an era in which a great deal has been discovered about the biology of behaviour, many of the cat's former secrets have been penetrated.

While many popular books on cats have appeared in recent years, the accounts of cat behaviour are usually based on the author's personal experiences with only a few individual animals. Cat owners often make careful observations on their own pets, but most people also appreciate that each cat has a distinct personality. It is difficult and often misleading to make sweeping generalisations about 'The Cat'. Scientists who study larger numbers of animals are also wary of generalising too much. They feel that they must wait until colleagues studying other individuals in other situations also publish their findings. If the results are different (as they often are), the reasons for the discrepancy must be found. However, the body of knowledge has grown sufficiently large in recent years, so that more confident statements can now be made both about the common features of domestic cats and about the origins of their differences.

A survey of cat behaviour based fully on the results of scientific studies and written by the active researchers has not appeared since Paul Leyhausen's book, *Cat Behavior*, which was first published in German in 1956 and partially rewritten for publication in English in 1979. Meanwhile, many studies have appeared in scientific journals, and the latest results from numerous investigations are only just going to press as we write. The time has come to pull

3

these new studies together. This book presents the cat in the light of the modern work on its behavioural biology. Particular emphasis has been placed on reviewing and integrating scientific research, in order to give an up-to-date picture of cat behaviour.

The book begins with a section on the emergence of behaviour in young cats. Chapter 2 describes the normal pattern of behavioural and physical development, which proceeds in a highly ordered and integrated fashion. Such development is not simply a matter of preparing for adult life, however. The young animal must be able to survive in the year-long period of growth and it must have adaptations for the special conditions it will meet on the way to adulthood. It must also have adaptations for acquiring information and skills that it will need later in its life. Finally it must be able to cope with variation in the environment, so that it can acquire the same skills in different ways. This flexibility is especially important in relation to the development of its predatory behaviour.

Chapter 3 examines the mother–kitten relationship in detail. As would be expected, the mother's behaviour changes as her kittens develop. Important influences on the relationship also include the mother's breeding experience, the size of her litter, and the presence of other adult females during the nursing period. Much depends on how well fed the mother has been, since the production of milk for her kittens places a great drain on her reserves.

For years behavioural differences between individuals were disregarded by many scientists as meaningless variation. Only recently have research workers begun to take interest in individual differences, inquiring about their causes and biological significance. The domestic cat is an ideal subject for studies on individuality and personality. Chapter 4 examines ways of measuring the differences and lists the questions which can be asked about the variability. Both the individual's genes and its experience influence its personality, but the ways in which the genes are expressed are likely to be critically dependent on the conditions encountered, particularly during early life.

The section on adult behaviour opens with Chapter 5 which presents the distinctive views of Paul Leyhausen. He makes two points about the autonomy of the cat's behaviour. The patterns concerned with different aspects of each individual's biological needs are parts of relatively independent systems which are often in conflict and which are not organised into a single hierarchy. A similar though logically separate point is made about the social behaviour of collections of individual cats, each of which 'walks by himself'. How solitary is the cat in fact?

Modern field studies, reviewed in Chapter 6, suggest that domestic cats are more gregarious than fable would suggest, although they show great variation in their sociality. Comparisons of different sized colonies of farm cats show that these are truly structured and functional social groups rather than loose aggregations of individuals around concentrated abundant sources of food. Chapter 7 concentrates on the spacing patterns of free-ranging cats and relates these to the different reproductive tactics of the two sexes. The density of the females in a given area is likely to be affected by the availability of food. On the other hand, the sizes of the much larger areas, over which the males range, are first and foremost determined by the density of the females. Many of the topics covered in the two preceding chapters are picked up in Chapter 8 which deals with the mating system of cats living in a market square of Rome. This shows what happens at the upper extreme when free-living cats are found at very high densities.

The fourth section of the book deals with the predatory behaviour of cats and the effects of ecological conditions on such behaviour. Chapter 9 reviews what is known about the hunting behaviour of free-ranging domestic cats, describing their methods and success rates, as well as when and where they do it. The differences in diet of feral cats around the world are revealed in Chapter 10. Cats have become established on many remote oceanic islands which had been visited by ships. As might be expected the latitude of the island affects the type of prey and therefore the diet of the local cat population. This chapter also raises a practical matter. The serious impact of cat predation on prey populations, particularly birds on oceanic islands, points to some important issues for cat management.

The fifth section of the book deals with the association between humans and cats, which has been a long one. Chapter 11 traces the origin, domestication and early history of the house cat. Although cats have been terribly persecuted at certain times in history, they were also treated with great affection bordering on reverence from the earliest stages of their domestication. Chapter 12 examines the many factors which can affect the relationship between cats and people.

An especially important matter is the existence of a sensitive period in early development when kittens are particularly likely to form attachments to humans. More general questions pertaining to the keeping of cats are covered in Chapter 13. The practical consequences of basic research on these animals are assessed for the pet owner.

Finally, as a postscript, Chapter 14 discusses the patterns of behaviour in the cat's repertoire which are particularly likely to intrigue cat owners. In doing so, many questions to which we still do not have answers are raised. This final section shows that while a lot has been learned in the last few years about the behavioural biology of the cat, a great deal more remains to be discovered. Whether or not the cat walks by himself, he still preserves some of his secrets.

II

Development of young cats

2

Behavioural development in the cat

Paul Martin and Patrick Bateson

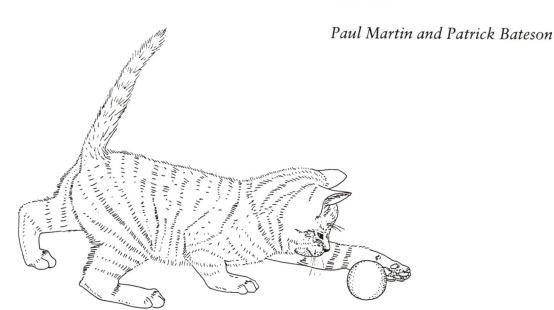

Introduction

In the course of every individual animal's development, from conception to maturity, highly organised anatomical structures and behaviour patterns appear with remarkable regularity and at remarkably consistent times. Most kittens open their eyes during their second week, for example, and start to eat their first solid food at around one month of age. At the same time, though, animals such as the cat are also adaptable and modifiable in their behaviour, responding sensitively to changes in their environments. Moreover, cats are astonishingly variable in their habits. Some cats spend much of their time hunting, while others seldom seem to wish to leave the comfort of their owner's armchair. Explaining how and why such differences arise during development is a major problem which we attempt to address in this chapter. We present a brief outline of the major changes that occur after birth in the domestic cat. We then consider how these events may be explained and what might be the origins of individual differences. We end by considering the general principles which are starting to emerge from the studies of behavioural development.

The normal development of the domestic cat

The time from conception to birth is usually 63 days in the domestic cat (Hemmer, 1979). This, according to Haltenorth & Diller (1980), is 3–7 days longer than in the supposed wild ancestor, *Felis silvestris libyca*. The mean birth weight is 100–110 g, which is of the order of three per cent of adult body weight (Leitch, Hytten & Billewicz, 1959). The kitten is born with its eyes closed and a poorly developed auditory system. Tactile sensitivity, however, is present in the embryo by day 24 of pre-natal life (Corionos, 1933) and the vestibular righting reflex has developed by about day 54 of gestation (Windle & Fish, 1932).

The cat is like many other vertebrates in that the tactile system develops first, next the vestibular system, next the auditory system and finally the visual system (Gottlieb, 1971). The sensory world of the kitten in the first two weeks of life is dominated by thermal, tactile and olfactory stimuli, and only from three

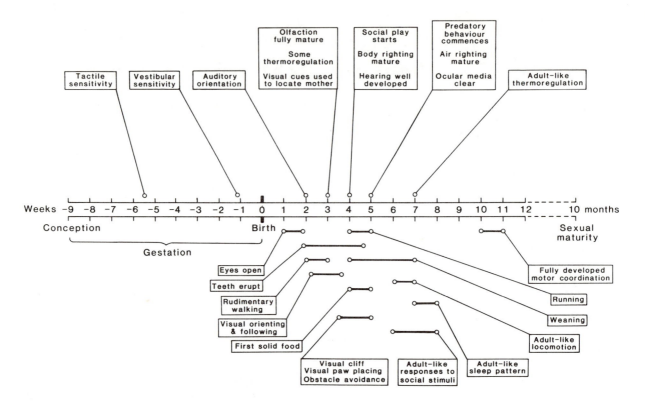

Fig. 2.1. A timetable outlining some of the major behavioural and physiological changes that occur during the development of the domestic cat.

weeks of age onwards does vision play a major role in guiding behaviour (Rosenblatt, 1976). A rough time-table of the kitten's sensory, locomotor and behavioural development is shown in Figure 2.1.

Sensory and physiological development

Olfaction, which plays a central role in the orientation of suckling in very young kittens, is present at birth, and more or less fully mature by three weeks of age (Villablanca & Olmstead, 1979). Hearing is also present early in life and is well developed by one month of age. Definite responses to sounds are seen by day 5; orientation to natural sounds by about two weeks; and adult-like orienting responses are seen in all kittens by the fourth week (Olmstead & Villablanca, 1980).

Kittens' eyes remain closed until, on average, 7–10 days after birth, although the age at which they open

ranges between two and 16 days (Villablanca & Olmstead, 1979). It takes, on average, two to three days for both eyes to open completely (Braastad & Heggelund, 1984). Following eye-opening, visually guided behaviour develops rapidly in the following weeks. By the end of the third week, a kitten is able to use visual cues to locate and approach its mother (Rosenblatt, 1976). Visual orienting and following develop between 15 and 25 days, while response to a visual cliff, usually guided paw-placing, and obstacle avoidance all develop somewhat later, between 25 and 35 days (Norton, 1974).

The kitten's visual acuity has improved markedly by one month after birth (Thorn, Gollender & Erickson, 1976), although the fluids of the eye do not become completely clear until about five weeks and some improvement in acuity continues until as late as 3–4 months (Ikeda, 1979). Overall, visual acuity improves

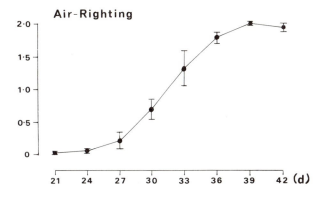

Air-Righting

Fig. 2.2. The development of the air-righting reaction. Kittens were held upside-down 40 cm above a padded surface and released. A score of 0 denoted a complete failure to right, while the maximum score of 2 was obtained if the kitten landed upright on all four paws. The graph shows the mean scores of 14 kittens, tested every three days between 21 and 42 days of age. No evidence of air-righting was seen at 21 days, whereas by 39 days all kittens showed complete air-righting on every trial. (From Martin, 1982.)

16-fold between two and 10 weeks after birth (Sireteanu, 1985). Kittens under two months of age can be trained to perform complex visual pattern discriminations (Wilkinson & Dodwell, 1980).

Kittens can regulate their body temperature to some extent by three weeks of age (Jensen, Davis & Shnerson, 1980). However, even one-day-old kittens can detect and attempt to move along a thermal gradient, avoiding cold regions and approaching warmth. By seven weeks of age a fully adult pattern of temperature regulation is attained (Olmstead *et al.*, 1979). Adult-like sleep patterns have also developed by 7–8 weeks after birth (McGinty *et al.*, 1977). Females become sexually mature between seven and twelve months of age (Hemmer, 1979). Brain weight at birth is about 20 per cent of adult weight, and reaches the adult level by about three months of age (Smith & Jansen, 1977a).

Motor and physical development

During the first two weeks after birth, kittens are relatively immobile and use a slow, paddling gait. Rudimentary walking appears during the third week, but not until four weeks of age can kittens move any great distance from the nest (Moelk, 1979). By the fifth week they show brief episodes of running, and by 6–7 weeks they have started to use all of the gaits found in adult locomotion (Peters, 1983). Complex motor abilities, such as walking along and turning around on a narrow plank, may not develop fully until 10–11 weeks after birth (Villablanca & Olmstead, 1979). The body-righting reaction is present at birth and fully mature by one month. The ability to right the body in mid-air while falling (the air-righting reaction) starts

to appear during the fourth week and develops smoothly over the next two weeks (Martin, 1982; see Figure 2.2).

Limb-placing reactions develop progressively over the first two months, with internally controlled responses present at birth and visually controlled responses developing later, in parallel with the development of the visual system. Some tactile contact-placing is present at birth, while visually guided paw-placing starts to develop at around three weeks and is mature by 5–6 weeks (Villablanca & Olmstead, 1979). Teeth start to erupt shortly before two weeks of age, and continue until the fifth week. The change from milk teeth to adult teeth starts at about three and a half months after birth (Hemmer, 1979).

Social and behavioural development

This topic is dealt with in detail by Deag *et al.* in Chapter 3 and we shall only touch on it briefly here. During the first three weeks after birth, the kittens depend entirely upon mother's milk for their nutrition, and episodes of nursing are initiated entirely by the mother, who returns frequently to the nest to nurse her kittens (Martin, 1986). Under free-living conditions, mothers start to bring live prey to their kittens from four weeks after birth onwards, and kittens may start to kill mice as early as the fifth week (Baerends-van Roon & Baerends, 1979).

Four weeks is also the age at which kittens normally start to eat some solid food and marks the onset of the weaning period (Martin, 1986). As weaning progresses, the kittens become increasingly responsible for initiating bouts of nursing (Schneirla, Rosenblatt

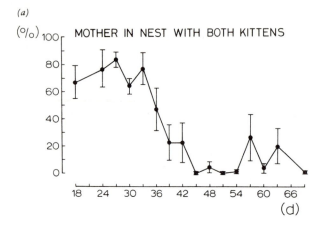

(a)

(%) 100

MOTHER IN NEST WITH BOTH KITTENS

80

60

40

20

0

18   24   30   36   42   48   54   60   66

(d)

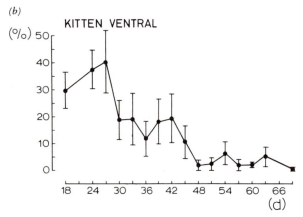

(b)

(%) 50

KITTEN VENTRAL

40

30

20

10

0

18   24   30   36   42   48   54   60   66

(d)

Fig. 2.3. (*a*) The average percentage of time spent by mother cats in the nest box with their kittens; and (*b*) the average percentage of time spent by kittens in the suckling ('ventral') posture. The results are for seven mother cats, each nursing two kittens. Each family was observed for 30 min every three days. In both cases the x-axis shows the kittens' age in days. (From Martin, 1982).

& Tobach, 1963). By 5–6 weeks of age, voluntary elimination has developed, and kittens are no longer dependent on their mother to lick their perineum in order to stimulate urination (Fox, 1970). Weaning is largely completed by seven weeks after birth (Martin, 1986), although intermittent suckling – without, necessarily, any milk transfer – may continue for several months, particularly if the mother has only one kitten (Leyhausen, 1979, p. 290). Figure 2.3 shows how the amount of time spent by mother cats in the

home nest site with their kittens, and the amount of time spent by the kittens in the suckling position, change as the kittens become older.

Social play becomes prevalent by four weeks of age and continues at a high level until 12–14 weeks, when it begins to decline (West, 1974; Caro, 1981a). Social play-fighting can sometimes escalate into serious incidents, especially during the third month (Voith, 1980a). Play with objects develops slightly later, as kittens start to develop the eye–paw coordination that enables them to deal with small, moving objects, and its incidence rises markedly at around 7–8 weeks after birth (Barrett & Bateson, 1978), while locomotor play also develops rapidly at around this age (Martin & Bateson, 1985a).

Many other major changes in behaviour have been recorded between one and two months of age. For example, at 4–5 weeks of age kittens first start to alternate spontaneously between entering one arm and then the other of a T-shaped maze (Frederickson & Frederickson, 1979). At about the same age, but not before, heart-rate can be conditioned to respond to a neutral event associated with an aversive one. One month is also said to be about the earliest age at which learned performance based on purely visual cues is possible (Bloch & Martinoya, 1981). However, conditioned responses to sounds are seen by 10 days of age (Ehret & Romand, 1981), and kittens show specific forms of learning – such as forming nipple preferences – shortly after birth (Ewer, 1961). Kittens under a month in age differ from older kittens in passive avoidance (shuttle box) learning, though not in active avoidance (step-up) learning (Davis & Jensen, 1976). According to Adamec, Stark-Adamec & Livingston (1983), a predisposition to respond defensively towards large and difficult prey such as rats – a defensive 'personality' – develops during the second month. By 6–8 weeks of age, kittens have begun to show adult-like responses to threatening social stimuli, both visual and olfactory (Kolb & Nonneman, 1975).

Different routes to the same end-point

In the latter parts of this review we shall consider how normal development can be upset by deliberate experimental manipulation and by naturally occurring events. We shall also consider the plasticity of developmental processes in greater detail. In many respects, though, the kitten's development is remarkably well ordered. Within limits the systems that generate the beautifully integrated behaviour of an adult cat have a goal-directed character to them and are resilient to both internal and external disturbances. Most cats eventually become reasonably competent predators, for example, almost irrespective of the type of experiences they have as young kittens.

In reaching an understanding of these sorts of effects, one useful principle is the system theory concept of equifinality. This states that in an open system, such as a living organism, the same steady state in development can be reached from different starting conditions and by different developmental routes (see Bateson, 1976; Martin & Caro, 1985). In behavioural terms, this principle means that the same state in behavioural development could be achieved through quite different developmental histories.

The notion of equifinality does seem particularly appealing when applied to the development of predatory skills in domestic cats. Individuals can differ very considerably in their predatory behaviour during early development – particularly during the second and third months. This variation lies not so much in the basic predatory motor patterns, which virtually all individuals develop, but in their integration and in the early stages of predation, such as identifying prey, assessing whether the prey can be caught and choosing the appropriate tactics (Baerends-van Roon & Baerends, 1979). Despite this individual variation among young cats, however, most eventually become competent predators, albeit with different preferences and specialisations for particular types of prey (see 'Social influences on predatory behaviour', below). Thus, at the crude level of overall predatory competence, much of the early individual variation in predatory skill disappears by the time adulthood is reached. Some measures of predatory skills made before three months of age are not related to those made at six months, because individuals who were poor predators as kittens have usually caught up by the time they are adults (Caro, 1979a, b).

We can make sense of this by considering experimental work with cats which has shown that various kinds of early experience can improve predatory skills. Adult predatory skills are improved by experience with prey when young, by watching the mother dealing with prey when young and, possibly, by the effects of competition between litter mates in the presence of

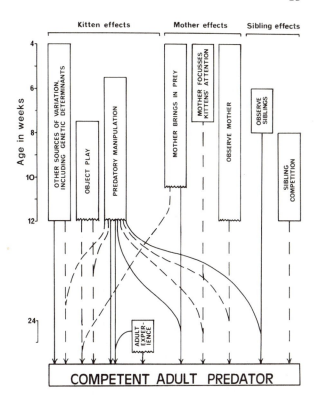

Fig. 2.4. Some known and some hypothesised factors that influence the development of adult predatory skills in domestic cats. Continuous lines refer to empirical results reported by Baerends-van Roon & Baerends (1979) and Caro (1980a, b, c). Dotted lines denote hypothesised influences. (From Caro, 1979b.)

prey (Caro, 1980a, b, c). Kittens which have never killed a rat, for example, can become rat-killers merely by watching another cat kill a rat (Kuo, 1930). In addition, experience of prey when adult can also improve adult skills, which means that adults who have lacked early experience with prey can, to some extent, catch up later in ontogeny (Caro, 1980b). Playing with prey or inanimate objects when young does not seem to improve adult predatory skills, however (Martin & Caro, 1985). These, and other possible influences on the development of adult predatory behaviour are illustrated in Figure 2.4.

The main point here is that a given set of adult behaviour patterns – in this case predatory behaviour – is affected by several different types of experience. Variation in one type of experience – say, experience of dealing with prey when young – may be compensated for by other forms of experience, such as watching the mother deal with prey when young, or experience with prey when adult. Thus, a given developmental outcome – competence as a predator – might be attained via many different types of developmental history. In functional terms, this type of process would clearly be of benefit to the individual, in that it allows the same type of behaviour to develop in a variable environment where individuals might have quite different types of early experience.

Of course, other processes may lead to apparently similar results. The effects of trauma or injury may disappear as the result of normal repair mechanisms. Where certain types of experience exert a facilitatory effect on development, it is also possible that considerable individual variation early in life will have disappeared by adulthood. In this case, though, the same developmental end-point is reached via the same developmental route, but at different rates. For example, exposing kittens to a cool environment during the first few days after birth hastens the development of temperature regulation. At two weeks of age, therefore, individuals may differ considerably as a result of differences in their exposure to low temperatures, but by four weeks of age they no longer differ (Jensen *et al.*, 1980).

Continuity and discontinuity in development

Attempts to trace particular patterns of behaviour back to the early action of certain genes, or to particular kinds of early experience, are often misconceived because of profound changes that occur at certain stages in development. Early influences may not necessarily exert detectable long-term effects on behaviour because of major changes in the organisation of behaviour that have occurred in between. Some early influences may simply be 'wiped from the tape' (Kagan, 1984). Such a possibility is, of course, in stark contrast to traditional views of development, which tend to emphasise the important and far-reaching consequences of all events that occur early in life (see Hinde & Bateson, 1984).

Play

Some evidence does indicate that reorganisation occurs in the behaviour of cats at around the time of weaning, towards the end of the second month. Play, in particular, changes markedly at around this time.

The frequency with which kittens play with inanimate objects increases sharply at around 7–8 weeks of age, and many measures of play before this age do not predict the same measures in the same individuals at 8–12 weeks, after weaning is over (Barrett & Bateson, 1978).

Correlations between different measures of social play also break down at the end of weaning, as do correlations between some measures of predatory behaviour (Caro, 1981b). Certain measures of social play become increasingly associated with some measures of predatory behaviour during the third month. This might indicate that motor patterns come under the control of new motivational systems as the kitten develops, some becoming controlled by the same factors that control predatory behaviour, and others by the factors controlling agonistic behaviour. Some playful motor patterns become increasingly associated with patterns of predatory behaviour, and some become associated with agonistic social behaviour (see Figure 2.5).

In passing, it is worth pointing out that the different developmental time courses and general lack of intercorrelations between measures of social play and measures of object play indicate that these two forms of play are separately organised and separately controlled (Barrett & Bateson, 1978). Even in terms of the motor patterns used, object and social play differ distinctly in a number of respects; for example, repetition of certain motor patterns occurs frequently during object play but seldom during social play (West, 1979).

Cats are, of course, formidable hunters and many of the motor patterns that appear in play resemble those used in catching and killing prey (Caro, 1979a; Leyhausen, 1979). Not surprisingly, many hypotheses about the function of play in cats have invoked links between play and later predatory behaviour, with play seen as a form of practice for adult predatory skills (e.g. Moelk, 1979). However, it must be said that little, if any, evidence has yet been produced to support this view (Martin, 1984a). Play experience is most certainly not necessary for at least the basic elements of predatory behaviour to develop (Baerends-van Roon & Baerends, 1979). For example, Thomas & Schaller (1954) reported that 'Kaspar Hauser' cats which were reared in social isolation and without opportunities for visual experience, let alone play behaviour, none the less showed 'normal'

THE SOCIAL PLAY PATTERNS BECOMING INCREASINGLY

DISSOCIATED WITH

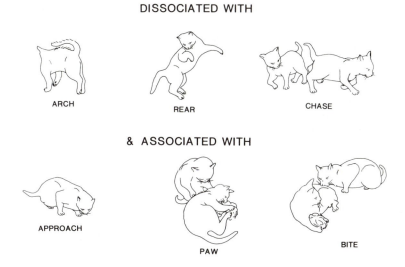

ARCH   REAR   CHASE

& ASSOCIATED WITH

APPROACH

PAW   BITE

PATTERNS OF PREDATORY BEHAVIOUR DURING KITTEN DEVELOPMENT

Fig. 2.5. Some social play patterns become dissociated from motor patterns used in agonistic social encounters, after the end of weaning at two months of age. At the same time, social play patterns become increasingly associated with predatory motor patterns such as Approach, Paw and Bite. Thus, different motor patterns appear to come under separate types of control after weaning: some motor patterns are increasingly controlled by the same factors that control predatory behaviour, whereas others become controlled by the factors that control agonistic social behaviour. (After Caro, 1981b.)

predatory responses when presented with a prey-like moving dummy at 11 weeks of age.

However, the possibility remains that play may have subtle beneficial effects on predatory skills. The one experimental test of this hypothesis so far carried out failed to find any relations between early object play experience and later predatory skills in domestic cats. Cats which had no opportunities for playing with small, inanimate objects when growing up did not subsequently differ from kittens which had regularly played with objects, when their predatory skills were measured at six months of age (Caro, 1980b). This failure to find an effect might have been due to insufficient differences in the experience of the normal and the deprived groups of cats, or to measures of predatory behaviour that were insufficiently fine-grained to pick up genuine differences in skill. Theories about the role of play in behavioural development remains, as yet, unproven (Martin & Caro, 1985).

The control of behaviour patterns and their biological functions are likely to change as development proceeds. Caution is, of course, needed before making sweeping claims for reorganisations in behaviour based on limited evidence. On the other

hand, it is undoubtedly true that measurements of behaviour at different ages may not be equivalent; activities that look the same at different ages may be controlled in different ways and may have different functions. The time a kitten spends in contact with its mother, for example, is influenced primarily by its need for milk early in life and by its need for comfort later. Some activities, such as suckling, are special adaptations to an early phase and drop out of the repertoire as the individual becomes nutritionally independent of its mother. Similarly, certain motor patterns and reflex responses that are present at birth have disappeared from the behavioural repertoire by the time the cat is a few weeks old (Villablanca & Olmstead, 1979).

Despite these indications that not all aspects of development are continuous, it is clear that many types of early experience can be related to what happens later in ontogeny. For instance, many measures of predatory behaviour at 1–3 months of age are positively correlated with the same measures taken at six months (Caro, 1979a). Similarly, measures of defensiveness towards prey early in life are predictive of attacking behaviour in adult cats (Adamec, Stark-Adamec & Livingston, 1980a). In both cases, individual differences in behaviour early in development can, to some extent, predict individual differences later in life.

Laboratory studies suggest that cats' choice of prey and their adult food preferences are strongly influenced by experience with their mothers when young (see below). For example, cats are more likely to kill prey species with which they are familiar from experience as kittens (Caro, 1980a). Similarly, cats which have had experience with a particular type of prey when young are more skilful at catching and killing the same type of prey when adult. This effect of early experience appears to be specific, in that early experience with one type of prey does not produce a general improvement in predatory skills when other prey species are considered (Caro, 1980a).

Sensitive periods

A sensitive period is an age range during which particular events are especially likely to have long-term effects on the individual's development (Bateson, 1979). The older term 'critical period' was abandoned because it implied a sharply defined phase of susceptibility preceded and followed by a complete lack of susceptibility. The supposition was that if the relevant experience were provided before or after the period, no long-term effects would be detectable. Experimental studies of imprinting in birds showed that the period was not so sharply defined and the term 'sensitive period' or 'sensitive phase' is therefore preferred by many ethologists (see Immelmann & Suomi, 1981). The sensitive period concept implies a phase of greater susceptibility preceded and followed by lower sensitivity, with gradual transitions. An example of a sensitive period that has been studied in depth is the development of visual cells in the cat's cortex (see Rauschecker & Marler, 1987). The response properties of neurons in the visual cortex are modified by visual experience during early development. Thus, certain types of visual deprivation – such as exposing kittens only to visual contours of one orientation – can exert long-term effects on the properties of the visual system.

Social influences on development

Under natural and semi-natural conditions, cats will form strong social relationships with familiar individuals, usually close kin. From an early age, the mother is recognised and greatly preferred to unfamiliar females. The young also recognise other adults in their own group and readily accept care from them (see also Chapters 3, 6 and 8). In groups of feral cats, the kittens are often allowed to suckle from females other than their mother (Macdonald & Apps, 1978). Social relationships such as these, which depend so much on familiarity, are most readily formed in the first two months after birth in domestic cats. When the process by which strong social attachments are formed was first described in precocious birds it was called 'imprinting', because it happens quickly and leaves a long-lasting effect on social preferences. Cats are much less well developed at birth and form social attachments more slowly than, say, mallard ducklings (see Karsh & Turner, Chapter 12).

Humans and members of other species may also be incorporated into the social group and responded to with affection if they were encountered by the cat when it was young. Despite a basic ability to respond socially towards people, adult cats and kittens show considerable individual variation in their friendliness towards humans, whether familiar or unfamiliar, and even kittens from the same litter can differ considerably in their friendliness (Turner, 1985a).

Social influences on predatory behaviour

The importance of social relationships in the behavioural development of cats is perhaps best seen in the development of predatory behaviour. Under natural conditions, cat mothers gradually introduce their young to prey, providing them with a series of situations in which their developing predatory skills can be expressed. Early on, the mother will bring dead prey to her young; later she will bring live prey and release the prey near the kittens, intervening only if the kitten starts to lose control (Leyhausen, 1979). Rather than 'teaching' her kittens to catch prey, the mother creates situations in which their own responses will lead them naturally to learn the right things (Ewer, 1969).

The predatory behaviour of a cat mother is beautifully meshed with the improving capabilities of her developing kittens and, as their predatory behaviour develops, so hers declines. In the short term, the mother's responses to prey she has brought back to the nest are finely tuned to her kittens' responses, as Caro (1980c) has demonstrated. The longer the kittens pause before interacting with the prey, the more likely the mother is to attack the prey, for example. Kittens show increased rates of predatory behaviour in the presence of their mother, and the mother's behaviour tends to lead the kittens to interact with prey (Caro, 1980c). When dealing with live prey, laboratory studies suggest that kittens tend to follow their mother's choice. For example, Kuo (1930) found that kittens almost invariably killed the same strain of rat that they had seen their mother kill, although they might also kill other strains of rat as well.

Social experience when young plays an important role in determining the range of stimuli that will elicit predatory, as opposed to social or fearful, behaviour. In a pioneering set of experiments, Kuo (1930) raised kittens and rats together in the same cages. Kittens raised with rats never killed rats of the same strain when they grew up, although some would kill rats of a different appearance. The implication of Kuo's results was that kittens whose social companions during early life were rats formed social attachments to rats, inhibiting later predatory responses to them. However, when given the opportunity to form social attachments to other kittens as well as rats, other kittens were preferred. Kittens raised both with siblings and rats formed clear social attachments to their siblings. None the less, these kittens did show a distinct tolerance of rats and a reduced predatory response towards them, although some eventually became rat-killers (Kuo, 1938). The presence of siblings also seems to be important in encouraging young kittens to interact with prey. Caro (1980c) found that pre-weaning kittens were more likely to watch prey if their siblings or mother were also watching the prey.

Willingness to try new foods, and preferences for particular types of food also appear to be strongly influenced by the mother. Wyrwicka & Long (1980) reported that laboratory kittens which were presented daily with a novel food, tuna or cereal, whilst their mother was present started to eat the new food on the first or second day of exposure. However, kittens which were presented with the novel food whilst on their own did not start to eat it until about the fifth day of exposure. These results do not, however, match our experience with the kittens in our own laboratory colony, who have been observed to eat a novel food voraciously on the first occasion, even without the

mother being present (R. Harcourt, personal communication).

Weanling kittens tend to imitate their mother's choice of food, even when this means eating food not normally eaten by cats. Wyrwicka (1978) trained mother cats to eat banana or mashed potato. She then tested their kittens' food choice. When offered a normally preferred food (meat pellets) and an unusual food (banana or mashed potato), most of the kittens imitated their mother and ate the unusual food rather than meat pellets. The kittens' preference for the unusual food persisted even when the kittens were tested on their own. The kittens started to imitate their mother's food choices soon after weaning commenced (at about five weeks of age), and imitation was most marked towards the end of the weaning period (7–8 weeks).

Observational learning

Young cats are well adapted to learning from their mother, and show a strong interest in, and ability to learn from, the behaviour of other cats (Adler, 1955). This general phenomenon, of being able to benefit from observing a conspecific's experiences, is found in many species (Pallaud, 1984) and is referred to as observational learning.

Chesler (1969) found that kittens which were allowed to watch their mother perform an operant response (pressing a lever to obtain food) were able to acquire the response quickly, whereas kittens who were given the opportunity to acquire the response by trial-and-error never did so. Moreover, kittens which watched their own mother acquired the response sooner than kittens which observed a strange female, suggesting that observational learning is facilitated if the 'model' cat is familiar to the observer kitten.

Adult cats also show observational learning, and can acquire some learned responses faster by observing another cat performing them than by conventional conditioning responses (John *et al.*, 1968). Observing another cat actually acquire the response is important, and has a more beneficial effect than watching another cat perform a skilled response that has already been learned (Herbert & Harsh, 1944).

The mother–kitten relationship

The mother–kitten relationship is described in detail in the chapter by Deag *et al.* (Chapter 3). This relationship is obviously crucial to the kitten's development, particularly in view of the domestic cat's relatively slow development and long period of dependence on maternal care.

From the outset, interactions between mother and kittens regulate suckling. During the first three weeks after birth, the mother initiates suckling by approaching her kittens and adopting a characteristic nursing posture in which her nipples are easily accessible. At this stage, kittens can orient towards the nest, using olfactory and, to a lesser extent, thermal cues (Larson & Stein, 1984). Nest orientation starts to decline during the third week, following eye-opening and the development of visually guided behaviour (Rosenblatt, 1972).

Kittens will suckle from a non-lactating female in the same way as from a lactating female until about three weeks of age, which means that milk reward is not necessary for either the initiation or maintenance of suckling. After three weeks of age, an absence of milk reward leads to a reduction in the duration of suckling, although the frequency with which suckling is initiated remains unaffected (Koepke & Pribram, 1971). Clearly, suckling is a rewarding activity in its own right, irrespective of whether the kitten obtains milk from so doing.

Later, as the kittens become more mobile, they become increasingly responsible for approaching the mother and initiating suckling. In the later stages of the weaning period, towards the end of the second month, the kittens become almost wholly responsible for initiating suckling and the mother may actively impede their efforts by blocking access to her nipples or by removing herself from the kittens' proximity (Martin, 1986). The increasing role of the kitten in initiating suckling develops in close parallel to the kittens' improving sensory and motor abilities.

Kittens which have been reared since birth on an artificial brooder are perfectly capable of suckling from a brooder nipple, but fail to suckle when given access to a lactating female because they show inappropriate social responses to her (Rosenblatt, Turkewitz & Schneirla, 1961). Kittens which are artificially separated from their mother much earlier than normal (at two weeks of age) subsequently develop a variety of behavioural, emotional and physical abnormalities (Seitz, 1959). They become unusually fearful and aggressive towards other cats and people, show large amounts of random and undirected loco-

motor activity, and learn less well. Some develop asthma-like respiratory disorders.

Siblings

The mother is, of course, not the only source of social experience during a kitten's development, and increasing evidence indicates that siblings play an important role in social development. During the early suckling period, for example, competition between litter mates for access to nipples can be an important regulator of suckling (Rosenblatt, 1971). Kittens establish distinct and consistent preferences for suckling from a particular teat during the first few days (Ewer, 1961). Teat preference is one of the earliest forms of learning shown by kittens.

Social experience with siblings also seems to play at least a facilitating role in the development of later social skills. Kittens which have been reared on an artificial brooder, with no experience of siblings when young, do eventually form social attachments, but are generally slower to learn social skills than normally reared kittens. Brooder-reared kittens do not appear to form substitute social attachments to their brooder (Guyot, Cross & Bennett, 1983). However, Mendl's (1986) work suggests that the mother may in some ways provide a substitute source of social experience for single kittens raised without litter mates. The main point here, though, is that social experience with litter mates is another potentially important factor influencing behavioural development, albeit in ways that are not yet well understood.

Variations in the age of weaning

In the domestic cat, weaning is a gradual process during which the mother progressively reduces the rate at which she is giving care and resources (notably milk) to her offspring (see Figure 2.6). Under favourable laboratory conditions, weaning commences at about four weeks after birth and is largely completed by seven weeks (Martin, 1986).

Weaning represents a period of major transition for young mammals, marking a change from complete dependence on parental care to partial or complete independence. This transition, which is shown most obviously by the change in food source, involves a whole range of behavioural and physiological changes on the part of both mother and offspring (Martin, 1986). If, as is likely for a variety of reasons, the time of weaning may vary according to factors such as

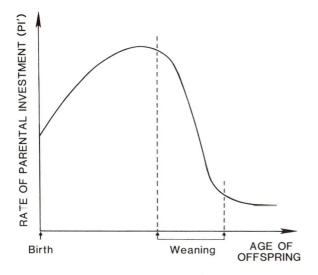

Fig. 2.6. One way of representing the process of weaning in general biological terms. Weaning is shown here as the phase of parental care during which the rate of parental investment (PI') drops most sharply. The term parental investment signifies any biological resources – such as time or energy in the form of milk, provision of solid food, protection against predators, etc. – invested by a parent in its current offspring, which increases the offspring's chances of surviving and reproducing at a cost to the parent of a reduced ability to invest in future offspring. (From Martin, 1982.)

maternal food supply (Bateson, 1981b), then the developing offspring must be able to adapt by altering its behaviour accordingly.

Evidence that kittens may alter their development in response to changes in weaning time comes from two sources. Tan & Counsilman (1985) looked at the development of predatory behaviour in kittens which had experienced early, normal or late weaning. Early weaning was simulated by gradual separation from the mother starting at four weeks, while late-weaned kittens were left with their mothers but were denied access to solid food until the ninth week. Tan & Counsilman found that early-weaned kittens developed predatory behaviour sooner than normally-weaned kittens and were more likely to become mouse-killers. Conversely, late weaning was associated with delayed development of predatory behaviour and a reduced propensity to kill mice, although these effects might have been due to non-specific debilitating effects of delayed weaning. In general, Tan & Counsilman's results fit with the notion that the development of predatory behaviour is linked in an adaptive way to the time of weaning; in other words, that it develops when needed.

A series of studies at our own laboratory has shown that the development of play behaviour is markedly influenced by the time of weaning. Under normal laboratory conditions, kittens' play behaviour undergoes a number of major changes towards the end of

the second month, most notably by showing a large increase in the frequency of object play (Martin, 1984a). This change in play coincides with the end of the weaning period, suggesting the hypothesis that the change from social to object play occurs in response to the kitten's increasing independence from the social environment of the nest (Bateson, 1981b).

To test this hypothesis, early weaning – or, more specifically, a reduction in maternal care – was simulated in a variety of different ways: by gradual separation from the mother starting at five weeks (Bateson & Young, 1981); by interrupting the maternal milk supply with the lactation-blocking drug bromocriptine starting at four weeks (Martin, 1982; Martin & Bateson, 1985b) or five weeks (Bateson, Martin & Young, 1981); or by slightly reducing mothers' food supply (Bateson & Mendl, unpublished). In all cases, the experimental manipulation led to the surprising result that the frequencies of certain types of play were increased. One tentative interpretation of the increase in play is that it marks a conditional response by the kitten to enforced early independence, by increasing play experience before complete independence (Bateson & Young, 1981).

Influences of multiple and varied factors

Whenever developmental processes are studied in detail it becomes obvious that they are influenced by many factors, some internal and some external. Furthermore, these factors act in different ways, some enabling a process to occur, others initiating the developmental change, others merely facilitating the process and yet others maintaining a character once it has developed. Finally, the influences on development may have highly specific effects or they may be general.

The expression of many genes depends upon prevailing conditions, and the conditions necessary for the expression of a particular gene may not occur in the case of any one individual possessing them. On the other hand, under most conditions of the environment and with most background genotypes, the actions of certain genes may invariably be detectable in the adult phenotype. Examples of both types are found in the genes affecting coat coloration in domestic cats, about which much is known (e.g. Robinson, 1977).

Unfortunately, remarkably little research has been done on genetic influences on the behaviour of domestic cats. Some strains of cats, bred for particular coat characteristics, have developed other peculiarities. Blue-eyed white cats, for example, are usually deaf, while in some lines females display unusual timidity and abnormal sexual behaviour (Beaver, 1976). In Siamese cats, the visual system develops abnormally, with a disrupted pattern of crossing-over of neural projections from the retina to the lateral geniculate nuclei (Partridge, 1983). Although the Siamese cat's deficit is a single enzyme (tyrosinase), the effects on its nervous system are rather general, even though the adaptive plasticity of the cat's visual system allows the Siamese to develop almost normal visual abilities.

General influences on development: early handling and nutrition

Some types of experience, as well as some genes, exert general rather than specific effects on behavioural development. Early handling, for example, has a number of effects on the behavioural and physical development of cats, the handled animals tending on the whole to develop more rapidly. In one study, Siamese kittens that were handled (held and lightly stroked) daily for the first few weeks of life were precocious in their physical and behavioural development compared with unhandled litter mates (Meier, 1961). They opened their eyes earlier, first emerged from the nest box earlier and even developed the characteristic Siamese coat coloration earlier than their litter mates. In another study, Wilson, Warren & Abbott (1965) reported that kittens which were handled for five minutes per day from birth to 45 days of age approached strange toys and humans more readily, but were slower to learn an avoidance task than unhandled kittens. They attributed both results to a general reduction in fearfulness resulting from the early handling. Karsh (1983a) notes that the precise effects of early handling on kittens' development depend on a variety of factors, including the number of different people who handle the kitten, and the frequency and duration of handling.

Nutrition is another factor with general effects on development which has been investigated in the cat. Several studies have found that kittens of undernourished mothers subsequently exhibit a variety of behavioural and growth abnormalities. In one study, mother cats were fed 50 per cent of their *ad libitum* intake during the second half of the gestation period and the first six weeks post partum (Smith & Jansen, 1977b, c). These undernourished mothers showed less active mothering than normal and were more irritable towards their kittens. Their kittens showed growth deficits in some brain regions (cerebrum, cerebellum and brain stem), although their overall brain composition was not affected. The undernourished kittens were 'rehabilitated' with *ad libitum* access to food from six weeks of age onwards, and eventually achieved normal body size. However, they showed a number of behavioural abnormalities and differences in brain development later in ontogeny. At four months, for example, they had more accidents during free play and performed poorly on several behavioural tests. Males showed more aggressive social play than controls, while females did less climbing and more random running (Smith & Jansen, 1977c).

Simonson (1979) found a wide variety of behavioural and physical abnormalities in kittens whose mothers had been restricted to 50 per cent of normal food intake throughout gestation. Delays were apparent in many measures of early behavioural development, including posture, crawling, suckling, eye-opening, walking, running, play and climbing. Predatory and exploratory behaviour were also delayed in development. In terms of both physical growth and behaviour the greatest effects of early undernutrition tended to show up later in ontogeny. Growth stunting, for example, did not become apparent until well after weaning, while the greatest delays in behavioural development tended to be in late-appearing behaviour patterns, particularly those requiring a high degree of motor coordination. Kittens of undernourished mothers showed poorer learning ability, antisocial behaviour towards other cats and heightened emotionality, characterised by abnormal levels of fear and aggression. Despite nutritional rehabilitation, some of these developmental delays, learning deficits and emotional abnormalities persisted into the next generation, albeit in a less severe form (Simonson, 1979).

Kittens of mothers fed on a low-protein diet during late gestation and lactation showed a variety of behavioural abnormalities (Gallo, Werboff & Knox, 1980, 1984). The kittens lost balance more often, indicating possible abnormalities in their motor development. Not surprisingly, social interactions between mothers and kittens were also affected by maternal malnutrition, with kittens generally showing fewer social interactions with their mothers and poorer attachment, as assessed by separation experiments.

Time of eye-opening

An illustration of multiple factors influencing a developmental characteristic comes from a study by Braastad & Heggelund (1984), who looked at several factors affecting the age at which kittens open their eyes. Under normal rearing conditions, the time of eye-opening varies considerably between individuals, ranging between two and 16 days after birth (Norton, 1974). A considerable amount of this variation was explained by four factors: the father's identity (paternity), exposure to light, the kitten's sex and the age of the mother. Dark-reared kittens opened their eyes earlier than normally-reared kittens; kittens of young mothers opened their eyes earlier than those of older mothers; and female kittens opened their eyes earlier than males. The number of siblings (litter size) and kittens' growth rate were not related to the time of eye-opening. Of all the factors influencing eye-opening, the one which explained most variance was paternity, indicating a strong genetic effect.

Multiple influences on predatory behaviour

The point about multiple influences on development is well illustrated by the development of predatory behaviour in cats, where it is clear that many different forms of experience contribute to development, as we have discussed earlier. To reiterate some of the main points, adult predatory skills are improved both by previous experience with prey when young and by observing the mother's predatory behaviour when young. A single experience of catching and eating a mouse can be enough to make a kitten a skilled mouse-killer thereafter, with a large increase in the success of subsequent predatory attempts. Kittens always kill the type of rat they have seen their mother kill when young, although they might also kill other kinds of rats. Early diet also exerts an influence; Kuo (1930) raised kittens as vegetarians and found that this early experience reduced their tendency to eat rats, although it had no effect on their readiness to kill rats. Another early influence on the development of predatory behaviour is competition between litter mates for access to prey; the approach of a litter mate often triggers an attack on the prey. Adult predatory skills can also be improved by experience with prey when adult.

A combination of hunger plus exposure to dead prey when young is most likely to produce an adult cat that will kill rats. Hunger also facilitates attack on prey in older kittens, by making them less defensive (Adamec, Stark-Adamec & Livingston, 1980b). In adult cats, prey-killing is jointly dependent on how long they have been deprived of food and the size and apparent difficulty of the prey, so hunger by itself is not a necessary condition for predatory behaviour to occur (Biben, 1979).

Concluding remarks

It is easy to suppose that development is merely preparation for adult life. However, the young animal has to survive and not everything seen in early life is a precursor of adult behaviour, the most obvious example being suckling. As some patterns of behaviour drop out of the kitten's repertoire and others come in we see something almost like the metamorphosis of a caterpillar into a butterfly.

The development of behaviour clearly depends both on internal factors (primarily genes) and external factors (environmental influences). However, to look at a cat's behaviour and ask, 'Is it genetic or is it learned?' is to ask the wrong question. All behaviour patterns require both genes and an environment in order to develop. They emerge as a result of a regulated interplay between the developing cat and the conditions in which it lives. Moreover, like the records in a juke-box, different genes may be expressed in different environmental conditions. For that reason the cat's behaviour cannot be divided into two types — those patterns caused by internal factors (often referred to as 'genetic' or 'innate' behaviour) and those caused by external factors ('acquired' behaviour). Many actions, such as suckling, are clearly present at birth (the strict meaning of 'innate') and many other behaviour patterns, such as some of the motor patterns used by the cat for catching prey, appear without opportunities for practice or for copying from other individuals. None the less, even such unlearned patterns of behaviour are often modified by learning and other forms of experience later in development. And other environmental factors, such as the quantity and quality of nutrition, can have general effects on behavioural development.

We are beginning to understand the dynamics of the processes which generate both the stable and the modifiable aspect of the individual cat's behaviour. These processes may often seem complicated, but it is becoming apparent that relatively simple rules for development can generate the variability found at the surface. For instance, at a particular stage in its development the kitten has something almost equivalent to a hunger for learning about certain kinds of things. However, once the knowledge is acquired, the kitten is resistant to further change. The most striking example of this is the way preferences are formed for social companions (which in the case of the domestic cat often include humans). Once formed, their preferences can be very hard to change.

It is easy to focus on how different cats are from each other. But it is as well to remember that the underlying organisation is often such that the animal seems to know where it is going in its development. The same skills found in adults have often developed in very different ways. The example which we considered at some length in this chapter was predatory behaviour. While cats show many of the components of stalking and catching prey without obvious pre-

vious experience of doing such things, they also greatly improve these skills. They may do so as a result of play or as a result of watching their mother. But if all else fails, they may become as good as other cats with plenty of early experience as a result of catching prey when they are forced to fend for themselves. Examples of versatility such as these demonstrate how well adapted is the cat to thrive in different environments. They serve to explain the similarities as well as the differences that are found in cats living in very different climates and conditions.

Acknowledgements

We are grateful to Tim Caro, Robert Harcourt, Mike Mendl, Jay Rosenblatt, James Serpell and Dennis Turner for reading and commenting on an earlier draft.

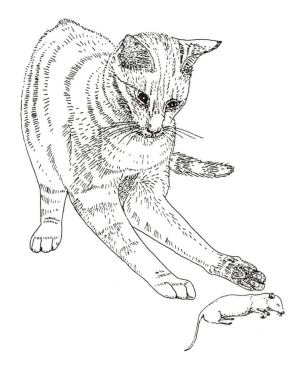

3

Factors influencing the mother–kitten relationship

*John M. Deag, Aubrey Manning
and Candace E. Lawrence*

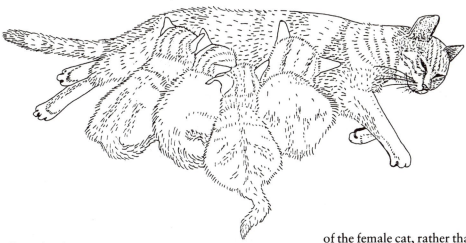

Introduction

Discussions of the mother–kitten relationship of the cat (*Felis s. catus*) often concentrate on the behaviour exchanged between a mother cat and her litter of kittens, and how this changes as the kittens pass from birth, through weaning to independence. Although we consider this to be a fundamental aspect of the subject, we propose here that the nature of the mother–kitten relationship can only be understood if it is examined in relation to other aspects of the animal's biology. For a domestic animal, such as the cat, this approach is not without its problems but we hope to show that it can be rewarding.

Studies of feral cats suggest that it might be misleading to consider the relationship between a mother and her kittens without examining the influence of other members of the population. For instance, the role of social organisation must be considered, for the success of the reproductive female may be influenced by her relationship with other members of the population. It is equally important to examine the whole life history

of the female cat, rather than to concentrate simply on what happens within one litter. This is because the cat, like so many other small mammals, has a series of litters of variable size over a number of reproductive seasons. It is quite possible that what happens between a mother and her kittens in one litter, may have consequences for her subsequent reproduction and may be determined, at least in part, by her earlier reproductive history.

The exchange of behaviour which characterises the relationship between a mother and her litter, is influenced by kitten age and a variety of other factors such as litter size and maternal condition. In captive animals the importance of litter size and maternal condition is easy to overlook since constant supervision can protect mothers and kittens from the ill effects of food shortage. However, lactation is a costly process to the female and in feral cats a large litter or low hunting success may have a dramatic effect on the competition between the kittens and on their survival.

For these and other reasons which will be examined, it is important to be cautious about discussing *the* mother–kitten relationship. A typical form of maternal behaviour is, of course, shown but, because of the numerous factors influencing a mother's behaviour and that of her kittens, no single, stereotyped pattern of relationship should be expected. Are the different styles of mothering and the different relationships seen, simply a consequence of the different factors (such as litter size, kitten sex) acting on a particular litter, or are they influenced by factors such as maternal experience or personality? We shall end our chapter with a discussion of this issue.

Sources of information

Most information on the mother–kitten relationship comes from laboratory or house cats. Studies of these may provide detailed, well structured information, but suffer from being artificial in several important respects. Mothers are usually kept alone with their kittens, thus excluding interaction with other cats, particularly other females who would often be present in the social group (see below). Mothers are usually confined with their kittens, limiting their freedom to control the time they spend with their litter. *Ad lib.* food is usually provided so that mothers do not have to partition their time between hunting and being with their kittens and as a consequence, a mother's response to low hunting success cannot be assessed. In house cats, a human caretaker may interact frequently with the mother and kittens, and become an unnatural focus of attention for the mother and the growing young. As a consequence, important aspects of the mother–kitten relationship may be concealed or inadequately expressed. Finally, litters may be artificially culled for convenience of study. This may particularly distort the situation when litters are culled to below the average litter size. It could be argued that these points are irrelevant because the cat is a domestic animal that has evolved alongside man for thousands of years. Many cats must, however, have survived and reproduced without constant human help and their behaviour will have been subject to natural selection. To understand fully the significance of the mother–kitten relationship, it is essential to relate studies of captive animals to broader aspects of the species' biology.

The context of the mother–kitten relationship
Social organisation

When not strictly confined by their owners or when feral, female cats tend to live singly or in small groups with a few other females, some of which are often daughters from previous litters. These groups are usually based at a farm or other human habitation, the females hunting in a home range which they share with other females from the group. Some groups include an adult, reproductive male but many males tend to live more solitary lives. Males typically use larger home ranges which may overlap those of several female groups and usually overlap with the ranges of other males (see Chapters 6 and 7).

The social organisation of the cat shows considerable variability (Kerby & Macdonald, Chapter 6) but two features relevant to the present discussion are regularly seen. First, while some females live alone, many live in small groups with other females. Litters from different females may be reared in the same nest and become mixed, the females giving maternal-like care, including severing umbilical cords and suckling, to kittens that are not their own (Baerends-von Roon & Baerends, 1979; Macdonald, 1981). This adds an additional level of complexity to any study of the mother–kitten relationship, since the latter cannot, in these cases, be considered in isolation from the relationship between the females involved. Unfortunately, all detailed studies of maternal behaviour have ignored communal rearing and have been made on single mothers isolated with their kittens. The second general point to emerge is that the mating system tends to polygyny (with one male living and mating with several females) or promiscuity (no long-term bonds between sexual partners) (Liberg, 1981). In these mating systems, males usually play no direct part in rearing their offspring and male cats can largely be discounted in studies of the mother–kitten relationship. In particular, males do not usually form a close bond with a single female (for a possible exception, see Corbett, 1979), do not usually provision the lactating female with food, and do not bring food to the kittens (Corbett, 1979; Liberg, 1980). Given the stress that lactation can sometimes place on a female, this lack of male care is significant.

Life history

A litter of kittens usually represents only part of a female's lifetime reproductive output. Females breed for a number of years and often have two litters in a year (Liberg, 1981) but this may depend on whether kittens from the first litter survive (Ewer, 1973;

Baerends-van Roon & Baerends, 1979). Litter size varies from one to ten (Robinson & Cox, 1970), the mean being between four and five. In small mammals gestation typically puts little strain on a mother but lactating mothers frequently call on their body reserves to supplement their food intake. The cat is no exception to this rule and large litters place a considerable burden on the lactating mother (Deag, Lawrence & Manning, 1987). We shall discuss the behavioural consequences of this later. These factors mean that a mother is expected to limit the amount of maternal care given to her *current* offspring, for giving too much care may affect her health and reduce her lifetime reproductive success. The mother–kitten relationship seen within any one litter is expected to reflect this interaction between the short- and long-term benefits and costs of maternal care. This approach underlines the importance of understanding the relationship between maternal behaviour, kitten growth and mortality.

Another aspect of cat biology to consider here is that the mating system dictates that adult male and adult female cats live different lives. Adult males are larger than females, a factor presumably linked with male–male competition for females and other resources. In the present context it is therefore interesting to ask whether male and female kittens place an unequal burden on their mother, and whether this is reflected in the mother–kitten relationship.

Behavioural measures of the mother–kitten relationship

The *relationship* between a mother and her kittens is revealed by the nature and frequency of the interactions between them. As the kittens grow from birth through to nutritional independence, their relationship with their mother changes dramatically. The nature and control of this change, which involves changes in behaviour by both mother and kittens, usually provides the focus for our attention (Lawrence, 1981). It is important to remember that as there are several kittens in a litter, there is really a *set* of changing relationships, rather than a *single*, standard relationship. Most people who have bred cats will appreciate this point, for kittens often show individual differences in behaviour from an early age (Moelk, 1979). For some measures, however, we are forced to ignore these differences and to use litter means. This is not just a matter of convenience; when

litters are compared statistically the variation (for example in individual weight or behaviour) within litters is small compared with the variation between litters. As a consequence individual kittens in a litter cannot be considered as independent data points in a statistical analysis (Martin, 1982; Deag *et al.*, 1987). In this section we summarise the main types of interaction and behaviour patterns which can be measured in order to compare mothers and to reveal developmental changes.

Behaviour related to the provision of a suitably sheltered nest site

Kittens are born blind and helpless, with limited ability to move and thermoregulate (Olmstead *et al.*, 1979; Jensen, Davis & Shnerson, 1980); they are totally dependent on their mother and any other caring female. The choice of a suitable nest site for parturition and early care is clearly vital to the kittens; without it the mother–kitten relationship may end abruptly with kitten death from predation, chilling or dehydration. Mothers make use of what shelter they can find; no real nest building is done (Lawrence, 1981). Protection from predators, which include male cats (West, 1979) is required throughout the dependent period and prior to and after parturition mothers may become aggressive to both strange and familiar males (Moelk, 1979; Liberg, 1981) and to other species such as dogs (Lorenz, 1954; Ewer, 1969; Leyhausen, 1979). Mothers occasionally move all or part of their litter spontaneously (perhaps because of fouling by faeces and the remains of prey), or if the nest site is disturbed, for instance, by a strange male (Corbett, 1979; Leyhausen, 1979). Nest site selection and changing of nest site are mentioned by several observers (e.g. Baerends-van Roon & Baerends, 1979; Corbett, 1979) but seem to have received little systematic attention.

Kittens that become displaced from the nest, for example by not loosening their grip on a nipple when their mother stands and moves, soon cool and cry. This alerts their mother and they are retrieved (Rosenblatt, 1976; Haskins, 1977, 1979). Even young kittens, for example of four days old, have some ability to return to the nest site should they become displaced a short distance (e.g. less than 0.5 m) from it. In these young animals, olfactory and thermal cues play an important role in this orientation behaviour, vision becoming more important as they get older

(Rosenblatt, Turkewitz & Schneirla, 1969; Rosenblatt, 1971).

Maternal behaviour at and shortly after parturition

The mother's behaviour at parturition provides important information for assessing the relationship. Prior to parturition the mother cleans herself, especially around the mammary glands (Ewer, 1969) and genitalia. As the kittens are born she cleans the birth membranes from them and severs the umbilical cord, lies with them to provide warmth, makes her ventrum accessible to facilitate suckling and calls to the kittens (Schneirla, Rosenblatt & Tobach, 1963; Moelk, 1979). She stays with them and is responsive to their calls, licking them and nuzzling the kittens towards her ventrum and adjusting her body posture to suit them. Individual kittens or whole litters may die at this time if the mother does not adjust her behaviour to the kittens' needs. A mother may, for example, kill and eat a kitten while severing the umbilical cord (Baerends-van Roon & Baerends, 1979) or may lie on some of the kittens as she settles down to nurse them and not respond to their calls by moving off them. Kittens may also be eaten later in lactation (perhaps having been killed by the mother), when the changes associated with parturition are over.

Body postures adopted by mothers when with their kittens

When with their kittens mothers use several postures. These include: stand, walk, sit, on-side-lie (one side of the body in contact with the ground, the ventral surface partially or fully exposed, the legs out to one side), half-sit (intermediate between sit and on-side-lie), crouch (ventrum in contact with ground, all four pads support the weight of the body with the pads in full contact with the ground) and lie (ventrum in contact with the ground and supporting the weight of the body, the legs are partially extended or tucked under the body) (Lawrence, 1981). These postures differ in the extent to which the mother's nipples are accessible to the kittens and the frequency with which they are used changes significantly as the kittens grow older (Figure 3.1, Table 3.1). The crouch and lie postures tend to be used by mothers (particularly during the period of weaning), in order to block access to their nipples (Lawrence, 1981). In other circumstances it can be more difficult to interpret the significance of a mother's posture. For example, if a mother is not

Table 3.1. *Two-way analysis of variance on maternal postures and other behavioural measures related to nursing*[a]

Measure	Source of variance		
	Main effects		Interaction effect
	Mothers	Weeks	Mothers × weeks
Sit	8.91***	19.24***	1.32
Sit-nurse	17.73***	5.64***	2.97***
Half-sit	14.97***	1.03	1.55**
On-side-lie	6.54***	46.01***	1.55**
Half-sit + on-side-lie	9.57***	33.05***	1.80**
Crouch	8.21***	6.61***	2.29***
Lie	6.41***	10.99***	1.79***
Crouch + lie	8.65***	15.98***	2.01***
Shift	3.90***	25.16***	2.08***
Degrees of freedom	16,288	5,288	77,288

[a] Based on seventeen mothers observed for the the first six weeks (see Figure 3.1). F ratios are given with significance levels indicated as follows: ** $p < 0.01$, *** $p < 0.001$.
From Lawrence (1981).

making her nipples readily available, is it reasonable to assume that she is unable to produce sufficient milk and therefore limiting suckling? Or could she just be what might colloquially be called a 'poor mother', one who is healthy and has milk but who for some reason is not making this available to her kittens? These alternatives cannot be separated by studying body postures alone; information is also required on the mother's physical condition and on behavioural interaction, both related to nursing and to other aspects of the mother–kitten relationship.

Behaviour seen between mothers and their kittens

Initially, the kittens' activities are restricted to crawling along the mother's body and nuzzling against the ventrum to locate a nipple, often in competition with other kittens. They suckle, lie still by the mother, move around near her and call. A call frequently given by the kittens is the cry (called the 'Type A Call' by Brown *et al.*, 1978) which is associated with the kitten being distressed. It is given when a kitten wakes and is presumably hungry, when a kitten's movement is restricted, for example, by being trapped under its mother, or if it becomes isolated and cold (Haskins, 1979; Lawrence, 1981). Suckling is accompanied by

(a)

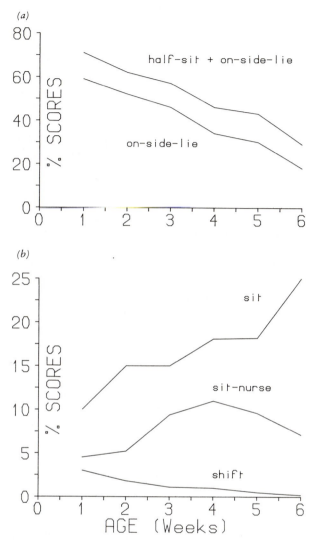

(c)

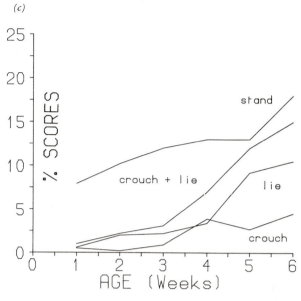

Fig. 3.1. Changes in the use of different body postures by 17 mothers (with two to four kittens) over the first six weeks after parturition. Based on instantaneous sampling of body postures with an interval of 90 sec. Four sessions, each with 50 samples, were made each week. The plotted scores are the percentage of scores for each of the postures defined in the text, together with some composite measures. Two additional measures are shown on Fig. 3.1 (*b*): Sit-nurse – kittens suckling with the mother in the sit posture. Shift – an adjustment in the mother's body posture while in sit-nurse, half-sit or on-side-lie when the kittens were in contact with the mother. From Lawrence (1981).

the kitten purring (Moelk, 1979) and treading against the mother's ventrum. It is thought that these treading movements stimulate milk ejection and that several ejections of milk may occur during one bout of suckling (Lawrence, 1981). Kittens may initially spend nearly eight hours a day suckling but this falls as they grow older (Rosenblatt, Turkewitz & Schneirla, 1962; see also Lawrence, 1981).

A mother's direct interaction with her kittens involves giving the 'brrp' call as she approaches them (Lawrence, 1981; called a 'mhrn' murmur by Moelk, 1979, and a 'chirp' by Bateson, Martin & Young,

1981), and nuzzling and licking the kittens to arouse them and stimulate urination and defecation. Nursing is often accompanied by the mother purring or giving 'brrp' calls and by the mother shifting her body posture in response to the kittens' nuzzling at her ventrum and in response to their cries (Baerends-van Roon & Baerends, 1979; Lawrence, 1981).

When the kittens are about four weeks old their mother brings prey to the nest site and the weaning process begins (see below). Over the next few weeks the mother plays an important role in the development of her kittens' predatory behaviour (see Chapter 2).

Mothers also play with their kittens but the extent to which this happens varies considerably (unpublished observations). During weaning, kittens take a particularly active role in approaching their mother in order to initiate suckling (see below) and may attempt to suckle when she is standing, feeding or moving (Rosenblatt, 1971; Lawrence, 1981). At this time mothers may respond to nuzzling by blocking access to nipples, moving away or with aggression (Lawrence, 1981; Martin, 1982).

As the kittens are now more mobile they also initiate a greater variety of interactions with their mother and each other, including play (Chapter 2) and rubbing against their mother (possibly a form of greeting [Moelk, 1979]). They become more and more responsive to external stimuli and from about six weeks of age start to show adult-like responses to visual social stimuli (e.g. a silhouette of an adult cat) and to odours (e.g. adult male cat urine) (Kolb & Nonneman, 1975). The kittens explore around the nest site and Hartel (1972, 1975) found that in this situation they give a call made up of pure ultrasonic components separated by low intensity, lower frequency components which are within the range of human hearing. The function of this ultrasonic call is unknown but, as the mother responds with a similar call, it appears to be concerned with communication between mother and kitten. Mothers watch over their kittens and continue to be vigilant and may give a sudden growl to warn their kittens of danger. The kittens scatter, hide and remain still until the danger has passed (Ewer, 1973).

The time spent with the litter

Important information on the relationship can be gained by recording the number of visits a mother makes to her litter and the time she spends with it. This will be dictated by the need to nurse the litter frequently and the need to feed herself to maintain body weight and to produce sufficient milk. Unrestricted mothers tend not to leave their kittens for two days following parturition (Baerends-van Roon & Baerends, 1979). In their studies of laboratory cats, Rosenblatt & Schneirla (1962), Scnheirla *et al.* (1963) and Martin (1982) found that mothers typically spend most of their time with their kittens until during the fourth and fifth week. After this a mother spends an increasing amount of time resting on her own until her freedom to isolate herself is eventually limited by the kittens' increasing agility. Our study (Deag *et al.*,

1987) has produced similar results. Each mother and litter were kept in a cage $1.06 \times 1.10 \times 0.46$ m, with a shelf 0.53×0.46 m positioned 0.55 m from the cage floor. Under these conditions the mother spent 95 to 100 per cent of the observation time with the kittens for the first four weeks. After this time there was a general but erratic decline in this measure as the mother spent more time on the shelf (Figure 3.2). Figure 3.3 shows the frequency with which the kittens went to the shelf, an indication of their increasing mobility.

Approaching and leaving

One way to demonstrate the changing roles of the mother and kittens in their relationship, particularly over the period of weaning, is to examine the relative frequency with which each approaches and leaves the other. This has been done using approaches that are specifically related to the initiation of suckling bouts (Figure 3.4; Rosenblatt *et al.*, 1962; Rosenblatt, 1971) or by measuring approaching and leaving without reference to the context of the behaviour (Martin, 1982). Hinde & Atkinson (1970) used the latter method in a study of rhesus monkey mothers and infants, to calculate an index representing the mother's or infant's responsibility for maintaining proximity. Although a similar index has been successfully used by Martin (1982) for mother cats with two kittens (by scoring each kitten separately), its use becomes more complicated in large litters where the mother may simultaneously approach and leave several kittens, which may or may not represent the whole of her litter. Martin (1982) found that as kittens grow older they become responsible for a higher proportion of approaches between their mothers and themselves (Figure 3.5a) and an increasing but smaller proportion of the departures (Figure 3.5b). As a consequence the kittens' responsibility for proximity index was positive over the period studied (Figure 3.5c). This means that at this time, the kittens played a greater part in keeping near their mother than vice versa.

Schneirla and Rosenblatts' measure concentrates on the initiation of suckling but ignores the termination of suckling, a feature that is important for assessing the willingness of the mother to continue nursing and for assessing the persistence of the kittens. Martin's measure gains from placing equal emphasis on approaching and leaving in both mother and kittens,

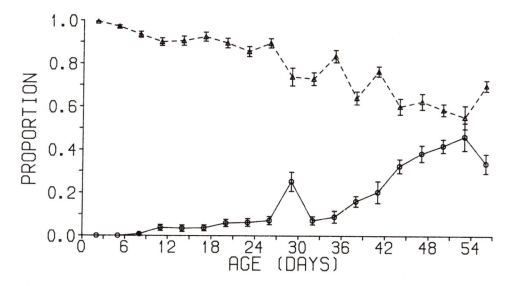

Fig. 3.2. The proportion of observation time in which a mother was with at least one of her kittens (dashed line) and a mother was on the shelf (line). Means and standard errors of the mean are given for 14 litters. The data were reduced to three-day blocks (days 1–3, 4–6, etc., day 0 = the day of birth), the centre of each block being plotted. The 30 min observations are described in the text.

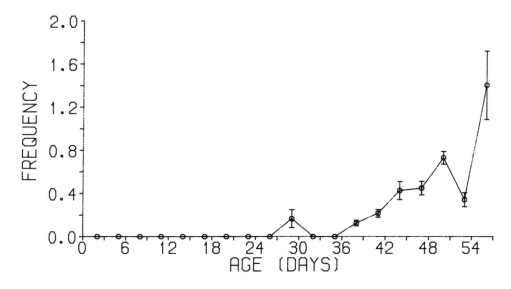

Fig. 3.3. The frequency each kitten went to the shelf in the 30 min observation periods. The mean score for the kittens in each litter was calculated and the mean and standard errors of these means are plotted. The peak in the curve at 28–30 days is due to the kittens in only one of the 14 litters. Other details as for Fig. 3.2.

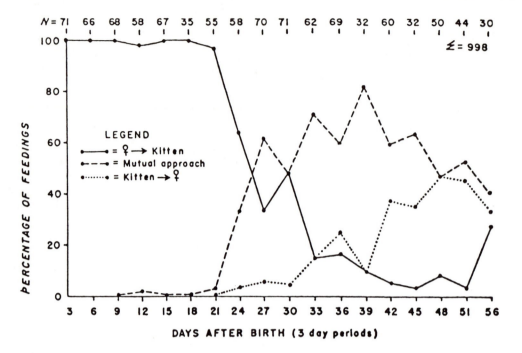

Fig. 3.4. The initiation of suckling in three litters of cats. Based on daily two-hour periods of observation which have been summed over three-day intervals. *N* is the number of feedings observed in each three-day period. From Schneirla & Rosenblatt (1961). Reprinted with permission, from the American Journal of Orthopsychiatry. Copyright (1961) by The American Orthopsychiatric Association, Inc.

so permitting the calculation of the index. The fact that the observer does not have to judge the reason for the approach or departure simplifies data collection but the method suffers from the drawback that interpretation can be difficult. A mother may, for example, indicate a reduced willingness to nurse by concealing her nipples, or being aggressive rather than by leaving the kittens. Similarly kittens may approach their mother for reasons other than for suckling, for example, to rest in contact or to initiate play. In spite of these drawbacks, both methods, when used in conjunction with other measures, may help us to understand the course of weaning and may provide a way of comparing the course of weaning in different litters.

Proximate factors influencing the mother–kitten relationship

Several good reviews are already available of the

behaviour typically shown by mothers and kittens from birth through to independence (e.g. Rosenblatt, 1976; Baerends-van Roon & Baerends, 1979). Accordingly we shall concentrate on some of the numerous factors that may influence the course of the mother–kitten relationship. For ease of discussion these will be treated separately but in reality many of them are interdependent. Little attention will be paid to the development of play and predatory behaviour as these are discussed by Martin & Bateson in Chapter 2.

Kitten age

The most critical factor, that dominates almost every part of the changing relationship, is kitten age. It takes about four weeks from birth for a kitten's motor and sensory abilities to develop and even then these show considerable modification and improvement over the

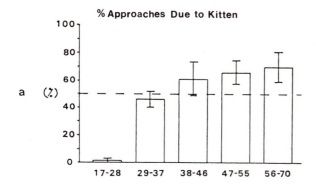

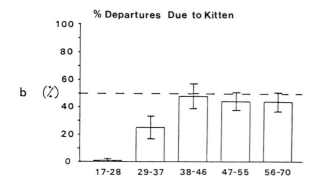

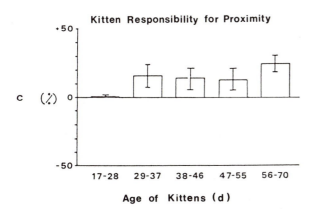

Age of Kittens (d)

Fig. 3.5. Kitten responsibility for maintaining proximity with its mother. (*a*) Per cent approaches due to kitten. The number of times the kitten approached its mother, expressed as a percentage of the total number of times the kitten approached the mother and the mother approached the kitten. Calculated separately for eiach kitten in seven litters of two kittens. (*b*) Percentage of departures due to kitten. Calculated as (*a*) but for kitten departures. (*c*) Kitten responsibility for proximity. Calculated as (*a*) − (*b*). A score of zero would indicate that the kitten and mother had equal responsibility for maintaining proximity. From Martin (1982).

subsequent weeks (Baerends-van Roon & Baerends, 1979; Martin, 1982; see Chapter 2). Studies typically divide the period of kitten dependence into several stages. Schneirla *et al.* (1963) split the first eight weeks into three periods. Birth to day 20, in which the mother mainly initiates suckling, the young kittens having only a very limited ability to approach their mother; day 20 to shortly after day 30, when the kittens and mother both initiate suckling; and the remaining period from shortly after 30 days onwards during which the mother becomes less tolerant of her kittens' suckling attempts and tends to avoid them rather than initiate suckling. Moelk (1979) divided the first eight weeks into two main blocks; the nest stage from birth to 32 days, and the period after this during which the kittens begin to handle prey brought by their mother and start to develop their prey-handling skills.

Temporal divisions like these may appear to be useful aids for organising our thoughts on the changing relationship. They should, however, be approached with caution, since they tend to suggest that during development there are discontinuities which may, in fact, not exist. The precise timing of development will also depend in part on factors other than age and so for some questions, for example those concerned with weaning, it is best to avoid thinking in terms of discrete, relatively fixed developmental stages.

Litter size

In our study (Deag *et al.*, 1987) the average litter size for 71 litters was 4.4 kittens (minimum = 2, maximum = 8), a typical figure (Robinson & Cox, 1970). Cats have eight nipples; however, the rear ones are used preferentially and so the nipples may not all be equally attractive to the kittens (Ewer, 1959). This may be because the rear ones are more readily accessible to new-born kittens and consequently become enlarged through repeated stimulation, or because the mammary tissue differs in its milk producing potential. Rosenblatt (1976) in fact stated that only three pairs of nipples are functional. Even if this is the case, there will be more than enough for the kittens in an average litter. Many kittens tend to select a preferred nipple or pair of nipples within a few days of birth but others show more variability in where they suckle (Ewer, 1959; Rosenblatt, 1976). Our observations suggest that in large litters, young kittens show proportionally more competitive scrambling and pushing

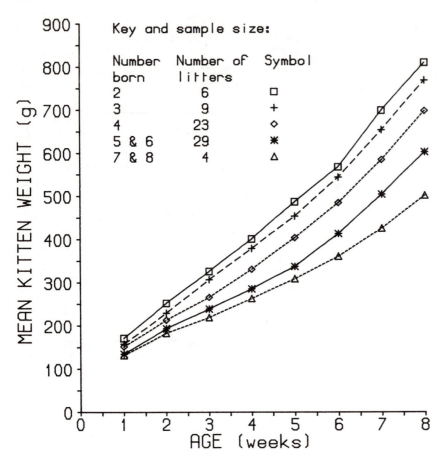

Fig. 3.6. The relationship between kitten weight and age for litters of different size. Kittens were weighed three times a calendar week and a mean kitten weight obtained for each of the 71 litters at each age. The mean of these means is plotted for each litter size (based on the number of kittens born). From Deag *et al.* (1987).

among themselves as they search for a nipple. It is also to be expected that such competition soon becomes less intense in litters in which the kittens develop clear nipple preferences.

Little difference is seen in the average birth weight of kittens born in litters of one to four kittens but in larger litters (five, six and seven), kitten birth weight is negatively correlated with litter size (Nelson, Berman & Stara, 1969, based on 169 litters, 662 kittens). Over the first eight weeks, kittens in small litters are generally heavier than those in large litters (Figure 3.6). The mean growth rate over the first eight weeks ranges from 7.3 g per day in litters of seven or eight, to 13.7 g per day in litters of two (Deag *et al.*, 1987). We have concluded from these and related measures that, as in other species with variable litter size, the mother's milk production increases with the number of young but not in direct proportion. There would therefore be

less milk per kitten in large litters than in small litters (Deag *et al.*, 1987). Schneirla *et al.* (1963) reported, on the basis of three litters (one each of one, two and three kittens) that the time spent nursing the kittens increases with litter size. We are currently checking this observation with a larger sample and a greater range of litter sizes. If confirmed, it would imply, as with the growth information just presented, that a mother finds it harder to supply adequate milk to larger litters.

Is being small and light weight disadvantageous to a weaned kitten? Although there is no evidence for this from feral cats, it does not seem unreasonable to suggest that kittens which are light at independence may have a reduced chance of surviving to breed. Male cats which are small and light are more likely to be low-ranking and less likely to reproduce (Liberg, 1981). This suggests that small male kittens may be at a distinct disadvantage and may suffer a delay in breeding. Further effects due to litter size are examined below when we discuss maternal health and weaning.

Kitten sex

Adult male cats are considerably larger than adult females and take about three, rather than two years to reach their full weight (Liberg, 1981). These differences can be related to the different selection pressures acting on males and females during the evolution of the mating system (Liberg, 1981). Are these differences in body size reflected in the relationship between the growing kittens and their mother? For example, are male kittens more demanding of their mother, do they take more milk and grow faster? It is easy to be impressed by the occasional large male kitten but the general answer to these questions appears to be 'no'. A graph presented by Latimer & Ibsen (1932) shows that up until eight weeks of age, male and female kittens are very similar in weight, after which males grow larger. We have recently been able to confirm this finding for the first eight weeks (71 litters, 312 kittens), and measures of maternal weight change during lactation also show no evidence for differential investment by mothers in male and female kittens (Deag et al., 1987). In the period between eight weeks of age and full nutritional independence, it is possible that the larger male kittens require more food and therefore that their mothers have to hunt more to support them, but this has not been established.

No published information appears to be available on the influence of sex on behavioural interaction between mothers and their unweaned kittens; however, in view of the finding reported above, we would not expect it to have a large influence. Barret & Bateson (1978) and Bateson & Young (1979) reported that, in the presence of their mothers during weeks eight to 12, male kittens made significantly more 'object contacts' during play than females. The sex differences were reduced when the female kittens had male litter mates. It might be expected that this object play would be associated in nature with the manipulation of prey items brought to the nest site by the mother but Caro (1980b, 1981b) could that kittens showed no sex differences in any aspect of predatory behaviour. During weeks four to 12, sex differences are not seen in social play (Barrett & Bateson, 1978) but differences do emerge during weeks 12 to 16, as

the frequency of play falls. The extent of the difference is influenced by the sex of the play companions; females playing with males become more male-like in their behaviour (Caro, 1981a).

Is it possible that the presence or absence of a male sibling during development could be responsible for some of the individual differences in the behaviour of adult females, including different styles of mothering (see below)? The probability of a female being born in a litter with only other females is surprisingly low, in the order of four per cent or less (Table 3.2) and this will be even lower if two mothers give birth together. Although some mothers will, for one reason or another, have a biased kitten sex ratio, the norm is for most kittens to grow up in mixed litters. The presence of a male litter mate may be an important envrionmental influence on the development of female kittens. Our calculation, however, shows that in practice females are rarely reared without males. This suggests that, while the absence of this experience may be important for four out of 100 females, it can normally play little part in producing the wide range of individual differences seen in female behaviour.

Parity of the mother

Schneirla et al. (1963) reported few differences between primiparous (first-time) and multiparous mothers during parturition. During the intervals between delivering foetuses, multiparous mothers were less restless and more likely to correctly direct their licking towards the kitten, their abdomen and genitalia. Primiparous mothers tend to have smaller litters (Robinson & Cox, 1970), irrespective of the age at which they become pregnant (Connelley & Todd, 1972), and are sometimes reported by cat breeders to lose more kittens and to be generally less effective mothers. Leyhausen (1956a, quoted by Ewer, 1969) recorded that young (by which we presume is meant primiparous) mothers may not use the correct neck grip when first picking up their young.

We have collected data on primiparous and multiparous mothers to compare them and to compare the behaviour of primiparous mothers with their first and second litters. We have yet to analyse the behavioural results but our study of growth indicates that, in the first eight weeks, parity had virtually no effect on kitten growth and mother weight change (16 first litters, compared with 55 later litters; Deag et al., 1987). One complication for studies of the

Table 3.2. *The probability of a female kitten being reared only with other females*[a]

	Litter size (L)							
	1	2	3	4	5	6	7	8
Number of litters recorded[b]	0	6	9	23	22	7	3	1
Probability of each litter size	0	0.085	0.127	0.324	0.310	0.099	0.042	0.014
Probability of all the other kittens in the litter being female[c]	—	0.5	0.25	0.125	0.0625	0.0313	0.0156	0.0078
Probability of a female kitten being in a litter of size L and only with female litter mates[d]	—	0.0425	0.0318	0.0405	0.0194	0.0031	0.0007	0.0001

[a] The last row shows that the probability of a female kitten being reared only with other females is 4% or less.
[b] Data from Deag *et al.*, 1987.
[c] On the basis of the evidence presented by Robinson & Cox (1970) we have assumed a 50:50 sex ratio at birth and that sex ratio is unrelated to litter size.
[d] More females than males tend to be stillborn and to die before weaning (Robinson & Cox, 1970), a point ignored in our calculation. We have also ignored the consequences of females being born into a litter of size one.

behavioural consequences of parity is that primiparous mothers tend to be younger than multiparous mothers and therefore any effects due to maternal age (e.g. playfulness) must be separated from effects due to parity.

Mother's body weight, health and food availability

In the next section we shall consider the timing of weaning and the associated behavioural changes in mothers and kittens. It is necessary, however, to precede this by considering the factors that may influence a mother's milk supply and, through this, the timing of weaning. As discussed above, milk production is a costly process for the mother and the restricted growth of kittens in large litters suggests there is a limit beyond which mothers cannot increase their milk supply. In other words a mother's mammary tissue can only produce enough milk to support a limited biomass of growing kittens. Once the suckling young have reached a certain weight they will be forced to find an alternative source of energy (solid food) simply because their mother cannot provide enough energy for them (Galef, 1981). Weaning is inevitable for this reason alone. Mothers, particularly in species producing more than one offspring per litter, are expected to push their offspring towards independence from the earliest suitable time, so that they can build up reserves for their next pregnancy and lactation.

What factors influence the upper limit of a mother's milk supply? Unfortunately, milk production in the cat has not been directly studied and we need to draw conclusions from other information. Mothers tend to lose weight when lactating, on average 5.7 g per day (Deag *et al.*, 1987; see also Martin, 1982) and this suggests that, as in many other mammals, a lactating female utilises her body reserves. Mothers with bigger litters are lighter (during the first eight weeks after their kittens were born) which suggests that they have to draw more on their body reserves to feed their kittens (Deag *et al.*, 1987). A female who stores more fat prior to parturition will presumably be able to produce more milk, all other influences being equal. We have evidence which suggests that milk production may be linked to maternal body weight; mothers of light basic weight (weighed when non-pregnant, non-lactating) tend to have light kittens, heavy mothers heavy kittens. Kittens only start to free themselves from this constraint in week 6, the effect being lost by week 8 (Deag *et al.*, 1987). Some of our mothers showed symptoms of what we shall call nutritional stress, during the eight weeks that they were with their kittens. The symptoms varied but typically a mother lost condition, was unsteady on her feet and sometimes lost her appetite. When this happened they were given special attention to improve their health. We have found that this is significantly more likely to happen in lighter mothers [stressed mothers mean basic wt = 2829 g (*n* = 18), unstressed 3048 g (*n* = 43)] and that stressed mothers had larger litters (4.80 kittens, *n* = 19, *vs* 3.63 kittens, *n* = 52). It also happens at an earlier kitten age in mothers with a light basic weight. It is clearly important to take these factors into account when considering the behavioural relationship between mothers and kittens during lactation and how these change at weaning.

In the first few days of lactation (a time when the kittens grow rapidly) a mother presumably relies heavily on her body reserves for milk production, so that she can spend a lot of time with the litter. As lactation proceeds, the growth and survival of the litter in nature would depend on the mother's hunting skills. No information is available on the weight of prey required to support litters of different sizes and the amount of effort required by a mother to catch it (see also Chapter 9). However, when prey are scarce mothers with large litters are likely to have difficulty rearing their kittens, particularly if the mother is small and in poor condition when she gave birth. We believe that this might be reflected in the age at which the litter is weaned, and in the duration of the weaning process (Deag *et al.*, 1987). Under these circumstances, mothers might be able to increase their lifetime reproductive success by culling their litter to a size that they can rear satisfactorily. Some kittens do die during lactation and they may be eaten by the mother, but it is as yet unknown whether such deaths should be interpreted as the mother reducing the size of the litter to a more manageable size.

The change from milk to prey

Weaning is the process during which the rate of parental investment falls sharply and the young move rapidly towards independence (Martin, 1984b, 1985). During this a kitten becomes less dependent on its mother's milk and more dependent (in feral cats) on eating the prey that she brings to the nest, until it is finally able to capture its own food. Weaning often appears to be a time of conflict between mother and offspring, and this becomes understandable when the process is viewed from an evolutionary point of view (Trivers, 1972; Galef, 1981).

Baerends-van Roon & Baerends (1979) reported that mothers brought back mice to the nest from the fourth week onwards and that in this way the kittens were introduced to solid food. Moelk (1979) picked out day 32 as the time when kittens are introduced to prey, while Ewer (1969) found in two litters that prey was first carried to the young at 35 and 36 days. At about this time both mother and kittens show changes in their behaviour. Schneirla *et al.* (1963), for example, found that mothers became less tolerant of their kittens from day 30. The typical picture that emerges from most studies is that from during the fifth week onwards, mothers take less initiative in initiating suckling. They make themselves less available for suckling by leaving their kittens when they attempt to suckle, using body postures to block access to their nipples (Lawrence, 1981) and moving to places that are inaccessible to their kittens. For example, Schneirla *et al.* (1963) and Martin (1982) found that from about day 33 the time the mothers spent on the shelf in the cage increased rapidly from its previous low value.

Some mothers respond aggressively to their kittens' suckling attempts during the weaning period and at least two factors may be responsible for this response. Suckling sometimes appears to cause the mother discomfort, because of the size and activity of the kittens pushing at the ventrum and because of the kittens' sharp teeth. Leyhausen (1979) considered that the extra discomfort caused by large litters may contribute to the family breaking up earlier than in small litters. Some mothers that respond aggressively to their kittens' advances appear to be out of condition and it is assumed that their milk supply is failing (Lawrence, 1981; Martin, 1982). Martin (1982) described one instance in which the mothers' aggression disappeared when their condition improved and the kittens were again allowed to suckle. Whatever the immediate cause of their aggression, mothers appear to be more tolerant of very small litters (e.g. one or two kittens) and in these the weaning process may be less traumatic and more gradual and prolonged (Martin, 1982). Indeed, in spite of all the rejection responses just described, kittens of up to eight weeks old and even older can sometimes be seen on the nipple, but it is unknown whether they are obtaining milk (Baerends-van Roon & Baerends, 1979).

While all these changes in the mother–kitten relationship are going on, the kittens eat more solid food, become more active around the nest, and start to play more vigorously in ways that seem associated with the development of prey capture and handling (see Chapter 2).

To understand the nutritional background to the weaning process we really need to know the proportions of the kitten's intake which are obtained from its mother's milk and from solid food over the weaning period. This information is not available. Unfortunately, behavioural observations of the proportion of time on-nipple are potentially misleading. If a kitten suckles a lot, for example, is it getting a lot of milk, is it suckling for a long time because milk let down is slow, or is it non-nutritional suckling which provides comfort (Lawrence, 1981)? Similarly, the decline in kitten nipple preference from about day 30, reported by Ewer (1959), could be interpreted in various ways. Do the kittens use more nipples, because, as they switch to solid food fewer kittens are interested in suckling at any one time (Ewer, 1959), or do they go from nipple to nipple because the milk supply of their preferred nipple is declining?

Studies of kitten growth provide a way of looking at this problem from another angle. When an individual kitten's weight is plotted against its age, a discontinuity in growth is often seen at around 30 days, after which the growth rate accelerates (Bateson & Young, 1981). We have investigated this phenomenon in both individual kittens' weights (266 kittens) and in the mean weights of kittens in a litter (71 litters). The discontinuity occurs in most kittens (78 per cent) and litters (86 per cent) and at a mean age (in both cases) of 31.6 days (Deag *et al.*, 1987). As noted above Schneirla *et al.* (1963) and Moelk (1979) selected, on behavioural grounds, days 30 and 32 as important times in development. The correspondence between these times, the time of decreasing nipple preference, and the mean age of the discontinuity in growth of 31.6 days is striking. It is assumed that this change in growth rate is associated with the weaning process and with kittens increasing the proportion of solid food in their diet (Bateson & Young, 1981; Deag *et al.*, 1987).

Kittens in large litters are significantly more likely to show a discontinuity in weight; the mean litter size for litters with a discontinuity was 4.09 ($n = 61$) and 3.06 ($n = 10$) for litters without a discontinuity. In large litters the discontinuity occurred at a lower mean kitten weight and the kittens grew proportionally faster after it. These findings all support the conclusion that the growth of kittens in large litters is restricted during lactation. The discontinuity occurred earlier in mothers with a low basic weight (weighed when non-pregnant, non-lactating), a finding which suggests a link between the discontinuity and the mother's ability to supply milk (Deag *et al.*, 1987). We suggest that the ability to locate objectively a discontinuity in growth is an important tool which will be extremely useful in studies of the mother–kitten relationship during weaning. In particular it provides an independent reference point for studies of individual or litter differences in behaviour during weaning and we are using it for this purpose in our current project.

The following preliminary results are based on the same sample of fourteen multiparous mothers referred to in Figure 3.2. Each litter was observed twice a week for the first eight weeks and on each observation day it was watched for three 10-minute periods, each separated by at least 30 minutes in order to control for gross changes in activity. Figure 3.7 shows, for a selection of four mothers, the relationship between the age of the kittens and the proportion of the observation time the mother was with them in the on-side-lie posture. In three of the mothers, C16, E09 and K03, note how the age at which the discontinuity in weight gain occurred corresponded with a marked dip in on-side-lie. This suggests a link between this change in kitten growth and the mother adopting this particular posture in which the kittens get easy access to the nipples. Our understanding of this relationship is still incomplete, for we have as yet no explanation for why mothers should return to using on-side-lie after the dip and why the relationship should be absent in some litters (e.g. Figure 3.7, I02). It is obviously necessary to investigate other postures and measures of kitten behaviour, such as the time spent nuzzling and on-nipple.

When all 14 litters are examined, it is seen that the time of the discontinuity in weight gain corresponded with a change in the ratio of kittens approaching and leaving the mother. Around this time the kittens rapidly switched from leaving much more than they approached, to an excess of approaching (Figure 3.8). This suggests that from that time on they took a greater role in trying to keep near their mother, presumably with a view to suckling. The first marked fall in the average time mothers spend with their kittens occurred just before day 30 and did not recover for a few days (see Figure 3.2). This again suggests an

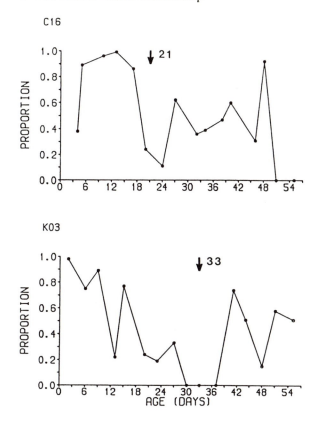

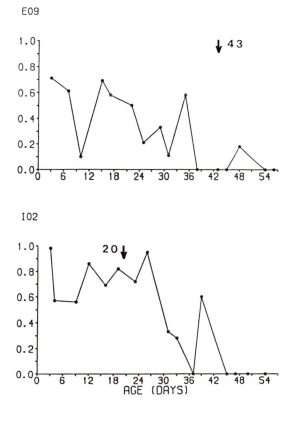

Fig. 3.7. The relationship between the age of the kittens and the proportion of the observation time the mother was with them in the on-side-lie posture. Graphs are shown for four mothers. The arrow indicates the age (in days) at which the discontinuity in weight gain occurred.

association between a change in behaviour and the discontinuity in kitten weight gain which occurred at a mean age of 31.5 days for these 14 litters.

The influence of other adult females on the mother–kitten relationship

No systematic investigation of this topic has been made but because of its potential importance we wish to draw attention to it here. As reported previously, kittens from more than one mother may be reared communally and females without young of their own may also give maternal-like care. In addition to the references quoted earlier, communal rearing has been reported by Ewer (1959), Leyhausen (1979), Lawrence (1981) and the Universities Federation For Animal Welfare (1981). Liberg (1981) found evidence for synchrony of oestrus within groups of cats and suggested that this would facilitate cooperation in the rearing and defence of the young.

Caution should be exercised in assuming that communal nursing is adaptive (see also Chapter 8). Possible costs might include the transmission of disease between litters and reduced transmission of passive immunity from the mother, if the kittens do not obtain colostrum shortly after birth. Unfortunately the information available on the immunoglobulins in cats' colostrum and milk, and on the absorption of these, is incomplete. A significant transmission of immunity from mother to young before birth does occur but the major transmission occurs via colostrum in the first

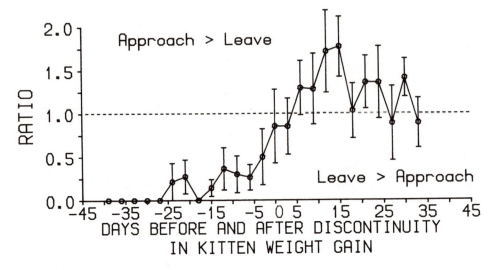

Fig. 3.8. The relationship between age at the discontinuity in weight gain and the ratio of the frequency of kitten-approach-mother/kitten-leave-mother. The mean and standard error of the mean is shown for 14 litters. The horizontal axis has been calculated as age minus the age at which the discontinuity in weight gain occurred. The day of discontinuity in weight gain is therefore represented by day zero for all litters; negative values are days before the discontinuity, positive values are days after it. When the ratio is one, the kittens make an equal number of approaches and departures.

one or two days postpartum. More information is required on the presence and function of the immunoglobulins which are often present in the milk of other species after colostrum production has ceased (Brambell, 1970; Watson, 1980). We conclude that new-born kittens who miss colostrum, through suckling a female who is in a later stage of lactation, may be at a severe disadvantage. It remains to be seen, however, whether in practice this is a problem, for during communal suckling kittens may first suckle from their own mother and only later from other females (P. Bateson, personal communication). A detailed investigation of communal suckling could be rewarding; it should include an analysis of the costs and benefits of the behaviour for all participants.

Different styles of mothering

Mothers show individual differences in many of the behaviour patterns used to measure the mother–kitten relationship (Lawrence, 1981). Differences are seen at all stages in the relationship. For example, mothers vary in the way they first settle down to suckle their kittens after parturition (Schneirla *et al.*, 1963) and in

the extent to which they respond to nuzzling and crying by changing their body posture to release a trapped kitten or to expose their nipples (Lawrence, 1981). In a study of litters from 17 different mothers (litter size two to four) Lawrence (1981) found that the mothers showed highly significant differences in their use of the body postures described earlier (Table 3.1). The interaction effects shown in Table 3.1 between the two factors (mothers and weeks) are significant but smaller than the main effects. This suggests that, although some mothers do change in relation to one another, there is overall consistency in the differences between mothers in terms of their percentage scores on each measure over the six weeks (Lawrence, 1981).

One possible explanation for these differences is that the behaviour shown by a mother reflects the particular combination of factors (e.g. litter size, maternal condition, experience with previous litters) acting on her at that time. We feel that this must be at least part of the answer and are currently making a detailed investigation of this possibility. One important question we are asking is whether mothers show consistent styles of maternal behaviour with consecutive litters, when any effects due to litter size, for example, have been taken into account.

Cats also show individual differences in many other aspects of behaviour, e.g. friendliness to people (see Chapter 4), a point well appreciated by those who keep them as pets and something which is now being systematically investigated (e.g. Feaver, Mendl & Bateson, 1986). Baerends-van Roon & Baerends (1979) found that their kittens started to show individual differences during the second month of life, as they started to become more independent, and attributed many of the differences to the contrasting environments the kittens had experienced. Differences in maternal care may possibly be associated with subsequent differences in kitten behaviour; for example, kittens which are experimentally weaned early play more (Martin & Bateson, 1985b). Whatever the source of such differences during development, it is possible that they contribute to the different styles of mothering discussed earlier. As an extreme and unnatural example, Baerends-van Roon & Baerends (1979) reported that two females who had been isolated from seven weeks of age, killed their kittens, one female treating them like prey. We are currently investigating whether there is any connection between the maternal style shown by a mother and that shown by her daughters when they have their own kittens.

Concluding remarks

We have seen that good descriptions of parturition are available. Several qualitative and quantitative studies have been made of the behaviour exchanged between mother cats and their kittens as they grow from birth through to independence. Most of this information has been obtained from cats kept under confined, laboratory conditions. Unfortunately, there are no comprehensive studies of mothers who cooperate to rear their young.

Quantitative information on the growth of kittens is available. The basic relationship between this, maternal condition and various factors such as litter size, has also been established. Kitten sex seems to have little influence on kitten growth and on the mother–kitten relationship in the first eight weeks.

The behavioural changes in both mother and kittens which are associated with weaning are known but the factors that influence the course of weaning are incompletely understood. An important dimension missing from all studies is the quantity and quality of milk transferred from mother to each kitten over the whole suckling period. Details of the relationship between this and the behaviour and body condition of both mother and kittens (in litters of different size) might help explain many of the behavioural changes that occur during weaning and permit us to assess objectively the relative roles of mother and kittens. One step in this direction has been taken by Bateson, Martin & Young (1981) and Martin & Bateson (1985b) who have simulated early weaning.

Some differences in maternal behaviour due to parity have been suggested. Individual differences in maternal behaviour are known to occur but the origin of these and their consequences for kitten development, are incompletely understood. Consideration of the mother–kitten relationship in the context of the cat's biology and natural history can be expected to shed new light on many of these unanswered questions.

Acknowledgements

We are grateful to the late Mr T. Graham-Marr and to Mr J. A. Woods for providing facilities at the University of Edinburgh Centre for Laboratory Animals. We thank Mr D. E. F. Hay, Miss A. Cave-Brown and the other staff of the Centre for technical help. Professor P. P. G. Bateson provided many helpful comments on the problem of measuring discontinuities in kitten growth. Our research was financed by the Science and Engineering Research Council.

4

Individuality in the domestic cat

Michael Mendl and Robert Harcourt

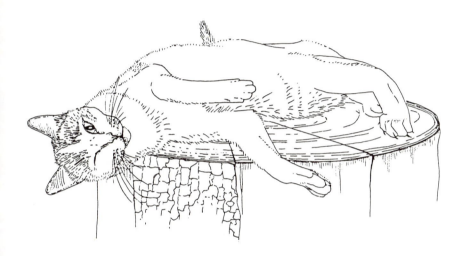

Introduction

Anyone who owns a pet cat and spends time observing it and interacting with it is likely to develop a strong impression of that animal's behavioural characteristics. From this knowledge of the cat's behaviour, the owner may come to view the animal as an individual with a distinct character, similar to other cats in certain respects, but different in others. The owner's perception of his or her animal as an individual with a unique character is reflected in the popular literature on the domestic cat in which references to individuality and personality abound. For example, Beadle (1977) writes the following.

Cats vary as much within their species as people do within theirs. Some cats are so dull-witted that never in their lives do they learn that a door which is ajar can be nudged further open. Other cats can open and shut doors as easily as if they had two hands with opposable thumbs. Some cats are born with unshakeably equable dispositions and others are so high-strung that they go all to pieces when a doorbell rings.

Similarly, accounts of people's relationships with

their pet cats and the surrounding 'cat society' are often peppered with detailed descriptions of the contrasting characteristics of the individuals involved. For example, Wilson & Weston (1947) describe three of their cats as follows.

Dolly was a long-haired silver tabby with the supercilious mannerisms of a pure-breed. Tivvy was short-haired, his coat grayish brown, his disposition most affectionate: he would jump on your lap if you sat reading, get between your face and your book, and, talking and purring prodigiously, pat your cheek with a curled paw until you agreed to stop reading and pet him. Nicky, whose short black fur was tinged with red, was a problem child from the start. He was the scariest, took the longest to tame, bitterly resented correction of any kind.

Many other popular books and articles also emphasise the personality and individuality of domestic cats (e.g. Chazeau, 1965; Necker, 1970; Rockwell, 1978; Johnson & Galin, 1979; Metcalfe, 1980; Alderton, 1983; Palmer, 1983).

However, despite the abundance of these references, this perceived phenomenon of clear and identifiable individual variation in the behaviour of domestic cats has received little direct attention in the scientific literature. Our aims in this chapter are to examine ways of measuring this phenomenon, to outline the sorts of questions of interest to psychologists and biologists that can be asked about individuality, to review the extent to which these have been investigated for the domestic cat, and to suggest areas for future work. We do not pretend to be able to answer most of the questions that we pose, but we do hope to present the phenomenon of individuality in the cat as one which touches on important conceptual issues in psychology and biology, and thus warrants attention.

What is meant by individuality and how can it be studied?

Before considering the questions that can be asked about individuality in the cat, it is important to outline what is meant by the term. From our reading of the popular and scientific literature it appears that when people refer to the individuality of a particular cat, they are using the term as a *descriptive* label for some sort of complex mental picture which they have of the animal. One way of describing this mental image is as an overall perception of the sum total of all the behavioural attributes which characterise the individual and which distinguish it from others of the same species. In this sense, the term personality is sometimes used in the same way. For example, Feaver, Mendl & Bateson (1986) state, 'We felt that each animal (cat) in our laboratory colony had a distinct personality in the sense that the sum total of its behaviour gave it an identifiable style.'

We feel that at the present stage we should not burden the term individuality with any explanatory power but rather should use it in this purely descriptive way to describe a phenomenon whose investigation may result in the elucidation of explanatory principles. Consequently, we also feel that the term individuality is preferable to the terms personality and temperament, the uses of which in the psychological literature have become equated with a variety of theoretical and conceptual approaches, and with the study of particular human characteristics which may or may not have obvious counterparts in the cat (see Pervin, 1980; Goldsmith *et al.*, 1987).

Returning to the statements of what is meant by individuality, two points can be made. The first is that individuality in the cat is seen as a complex emergent perception of 'the sum total' of an animal's behaviour.

The second is that the salient features of a cat's individuality are those which 'distinguish it from other's' or give it an 'identifiable style', in other words those which differ between individuals.

From this it should be clear that to study the phenomenon of individuality in the cat, we must examine individual differences in behaviour and, in particular, individual differences in more general overall descriptions of the ways in which animals behave. (The term individual differences refers to differences between rather than within animals.) But how can individual differences in the ways in which cats perform specific behaviour patterns be related to that complex overall perception of an animal's behaviour which we call individuality? To answer this we must examine how a mental picture of individuality is built up.

Consider an observer watching several cats. Through time he or she may interact with the animals and watch them behave in a variety of situations. Differences in how particular individuals perform specific behavioural actions and in how they interact with one another may become evident. Through observation of these differences, the observer gains an impression of the general patterning and nature of each animal's behaviour in relation to that of others. The general features that distinguish the behaviour of the individuals can be given names. For example, adjectives such as 'friendly', 'curious', 'nervous', 'bold' and so on may be used to refer to the overall patterns of each animal's behaviour which remain elusive when discrete events are considered on their own. These perceived characteristics may be called aspects of behavioural style (see Feaver *et al.*, 1986), and each such aspect, for example 'friendly', may be more characteristic of one cat than another. Finally, the various aspects of behavioural style perceived to be typical of a particular cat are assimilated in the mind of the observer to achieve the overall perception of that animal's behavioural individuality. Thus the perceived individuality of a cat is the result of a mental abstraction from direct observations of the animal's behaviour in relation to that of others. This complex mental process is represented in a very simplified form in Figure 4.1.

It is clear from this that, as we move from individual differences in behaviour patterns to individuality (from left to right in Figure 4.1), the role that the observer plays in describing the cats' behaviour

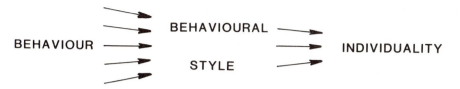

Fig. 4.1 A simplified representation of the levels of perception of individuality. Through observation of many discrete behavioural events (left hand side), the observer may come to view the cat as having certain aspects of behavioural style (centre). The cat's various behavioural styles contribute to the overall perception of its individuality (right hand side).

becomes increasingly complicated. Perception of the individuality of a particular cat may vary between observers according to the nature of their interactions with the animal, their knowledge of other animals (with which they can compare the cat in question), the weight they give to particular aspects of behaviour and behavioural style and so on. On the other hand, description of individual differences in a specifically defined behaviour pattern is likely to be achieved with reasonable agreement amongst observers. This difference is reflected in the fact that at present scientifically rigorous methods have been developed to rate, describe and distinguish individuals according to the way they perform specific behavioural acts and also in terms of aspects of their behavioural style, but not in terms of their overall individuality. Therefore, throughout this chapter we will need to draw on examples of individual differences in behaviour patterns and aspects of behavioural style in our attempt to examine the phenomenon of individuality.

In this respect it is clear that differences in aspects of behavioural style are more directly relevant in an examination of individuality than are simpler differences in behaviour patterns. However, examples of such differences in the scientific literature are few and far between. This is primarily because the study of individuality in the domestic cat is at a very early stage and few scientific papers specifically addressing this problem have been published. Consequently we have been forced to take many of our examples from papers whose specific interests were not individuality or even individual differences. Nevertheless, many of the behaviour patterns described in these papers can be thought of as contributing to our perception of aspects

of behavioural style and, where appropriate, we have categorised them as such. (For example, the time taken for cats to investigate a novel object in a test situation may be perceived in terms of their relative 'boldness' and 'curiosity'.) Our aims in doing this have been to emphasise how our perception of aspects of behavioural style may be affected by consideration of a wide variety of behaviour patterns. We have used adjectives such as 'friendly' or 'curious' in a colloquial way simply to indicate various aspects of behavioural style which can be identified in the cat. Precise definitions of such adjectives have been formulated by Feaver *et al.*(1986) and are necessary when distinguishing individuals, for example by rank-ordering them, according to the adjectives.

Can we be more specific about what types of behaviour we should examine in our study of individuality? We feel that until we understand exactly how we perceive individuality in the cat, and what sorts of behaviour are particularly salient in our perception, we must be open to the possibility that all behaviour patterns which are performed in different ways by different individuals may influence how we perceive the individuality of these animals. Therefore, at the present stage we should be prepared to consider a wide variety of individual differences in our study of individuality.

What questions can be asked about individuality in the cat?

Given the present paucity of our knowledge about what types of behaviour are perceived as characteristics of cat individuality, we prefer to present the study of individuality in terms of the particular questions that can be asked about this phenomenon. It is our contention that, at the present time, these questions rather than particular sorts of behaviour should define the limits of the study of individuality in the cat. The questions are briefly outlined below.

Two general approaches to the study of individuality can be identified. One involves examining the proximate *causes* of individual variation and the other involves studying the *consequences* of behaving in different ways.

The first approach encompasses a variety of questions. For example, can individual variation be directly related to variation in genetic and environmental factors? In other words, can we identify the origins of individuality? How do individual characteristics develop and change across time? How consistent are they as the animal grows older? Are individual differences in behaviour purely a result of differing responses to the immediate environment or are individuals consistently different in a variety of contexts? These problems are of particular interest to developmental psychologists and represent some of the fundamental questions that are asked about human personality and temperament (Pervin, 1980; Goldsmith *et al.*, 1987).

The other approach, favoured by evolutionary biologists (Davies, 1982; Dunbar, 1982), is to focus on the *consequences* of behaving in different ways. How do the particular individual characteristics of an animal affect its interactions and relationships with others? How might such effects have an influence on the individual's abilities to survive and reproduce?

In the cat we have an animal which displays clear and identifiable individual variation in behaviour. Through the process of domestication we have been allowed to become intimately acquainted with the behaviour and habits of this animal and interact with it in various ways. This first-hand knowledge of the cat's behaviour, experienced through living side-by-side with it, allows us to identify complex features of the behaviour of particular individuals and to see subtle differences in how these are expressed by different animals.

In addition, the process of domestication is likely to have relaxed the constraints imposed upon the cat's behaviour by natural selection and to have allowed it to express more variation in behaviour than is seen in non-domesticated species. The cushioned existence of many domestic cats alleviates the constant need for

behaviour to be continually directed towards catching prey, mating, avoiding predators and so on and consequently allows them more time in which to perform other behaviour such as exploration, play, hunting for prey which is left uneaten and so on. Variation in these forms of behaviour are probably not strongly selected against and so are displayed in a pronounced form.

The amount of variation displayed in the behaviour of the cat and the complexity with which we are able to describe this variation, coupled with the relatively short lifespan and maturation rate of this animal (in comparison to humans and other primates in which individuality has been studied), its availability and handleability, and the potential for performing controlled experimental manipulations make it an attractive animal for research into the phenomenon of individuality. In particular, identification of general aspects of behavioural style make the cat a potentially useful animal model for the study of issues which are commonly addressed in human personality and temperament research, fields which focus on more general descriptions of an individual's behaviour. In the following sections we examine methods of measuring individuality in the cat and the extent to which these questions have been investigated for this animal.

How can we measure individuality in the cat?

In the study of non-human primates, three methods of measuring individual characteristics have been used (Stevenson-Hinde, 1983). First, behaviour in a free situation may be recorded using standard ethological techniques. Second, behaviour in structured test situations may be recorded in the same way. Third, individual animals may be independently rated according to specifically defined criteria by two or more observers. To this list we can add a fourth method relevant to the study of the domestic cat: written or verbal reports about cat owners' perceptions and impressions of their pets.

Recording of behaviour in a free situation

The recording of behaviour in a free, uncontrolled situation (in the sense that no particular activities or tasks are required to be performed by the animal, and it is left in its home environment) may provide a useful way of distinguishing between individuals in terms of the frequencies, durations and patterning of their behaviour. This method is accepted as scientifically rigorous since the reliability of measurement can be established (e.g. Caro et al., 1979). However, although this method is useful in measuring individual differences in particular behaviour patterns, it is unable to provide direct measurement of differences in more general features of behavioural style (e.g. 'nervousness', 'excitability'; see Feaver et al., 1986). Furthermore, the uncontrolled nature of the situation means that there is no easy way to assess the effects of changing context on individual behaviour. In addition, to determine cross-time consistency of individual differences, several recordings must be performed and it is possible that the meaning of a particular behavioural item may change with age (Stevenson-Hinde, 1983). Also, a distinction must be made between measurement error and true individual variation (Martin & Kraemer, 1987).

Recording of behaviour in a structured test situation

The use of a structured test situation introduces some control into the context in which behaviour recordings are being made. However, when particular test situations are implemented, it is often difficult to know which sorts of measures (e.g. latency, duration, frequency) should be recorded (Spencer-Booth & Hinde, 1969) and how to interpret performance in terms of individual differences in other, less constrained, situations (e.g. Mendl, 1986). Generalisation of performance to another test or a free situation may be low (e.g. Stevenson-Hinde, Stillwell-Barnes & Zunz, 1980a). In addition, the problems of measuring cross-time consistency and general features of behavioural style, together with the problems of distinguishing measurement error from true differences, as mentioned above, also exist.

Observer rating

This method allows two or more observers who know the animals well to provide independent ratings of each individual on a series of behaviourally defined categories (see Stevenson-Hinde & Zunz, 1978; Feaver et al., 1986). The categories can include aspects of behavioural style such as 'equable' and 'excitable' which cannot be easily measured using conventional ethological recording techniques, because the combination of measures of discrete behavioural events to provide a description of an individual's behavioural style is very difficult (Feaver et al., 1986). The reliability of such ratings can be statistically determined by calculating the correlations between observers' ratigs. In addition, where possible, the method can be compared to more standard recording techniques by correlating observers' ratings with the results of direct recording methods that focus on behaviour patterns related to these categories (Feaver et al., 1986).

The value of this method lies not only in its ability to get at subtle features of an individual's behavioural style, but also through the role that the observer plays as an active instrument, filtering, accumulating and integrating information over a period of time (Block, 1977; Stevenson-Hinde, 1983; Feaver et al., 1986). Although this may mean that the observer introduces a personal bias into his ratings (see Stevenson-Hinde & Zunz, 1978) it also means that, for example, rare but important events which pass by unnoticed using conventional techniques, are given appropriate weight in the ratings (Stevenson-Hinde, 1983). However, to use this method effectively, two or more observers should have a detailed knowledge of their subjects (usually over several weeks or months) and this may result in practical limitations to the applicability of the technique. In addition, certain differences in behaviour may be more easily and accurately identified using standard recording techniques.

Owner report

The fine detail and clarity of authors' writings about their pet cats in the popular literature (e.g. Wilson & Weston, 1947; Chazeau, 1965) is an indication of the understanding and perception that cat owners show about their pets. Owners' reports can be harnessed (as they have been for dogs; see Serpell, 1983) through the use of interviews, free-written reports and questionnaires, to provide a useful source of information for behaviour ranging from individual eccentricities and quirks to global descriptions of aspects of behavioural style and overall individuality. (Within the realm of psychology, self-report questionnaires are widely and reliably used for assessment of individual characteristics.) However, descriptions of behavioural style and individuality may be affected by a variety of factors such as the environment of the owner and pet (town vs country), the nature of any restrictions imposed upon the cat's movements and behaviour (e.g. neutered vs intact, access to outside, presence of other cats, etc.) and the nature of the owner's personality and his or her attitude towards, and relationship with, the companion animal (e.g. Brown, 1984).

Although similar problems arise with the observer rating method, the potential enormity of the variation between owners and the usual lack of independent verification of owners' reports mean that this method of measurement is particularly difficult to use in a rigorous way.

Examples of individual variation in cat behaviour

All four methods of measurement outlined in the previous section have their practical and theoretical advantages and disadvantages when used in the assessment of individuality. The first two are easy to use but only provide information about individuality at the level of simple measures of behaviour. The second two are more difficult to use in a rigorous way (especially Owner Reports) but potentially provide information about more complex behavioural characteristics. As the study of individuality in the cat progresses, we expect methods like the observer rating technique to be used more often since these provide ways of rating cats according to more general aspects of behavioural style which, as is clear from Figure 4.1, are more closely related to overall individuality than are simpler measures of individual differences in particular behaviour patterns. However, at present the usage of these methods has been limited and so, for the purpose of this chapter, we must also draw on examples of simpler individual differences in behaviour. In the following two sections we illustrate how all four methods of measurement described above have been used to provide direct evidence of individual variation in cat behaviour. We go on to consider how the findings of these different measurement techniques can be related to one another such that measurements of simple individual differences in behaviour patterns may be interpreted in terms of differences in aspects of behavioural style, and measurements of aspects of behavioural style may even be interpreted in terms of overall individuality. Later on in the chapter we ourselves categorise simple individual differences in the performance of behaviour patterns (many of our examples being of this nature), in terms of more general aspects of behavioural style.

The method of direct behavioural recording was used by Lawrence (1981) to describe individual variation in maternal behaviour or maternal style in the cat (in terms of maternal posture and accessibility for suckling, timing of weaning, etc.). Similarly, Panaman (1981) recorded clear individual differences

in the time spent hunting and the hunting efficiency of five adult female farm cats, and Baerends van Roon & Baerends (1979) recorded individual differences in the development of predatory behaviour (the degree of skill shown and the time taken to develop these skills) during the second and third months of kitten life.

Standard ethological recording techniques of cats were used by Meier & Turner (1985) in a structured test procedure to demonstrate individual differences in the responses of cats to a strange person. The same type of technique was used by Mertens & Turner (in press) to demonstrate high individual variation in the responses of cats to several encounters with different human beings. A number of workers have also used structured test situations to investivate various aspects of dominance in the cat and some have demonstrated consistent individual differences over time in competitive ability (e.g. Baron, Stewart & Warren, 1957; Cole & Shafer, 1966).

Moving on to more general measures of behavioural style, Feaver *et al.* (1986) demonstrated the reliability and validity of using observer rating techniques as a method for measuring individual differences in certain characteristics in the cat (the categories used are displayed in Table 4.1). Turner *et al.* (1986) subsequently used this method to assess individual variation in the 'friendliness' of kittens to people.

Although owner reports of cat individuality are still largely confined to the popular literature, we have recently begun to use owner report questionnaires in an investigation of owners' perceptions and likes and dislikes of their cats' individuality. The questionnaire used is of the same design as that used by Serpell (1983) for dogs. Similarly, Meier & Turner (1985) used interviews with cat owners to provide additional evidence for their classification of the owners' pets into one of two 'personality types'.

Relating different types of measurement of individuality

We have shown how various methods of measurement have been, and are being, used successfully in the scientific literature to demonstrate the existence of individual variation in a variety of behavioural characteristics in cats, ranging from straightforward measures of behaviour in free or test situations to observer ratings of behavioural style. The results obtained using the different techniques may be related

Table 4.1. *Categories used in rating cats' behavioural characteristics*

Active
Aggressive
Agile
Curious
Equable with cats
Excitable
Fearful of cats
Fearful of people
Hostile to cats
Hostile to people
Playful
Sociable with cats
Sociable with people
Solitary
Tense
Vocal
Voracious
Watchful

Table 4.2. *Three uncorrelated groups of cats' behavioural characteristics*

Alert:	Active, curious
Sociable:	Sociable with people, fearful of people, hostile to people, tense
Equable:	Equable

to each other, and thereby give us a better overall picture of cats' individuality. For example, by measuring the responses of cats to a strange person using standard recording techniques, Meier & Turner (1985) were able to use specified criteria to divide their sample up into individuals whose behaviour could be classified as 'trusting' or 'shy'. Thus, standard recording methods may allow the observer to distinguish between animals which score high or low for particular behaviour patterns. Individuals may be assigned to different observer-defined groups according to their behaviour scores. The observer may then classify each group according to salient general features of the behaviour of its members (e.g. 'nervousness', 'curiosity'). This approach of categorising individuals according to their behaviour scores is described by Simpson (1985).

In a similar way, Feaver *et al.* (1986) used a statistical method to construct personality or individuality profiles from measures of behavioural style. They selected categories of behavioural style used in their rating method which showed high inter-observer reliability (inter-observer correlation, Spearman $r > 0.70$), and calculated the mean of the observers' ratings for each cat for these items. They then performed inter-item correlations of these mean rating scores. The correlations were examined and those

items which appeared to be strongly positively or negatively correlated (Spearman's $r > 0.70$ or < -0.70) were assigned to a particular group. Three relatively unrelated (uncorrelated) groups were identified in this way (see Table 4.2) and the scores of each individual on the behavioural items within each group were calculated to give the individuals a personality score for each group of items and an overall personality or individuality profile (Feaver *et al.*, 1986).

In this case a measure of overall individuality was achieved through measures of aspects of behavioural style. This procedure is similar in its effects to principal components analysis which has been used on ratings of rhesus monkey behavioural style (Stevenson-Hinde & Zunz, 1978), on direct recordings of social behaviour in this species (Chamove, Eysenck & Harlow, 1972), on recordings of rat behaviour in test situations (Denenberg, 1970) and on direct recordings of maternal behaviour in the cat (Lawrence, 1981), to generate emergent groups (or components) of related measures on which individuals can be distinguished.

Using these sorts of statistical methods it is possible to pick out overall scores of behavioural style or individuality from measures of specific behavioural characteristics. However, as Stevenson-Hinde & Zunz (1978) point out, it must be remembered that the scores produced by these methods are *not* independent of the method of assessment. Addition of new behavioural items or rating categories may alter the composition of the emergent groups of measures (or principal components). None the less, the methods are useful in helping to point out clusters of correlated measures on which individuals can be distinguished, and in reducing the sometimes large amounts of initial data to manageable groups.

We have shown here that the tools for measuring individual variation in cat behaviour can be related to each other using various techniques. Since some of these tools measure simple individual differences in behaviour patterns while others measure aspects of behavioural style this allows bridges to be formed between the different levels depicted in Figure 4.1, and thus allows us to study individuality at various levels of description. However, on their own, these techniques answer no questions! The rest of this chapter is devoted to a consideration of the types of question that can be asked about individuality in the domestic cat, as outlined earlier on, and that can be addressed through research into individual variation using some of the measurement instruments described above.

The origins, development and stability of individuality in the cat
Origins

In the study of temperament in humans, investigation of the relative heritability of various temperamental characteristics forms a prominent area of research (see Buss & Plomin, 1986; Goldsmith *et al.*, 1987). The prominence of this issue reflects the general interest, of behavioural geneticists in particular (Plomin, Defries & McClearn, 1980; Plomin, 1981), in the role that genetic and environmental factors play in contributing to variation in the behaviour of individuals. This interest in the origins of individual variation can be extended to the study of individuality in the cat.

Although little attention has been given to the role that genetic variation may play in the appearance of behavioural variation in the cat, there is some evidence that inter-individual differences in certain behaviour patterns or aspects of behavioural style may be related to genetic variation. A simple example comes from the considerable literature on the genetics of coat colour variation in the cat. Blue-eyed white cats and, to a lesser extent, white cats with orange eyes are often deaf. It appears that the gene involved in the production of the white coat colour may also induce deafness in one or both ears (Robinson, 1977; Pond & Raleigh, 1979). This genetically induced defect obviously has a marked effect on behaviour and caused breeders to regard such animals as 'dull of intellect and slow in thinking' (Pond & Raleigh, 1979, p. 183). In addition, and of more direct relevance to the issue of individuality, is the finding that in some lines of blue-eyed white cats, the females are unusually timid (Beaver, 1976) suggesting a possible genetic effect. The mechanism and process of this effect are, however, unknown.

Further indirect evidence that genetic factors may exert some influence over aspects of behaviour which contribute to our perception of individuality comes from reports of behavioural differences between various cat breeds; such differences are well documented for dogs (Scott & Fuller, 1965). In many popular books mention is made of the behavioural distinctiveness of different breeds. For example, the Siamese cat is repeatedly referred to as demanding considerable affection (Johnson & Galin, 1979), liking attention and involvement, talkative (Loxton, 1981), enjoying the sound of its own voice (Palmer, 1983), enormously talkative (Pond & Raleigh, 1979), probably the most demanding of all breeds (Alderton, 1983) and more talkative than any other breed of cat (Beadle, 1977). In contrast the Russian Blue is consistently described as downright quiet (Johnson & Galin, 1979), very silent (Palmer, 1983), quiet (Alderton, 1983), quite and gentle (Beadle, 1977) and as having a quiet voice (Loxton, 1983). Where the authors obtained their information is not always clear and it is conceivable that a common source explains the consensus.

However there is independent support for the breed characterisations. Hart & Hart (1984) conducted a survey amongst cat show judges and found that these judges, with their wealth of experience of many cats and many different breeds, reported remarkably similar and distinctive breed characteristics. Siamese cats, for example, were reported to be the most outgoing with strangers and the most demanding of attention and affection. Their vocalisations were often described as similar to talking. On the other hand, the Russian Blue was generally reported to be shy and withdrawn. A variety of other breeds were described in this way, most in agreement with the popular literature. In the context of this paper, it is noteworthy that Hart & Hart report that many of the judges, despite their characterisations of the different breeds, were also emphatic that within breeds there are large individual differences.

Further evidence supporting the suggestion of breed differences, comes from the naming of a recently developed breed after a notable behavioural characteristic of that breed. The Ragdoll (Loxton, 1981, 1983) is so called because of its extreme placidity and its tendency to hang limply like a ragdoll or bean bag when picked up.

We are not suggesting that breed differences are an

important scientific problem in their own right. However, given that cat breeds are genetically distinct at certain loci, the reported differences in aspects of their behavioural style may be an indicator of the influence of genetic factors on individual variation.

Evidence supporting an effect due to genetic variation comes from the work of Turner *et al.* (1986). Using observer ratings of kitten 'friendliness', Turner and his coworkers demonstrated that one factor which helped explain the variation in 'friendliness' scores was kitten paternity. Kittens of different fathers differed significantly in their 'friendliness' scores. Since the kittens never saw their fathers it is likely that genetic factors mediated this effect.

However, although these various studies do suggest that genetic variation influences behavioural characteristics, the mechanisms are unknown. As mentioned by Martin & Bateson (Chapter 2), it is important to remember that genes do not code for behaviour patterns (see also Bateson, 1987b). Therefore any genetic effect on behaviour will be mediated via complex interactions between gene products (polypeptides), other gene products, intermediaries such as organs and physiological processes, influences from the environment and so on (see Plomin, 1981).

Environmental influences on the development of individual characteristics have been indirectly examined during the many experiments aimed at elucidation of the developmental process. These experiments have repeatedly demonstrated that manipulating a kitten's environment can result in changes in the animal's behaviour which are directly attributable to the manipulation. Several of these experiments are described in Chapter 2 and therefore in this section we will concentrate on one group which they do not consider in detail, where the behaviour patterns studied can be related in a relatively straightforward way to aspects of behavioural style or individuality.

Behavioural measures which are indicative of the characteristics 'boldness' and 'nervousness' may be influenced by early experience. Konrad & Bagshaw (1970) showed that kittens isolated from birth to seven months and then kept with other individuals, were slower to explore or settle down and show relaxed play behaviour in a novel environment at 15 months of age than were normally-reared controls. In addition the animals displayed an exaggerated autonomic response (galvanic skin response and

disruption of regular respiratory rhythms) when presented with an auditory tone and when restrained.

Early handling also appears to affect the 'nervousness' or 'boldness' of the developing cat. Wilson, Warren & Abbott (1965) found that kittens handled regularly during the first 45 days of life approached unfamiliar objects more rapidly, and spent more time in close proximity to them at four to seven months than did non-handled controls. The same authors also showed that kittens exposed to topographically complex environments from 45 to 90 days of age were more active in an open-field at four to seven months than unexposed individuals. Mendl (1986) demonstrated that singleton kittens, reared with their mother alone, were quicker to emerge from a nest box into an unfamiliar room at three to seven weeks, than were kittens with their mother and a sibling.

As mentioned earlier, our perceptions of characteristics of individuality are influenced by our observations of a wide range of behaviour patterns. The different measures of behaviour taken in the experiments described above could all be thought of as contributing to our perceptions of 'boldness' or 'nervousness' in the domestic cat and, in this sense, it is clear that variation in these characteristics may be directly related to variation in early experience. There is therefore little doubt that controlled manipulation of features of a kitten's rearing environment can have effects on that animal's behaviour and behavioural style at a later date.

Further aspects of individuality in the cat such as 'friendliness' have also been shown to be affected by a variety of environmental factors. The timing and amount of early handling that a kitten receives (Karsh, 1984), and the number of handlers a kitten has (Collard, 1967) may influence its later 'friendliness' towards humans (see Chapter 12).

In most of the experiments described here the rationale has been to manipulate one feature of early experience while holding as many others as possible constant. This often results in the creation of a bimodal distribution of animals in terms of their subsequent behaviour, the two modes being related to the type of experience that was received. However, many features of individuality are likely to show a continuous, rather than a discontinuous distribution. For example, cats may be described as 'tense' and 'highstrung' or 'calm' and 'equable' or anything between. This continuity of variation probably reflects a fact that is also evident from the experiments described above, namely, many different types of early experience may exert some influence on the expression of a particular behaviour pattern at a later date.

In this section we have seen how individual variation in behaviour patterns and aspects of behavioural style can be related to variation in genetic and environmental factors. Although the evidence for direct effects of genetic variation is sparse, it is clear that both factors can exert an influence on the expression of particular types of behaviour and, in some cases, a direct correspondence is found between variation in these factors and variation in the behaviour. In uncontrolled situations, the influence of many independent factors, and the interaction of their effects, may make a one to one relationship between variation in these factors and individual differences in aspects of behavioural style very difficult to discern.

Development and cross-time consistency

The study of development provides a way of examining the interplay between various factors that give rise to individual variation in behavioural style. Longitudinal study of individuals also allows us to evaluate the stability and consistency of individual differences across time.

In Chapter 2, Martin & Bateson give a comprehensive discussion of behavioural development in the cat. One example concerns the study of the development of predatory behaviour. This is a pertinent example as it demonstrates how particular factors may interact across time and influence the expression of individual differences in what could be called 'predatoriness'.

To summarise briefly, the work of Caro (1979a, b; 1980a, b) and Baerends-van Roon & Baerends (1979), showed that between two and three months of age, individual kittens varied considerably in predatory ability. However, by six months and on into adulthood, many of these differences had vanished, although some forms of predatory skill still varied. In terms of the 'catch-up' effect of previously inept kittens, it was found that a variety of factors influenced predatory ability. Individual differences probably arose due to interactions between these and other factors, but adult experience may have been resposible for the 'catch-up' effect. Thus individual variation in kitten predatory skill was a transient phenomenon which subsequently disappeared, probably due to the effects of later experience. As Martin & Bateson note

in Chapter 2, a given developmental outcome (competence as a predator) might be obtained via many different types of developmental history. Perceived individual variation in aspects of behavioural style may thus sometimes be the product of 'alternative developmental routes' to the same outcome.

However, it is also clear from this example that certain forms of experience related to predatory behaviour also have longer lasting effects. Kittens which had experience of particular prey species were more adept at handling and killing these species (when tested at six months) and did not easily generalise the skill to other species (Caro 1980a).

Thus, a characteristic of individuality such as 'predatoriness' may comprise a variety of attributes which are affected in different ways by different variables. The study of developmental processes gives us an insight into how these variables interact and influence the appearance of individual variation in the various forms of behaviour.

Developmental studies can also be used to trace the emergence of individual variation in behavioural style, and their consistency across time. Moelk (1979) distinguished slow/quiet and quick/noisy kittens in her study of the development of friendly approach behaviour in the kitten. She suggested that these differences were present from birth, although the origins of such differences (e.g. pre-natal or peri-natal factors or genetic factors) were not considered. She also contended that they were related to subsequent variation in individual behaviour. For example, quick/noisy kittens were said to be generally more exploratory and tended to be the quickest to investigate unfamiliar stimuli, differences that persisted into adulthood. Karsh (1984) observed similar differences in developing kittens and found that 'excitable' and 'reactive' animals were less easily socialised to humans through the experience of handling treatment than less excitable animals (see also Chapter 12). Thus, individual variation in these characteristics appeared to persist across time and also influenced the effectiveness of certain environmental factors in bringing about further changes in individual behaviour.

The existence of individual variation in 'fearfulness' and 'anxiety' at, or shortly after birth, has been noted in species other than the domestic cat, and related to so-called constitutional differences in the physiological characteristics of the individuals. For example, Suomi (1983) found that young rhesus monkeys varied in the magnitude of physiological response shown (heart-rate change and rise in plasma cortisol level) to various situations, and that the magnitude of the changes was related to the degree of behavioural response shown in mildly stressful situations later in development. Similarly, the dominant wolfcub in a litter (as defined in behavioural tests and observation) was found to differ from its litter mates in heart-rate and other autonomic measures in particular test situations (Folk, Fox & Folk, 1970; Fox, 1972; Fox & Andrews, 1973).

The use of physiological correlates of individual differences in behaviour provides us with a further tool for studying the development of such differences. It may be possible to demonstrate a physiological basis for certain aspects of individuality, particularly those that appear to be present at birth, to examine how such characteristics influence the individual's susceptibility to the effect of environmental stimuli and how they can be changed by the stimuli, and to relate behavioural stability across time to stability at the level of physiological systems.

Stability across situations

A major issue in the study of human temperament is the extent to which temperament is a feature of the person or the situation (Goldsmith *et al.*, 1987; Stevenson-Hinde, 1988). This issue is often examined through an assessment of the cross-situational consistency of particular temperamental characteristics. For example, temperamental ratings of a child by its father and mother may be compared in an attempt to elucidate whether perception of a particular temperamental characteristic is influenced by the nature of the parent–child relationship, which may differ between the two parents, or whether it is relatively unaffected by this. Stevenson-Hinde (1988) suggests that some aspects of temperament may be thought of as lying at one end of a 'person–situation' continuum while others lie at the other end or at points ranging in between. Thus activity may be nearer the person end (relatively unaffected by situation or context) than negative mood (more dependent upon the situation).

This approach to the study of temperament can be extended to the study of individuality in the cat. For example, there is some evidence that certain measures of behaviour may change quite dramatically according to the context in which they are observed.

In their study of social dominance in cats, Cole &

Shafer (1966) performed two types of tests of competitive ability. In one test two cats were placed together to compete for one food reward while in the other several animals had to compete for access to a food bowl from which only one animal could feed at a time. Both tests were conducted using hungry cats. The authors found that reliable dominance hierarchies (in terms of access to the food) developed in both tests, that these were unaffected by time since last feeding, but that they differed between the two tests. For example, one of the most 'aloof', 'placid' and low-ranking cats in the group test was actually the most 'aggressive, 'energetic' and dominant in the two-cat test. The context of the test situation had a marked effect on the behaviour seen in social competition, even by the same individuals. Therefore, aspects of behavioural style which are measured through an assessment of relationships between cats (and between cats and people) may be especially open to contextual influences.

Mendl (1986) provides another example of the effects of context on behaviour. When siblings from a two-kitten litter were tested together in a novel room, they showed few signs of distress or nervousness (as measured by mew calling). Similarly, single kittens (reared without a sibling) appeared relatively calm in the same situation provided they were with their mother. When the kittens were tested in the same way but alone, those from two-kitten litters displayed significantly more calling than the singleton kittens. This difference only emerged under the more stressful condition of being tested alone.

Various anecdotes also indicate the importance of context on the expression of certain aspects of behavioural style. One example comes from our cat colony: certain mothers who are usually very friendly to humans, become extremely hostile once they give birth. The presence of young kittens and the onset of lactation appear to induce a more 'protective' and 'defensive' style of behaviour that overrides the previous 'friendliness'. Another example is the report that certain cat breeds may display particular types of aggressive behaviour at cat shows, but nowhere else (P. Bateson, personal communication).

Clearly the situation may have pronounced effects on measures of behaviour and aspects of behavioural style. Further research may tell us which sorts of characteristics are more stable across situations and which are easily affected, and may thus help us to construct a 'person-situation' continuum for individuality in the cat.

An evolutionary based approach to the study of individuality in the cat

So far we have considered ways of explaining the occurrence of individual variation in aspects of behavioural style in terms of proximate causal factors and processes of development. A complementary approach, and one favoured by evolutionary biologists, is to explain the existence of individual variation in terms of the actions of natural selection, and to consider the consequences of behaving in different ways.

Evolutionary biologists are interested in the functional significance of different behaviour patterns. They seek to understand the benefits and costs of behaving in certain ways in terms, ultimately, of the effects on survival and reproductive success (RS). This interest stems from the principle that natural selection will tend to favour individuals whose behaviour and morphology allows them to achieve a greater lifetime RS in comparison to other individuals who are built, or behave, in different ways. This being so, if a particular aspect of behaviour, or behavioural style, is found to vary between individuals of the same species, several different evolutionary based explanations may be put forward. First, the variation may simply be 'noise', or variation in behaviour that has no effect on RS and is thus selectively unimportant (Slater, 1981). Second, the behaviour under consideration may have effects on survival and RS such that one way of performing the behaviour is more beneficial than another. If this is the case, why do individuals perform in the less advantageous way at all? One possibility is that their behaviour is dependent upon environmental conditions. In certain conditions the benefits of behaving in different ways change, and so a different type of behaviour becomes most advantageous (Davies, 1982). Another possibility is that behaviour is conditional upon aspects of body size or weight. thus, the larger or heavier individuals behave in the most advantageous ways, while the smaller animals cannot compete and so make the 'best of a bad job' by behaving in alternative less advantageous ways (Howard, 1978; Davies, 1982). A third explanation for the existence of intraspecific variation in the expression of a behaviour pattern is that the different ways of behaving are, on average, equally successful

and represent a stable mix of 'alternative tactics' (Davies, 1982; Dominey, 1984). These theoretical explanations can be tested by examining the costs and benefits of behaving in different ways, and they draw our attention to the functional significance of variation in behavioural style.

In the domestic cat, the functional significance of individual differences in behaviour has received little attention. One possible reason for this is that certain differences appear to show continuous variation across the population. The existence of specific and qualitatively distinct alternative modes of behaviour is therefore difficult to demonstrate. Additionally, the functional significance of certain aspects of behavioural style such as 'excitability', 'playfulness' and 'nervousness' is not clear. Variation in these particular characteristics may have no influence on survival chances or RS and thus, in evolutionary terms at least, is 'noise'.

However, certain characteristics may have direct effects on chances of survival and RS. Variation in male 'aggression' and social dominance in the cat (Cole & Shafer, 1966; De Boer, 1977) has been shown to be related to the male's abilities to monopolise a group of oestrous females and to father offspring (Liberg, 1981). In a field study, dominant 'aggressive' and 'self-confident' males maintained mating priority in groups of females and fathered more litters than subordinates (Liberg, 1981). If these two distinct modes of behavioural style have differential payoffs, why didn't all makes adopt the 'aggressive', 'self-confident' style? Liberg found that the dominant animals tended to be the larger and also the older (more experienced) males. It could be suggested that the different modes of behaviour were conditional upon the relative physical attributes and age of the animals. Aggression tended to result in dominance most often in the heavier and older animals. The lighter and younger males made the 'best of a bad job' although it was likely that they would achieve dominance at some stage in their lives and thus would ultimately have a similar lifetime RS to the older animals (see also Dunbar, 1982).

Although more study of the functional significance of individual variation in behavioural style is required, it should be emphasised that such study is greatly facilitated if the behaviour under consideration is expressed in a limited number of ways (preferably two) in the population, so that clear cut alternatives can be distinguished. At present, there is little evidence that individual differences in aspects of behavioural style in the cat can be easily categorised in this way. In addition, the problems of measuring costs and benefits are substantial (Davies, 1982). Further work is necessary simply to be able to ascertain whether the domestic cat is a useful animal for this sort of evolutionary based analysis.

Concluding remarks

In this chapter we have examined the phenomenon of individuality through a consideration of a wide variety of individual differences in cat behaviour. If the study of individuality is to become distinct from the study of all individual differences, and, it must be said that we have not attempted, nor did we feel able, to make any such distinction here, then future research will need to investigate what types of behaviour are perceived as characteristics of cat individuality, and what distinguishes these from other sorts of behaviour. A start could possibly be made by utilising the list devised by Feaver *et al.* (1986) as an inventory of characteristics of individuality. To this list we could straight away add characteristics such as 'boldness' and 'predatoriness'.

Although attempts to distinguish characteristics of individuality from other sorts of behaviour and behavioural differences may be of use in defining a field of individuality study, we feel that they will not alter the types of question which are asked about such characteristics. It is these questions that we have considered in this article and which we feel are as characteristic of the study of individuality as are particular types of behaviour. In fact, these questions themselves may be used as tools for distinguishing between different characteristics of individuality. For example, a consideration of the origins, development and stability of behavioural differences would allow us to categorise these differences into various classes. Some might be relatively stable across time and situation and affected mainly by genetic variation, while others might be less stable and more easily influenced by environmental factors. Indeed some might show so little cross-time or cross-situational stability that we could exclude them from our categorisation of individuality altogether. In addition, individuals could be characterised in the same way. Some individuals might be very consistent in their behavioural style across time and situation, others not so. Defining different

types of individuality and behavioural style is thus a useful goal for future research.

Throughout this chapter, we have seen that cats show variation in behaviour which can be quantified using techniques which allow us to measure not only differences in frequencies and durations of particular behaviour patterns, but also differences in more general features of behavioural style. In this sense, and as mentioned earlier, the cat is a potentially useful animal model for the study of issues which are commonly addressed in human personality and temperament research. More work could be put into this area in an attempt to elucidate basic principles relating to characteristics of cat individuality which may have parallels in the study of humans. For example, cross-fostering experiments would allow us to perform direct assessments of the influences of genetic and environmental factors on variation in behavioural style, a problem often considered in the study of human temperament (Buss & Plomin, 1986). These would be particularly powerful if genetically distinct breeds were used.

Longitudinal studies of development would allow us to assess the timing of the emergence of aspects of behavioural style, their degree of stability across time and the factors that contributed to this stability or change. For example, physiological differences between young kittens in autonomic responses to a particular situation could be related to differences in behaviour. The stability of both physiological and behavioural characteristics could then be assessed.

Manipulation of various features of the situations in which we observe cats would allow us to assess the extent to which different aspects of behavioural style are affected by environmental changes, an issue often referred to in the temperament and personality literature (e.g. Goldsmith *et al.*, 1987; Stevenson-Hinde, 1988).

From the evolutionary biologist's viewpoint, the study of individuality in cat behaviour would focus on attempts to measure the consequences of behaving in different ways and attempt to determine the functional significance of such differences. For example, much inter-individual variation in behaviour may reflect animals making 'appropriate' responses to different situations and contexts. It would be interesting to know the immediate consequences of behaving in particular ways and to find out if animals differed in their ability or propensity to behave 'appropriately'.

However, this would require having an idea of utility or 'appropriateness' which might be difficult to achieve.

These sorts of study might all be focused on specific characteristics of individuality in the cat, such as 'friendliness' to people (which has received some attention already, see Karsh & Turner, Chapter 12), 'nervousness' or 'anxiety' (which might correlate to measures of autonomic response, see Suomi, 1983), and 'predatoriness' (a characteristic which has clear functional significance). Future research has the potential to contribute to a more thorough understanding of the well known phenomenon of individual variation in behavioural style, observed in several species but, at present, little understood.

Acknowledgements

We are grateful to Patrick Bateson, Saroj Datta, Paul Martin, Elizabeth Paul, Michael Simpson, Carel ten Cate and an anonymous reviewer for reading and commenting on an earlier draft.

III

Social life

5

The tame and the wild – another Just-So Story?

Paul Leyhausen

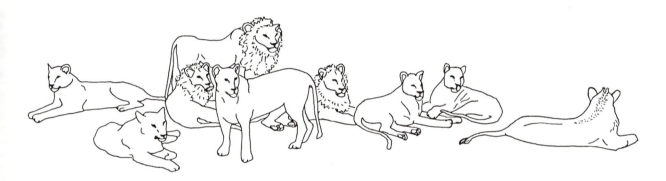

Introduction

In his delightful book, *Just-So Stories*, Rudyard Kipling tells us his version of how the cat became domesticated. He does it with imagination and humour, and quite unencumbered by any factual knowledge. And yet, when he lets his cat hero speak 'I am the cat who walks by himself . . . ', he perhaps tells us more about the background of the house cat than all the learned treatises on the subject written so far. 'Walks by himself' is usually taken as an allusion to the solitary existence cats are supposed to lead. However, I hope to point out that there is more to it than just that.

Anything that walks by itself must find within itself a source of energy to set it in motion. In the case of any animal, that source is, of course, provided by its metabolism. In all cases where the rate of energy gain and the rate of its expenditure are not running exactly in parallel, there is a need for energy storage devices; reserves must be built up while expenditure is low to meet future requirements in excess of current

production. All this is commonplace, and the devices which provide the functional systems of an organism with appropriate storage facilities can be read about in any physiology textbook.

With respect to an animal's ecology and behaviour, the demands of the animal on its environment and the demands of the environment on the animal are rarely synchronous, equidirectional and/or equal in any conceivable way. In order to survive, the animal must at times deny the demands of the environment, refuse to rise to the bait of an alluring stimulus, and on other occasions it must force its own demands on the environment and wrest fulfilment from it. In other words, the processes of evolution have endowed the animal with a certain degree of autonomy, a capacity and even a constitutional necessity to act independently of, even contrary to, current environmental conditions and, if necessary, to evade or change those conditions. Since I cannot detect any other theory dealing with these phenomena adequately and without subterfuge, for the purposes of this paper I shall assume that Lorenz's concepts of instinct, action-specific energy and appetitive behaviour are basically correct and need no further justification (Leyhausen, 1985a).

The autonomy of behaviour from the immediate conditions of the environment apparently increases as we follow the course of evolution up its ladder. A rat seems to enjoy more 'freedom of action' than does a termite. Traditionally, we believe the rat's greater and more flexible behavioural repertoire to be a result of its individual adaptability, its ability to learn. The time honoured conclusion was, and for many still is, that the more an animal can learn, the less it is in need of pre-adapted mechanisms and the better it is able to adapt to environmental conditions as it meets them. Pre-adaptations of the kind formerly called instincts could only be a hindrance to this minute-to-minute adaptability. Consequently, they were reduced as more and more learning capacity emerged. However plausible this reasoning may appear, it neglects a fact and a question: adaptation works both ways, and even when an animal is capable of learning, why should it do so? While it is true that an animal adapts to its surroundings and reacts to environmental stimuli, it also will effect changes in that environment to adapt it to its needs. Whatever kind of learning ability we deal with, it is but a tool. What is it in the animal that decides to use the tool, and in which way?

The organisation of behaviour

Both the fact and the question lead to the problem of how the elements or components of behaviour are organised into complex, seemingly goal-directed sequences of behaviour. In classical ethology, two attempts were made to answer this question besides that of Lorenz: the 'hierarchy of moods' model of G. P. Baerends (1941) and the 'hierarchy of instincts' model (see Figure 5.1) of N. Tinbergen (1951). Both models, though differing in some important details, are similar to each other. Both are fundamentally one-way systems. They proceed from generalised levels of behaviour down to increasingly specialised ones. This is the point where, for my part, the cats walked in – all by themselves – to correct the picture.

I had been studying cat behaviour for many years with a view to testing the validity of the above-mentioned Lorenzian concepts in a highly evolved mammal. I found them valid, but then I attempted to arrange the units or elements of behaviour thus established according to Tinbergen's hierarchy model. The

result looked artificial, but I contented myself with it for a while (Leyhausen, 1956b). In the end, however, the cats themselves walked right out of that picture. While I was writing the purely descriptive part of a paper on the basis of a great deal of recorded material, the cats told me that neither Baerends' nor Tinbergen's model would fit their behaviour.

Traditionally, the behavioural repertoire of an animal is considered to be divided up into a number of spheres which are defined by their observed or supposed biological function: reproductive, ingestive, predatory, agonistic and so forth. Von Uexküll's '*Funktionskreis*' might be best translated as 'functional sphere'. Without neglecting the others, I concentrated my studies on predatory behaviour in the cat.

It appeared that a cat possesses a number of discernible and recognisable behavioural units which it may employ while attempting to catch prey, such as watching, pouncing, hitting, grasping, pulling down, kicking with hindlegs, tossing and biting; some of them are always employed, others vicariously or depending on circumstances. They all mature in the young cat without any need for training or relevant experience. This is proven, among other things, by the fact that complete sequences of prey-catching can be elicited by electrical brain stimulation, the very first time the electrical stimulus is applied, from cats which have had absolutely no relevant experience or exercise.

Although the elements are normally arranged in a kind of routine sequence, the sequence is by no means as rigid as Fabre and others found in insects or even Tinbergen found in the stickleback. Under the experimental conditions of prolonged deprivation, the elements are independent of any sequential order and also of hunger. Satiated cats will then catch and kill as many prey as will hungry ones. This is of survival value since cats must be opportunists. They cannot know when they will meet the next prey. So they take what they can while the opportunity is there and do not forego a lucky chance just because they are not hungry. Of course, this does not mean that, in the normal course of events, hunger does not activate prey-catching. But if left unused for some considerable time predatory behaviour spontaneously activates itself in the non-hungry animal. More importantly, the units of behaviour may be expressed out of context and vary in strength and frequency, and each will then activate

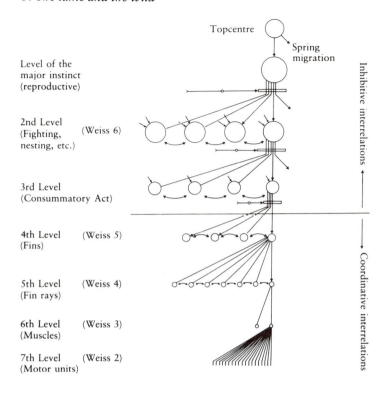

Topcentre

Spring migration

Level of the major instinct (reproductive)

2nd Level (Fighting, nesting, etc.) (Weiss 6)

3rd Level (Consummatory Act)

4th Level (Fins) (Weiss 5)

5th Level (Fin rays) (Weiss 4)

6th Level (Muscles) (Weiss 3)

7th Level (Motor units) (Weiss 2)

Inhibitive interrelations

Coordinative interrelations

Fig. 5.1 Tinbergen's (1951) model of the hierarchy of instincts, proceeding in a one-way direction from the general to the specific.

its own appetitive behaviour. This is particularly well demonstrated in a film I took of a female serval cat who caught a rat, put it down in front of a crevice and, when the rat refused to crawl in, deposited it there again and eventually pushed it in. Then the serval proceeded to hook it out once more, and repeated this game over and over again. Servals are very 'fond' of hooking or angling things out of a hole or crevice, and sometimes do the same with a piece of bark or similar plaything. The significant part of this behaviour pattern is that the animal disregards all stimuli emanating from the rat which at other times would elicit biting and killing or eating. When picking up and carrying the rat, the serval was careful not to hurt it. Thus, in this case grasping and carrying are appetitive acts which serve only to get the rat back in the hole so that it can be hooked out again. While the animal is in this mood, 'hooking out' or 'angling' is the 'consummatory act' which activates and coordinates every preceding activity that may lead up to it.

It becomes apparent that Tinbergen's hierarchy model does not fit this case because it is, so to speak, upside-down. The temporal sequence of events is not also the coordinating principle. On the contrary, what is performed last determines what is done first. There is no general 'first order instinct' which is then channelled down to ever more specific activities. What appears to be a generalised model is the overall balance of all 'third (or fourth) order' instincts which may, according to the momentary state of that balance, serve as appetitive or consummatory acts or be completely suppressed. The strongest mood among them will take the lead and order all else towards its own successful performance.

A system of this kind possesses a very high degree of built-in flexibility prior to all individual experience that changes behaviour by processes of learning. This flexibility does not exclude change by learning. Indeed, it may actually promote it. For instance, while attempting to push a live rat or a piece of bark or wood into a crevice, the serval in the above example learns a lot about manipulating such objects and about their physical properties. The animal could gain this kind of experience in no other way. And it would not be motivated to learn about it if the individual units or components did not, at times, waken to a 'life of their own' outside the strictly utilitarian context of killing and eating a prey. Thus the animal learns a great deal about its environment which it would never learn if the 'subordinate' components of prey acquisition were not occasionally liberated from their 'normal' context. Experience and the effects of learning do not, indeed cannot replace instinct because they depend on it for their scope, direction and intensity of motivation. The richer and more diverse the instinctual systems of an animal, the richer and more diversified the store of this animal's experience and knowledge can become. It is a myth that mammals have fewer instincts than fishes or insects; in fact, they have many more, and that is why they learn more. It is another myth that instinctual systems are rigid and keep their owners in a kind of strait-jacket. The individual instinctive movements (in the sense in which Lorenz used the term) are rigid (apart from their considerable fluctuations in readiness and intensity of performance), but the system they form is not: like the human hand, the individual bones of which are rigid while the way they are joined up provides immense flexibility and versatility. A behavioural system, however, is even more flexible than the hand. The instinctive components or units are not tied fixedly to one system as are the bones of the hand. Some units, for instance, which I first encountered when studying predatory behaviour in the cat, are also part of agonistic, social, courtship and maternal behaviour systems, and all this without in the least changing their identity and basic properties. This is also important because it favours and facilitates cross reference between stored experiences gained in different contexts.

One may ask how this kind of self-activating and self-regulating system works. What are its conditions at the neurophysiological level? We do not know yet, but we have a model in the mechanisms of 'relative coordination' in the spinal cord discovered by Erich von Holst (see Leyhausen, 1954). They produce at the spinal cord level phenomena exactly corresponding to those I have described for instinctual systems. By analogy, I referred to them as the 'relative hierarchy of moods' (Leyhausen, 1965a).

A very interesting feature of the relative coordination of spinal motor output is that certain phasic relationships between spinal motor units show perseverance or stability which renders them relatively resistant to internal and external disruption. Once established, these coordinations may remain stable and unchanged for longer periods than would be the case if they exactly followed all the tiny changes or fluctuations in the physiological states of their components. A similar phenomenon is observable in organised systems of behaviour, which is why we are able to identify such higher level units as predatory 'drives', aggressive 'drives', and so forth. 'Drives' in this, the Lorenzian, sense are ordered, sometimes enormously complex sequences of appetitive and consummatory behaviour which are self-stabilising within limits and therefore may persist for a time while, as mentioned above, the participating units do not show the same degree of stability. Only when one or more of them change their activity level too drastically will the 'drive' coordination break up. Thus a 'drive' is still a higher order 'unit', although it is not permanent and certainly not 'higher' in the sense of 'dominant'. The higher order unit is always subordinate to its members in that it is entirely dependent on their majority 'vote' or what I described as their internal balance.

Burned child as I am from being oft misunderstood, I should like to add that when speaking of a 'unit' I certainly do not mean anything 'unitary' or indivisible. But an atom is still a unit in many respects, although unlike Herakleitos we can no longer regard it as indivisible. So we may speak of units of varying degrees of complexity as long as we do not confuse the levels.

Undoubtedly, the inherent flexibility of the motivating system of instincts increases in vertebrates from fish to mammal and, in mammals, from marsupial to man. Hence it might seem plausible to assume that behavioural systems, based on a rigid carapace of instincts held together by few links with limited flexibility, stood at the beginning of animal evolution. However, the study of coelenterates suggests that this is a doubtful conclusion. Von Uexküll (1921) called the kind of behavioural organisation which characterises them 'reflex republics', meaning that each element was equal to all others and not bound into a fixed, unalterable order. This and many other facts reveal that rigid behaviour systems are an acquisition which appeared rather late in animal evolution. In their extreme form they probably represent an evolutionary cul-de-sac. Somewhere along the road from almost amorphous equality to sequential order of elements, some organism(s) must have 'discovered' that it is possible to arrange the same elements in different ways and in different combinations which then enables them to serve various purposes. Thus, before rigid one-way hierarchy was cemented too firmly, these organisms started to develop coordinating mechanisms which, though subject to certain rules, allowed for the flexible use of elements previous to any insight by the subject into the purpose of the flexible arrangements. That is what I called 'Relative Hierarchy of Moods'. In the higher mammals this kind of organisation of the motivational system of an animal has attained its greatest success, not by reducing but by increasing the number of rigid elements in the system. Von Uexküll has put it very succinctly: 'The amoeba is less of a machine than the horse'.

The design principle has been successful not only because it instigated learning in the way explained above and thus played a decisive, perhaps indeed *the* decisive role in the evolution of learning abilities and capacities of all kinds. It has been successful because, contrary to all traditional thought, it has opened up the road to an ever increasing freedom of action. If the organism were entirely at the mercy of environmental influences, it could neither resist them nor attempt to change them. It could never conceive of such a course of action. As it is, even a fish can virtually say 'No' to a stimulus that is offered or forced upon it and swim away in search of another more suitable to his present mood. The built-in motivational system frees the higher animal from the tyranny of its past and present environment. The animal may use its experience but is not its slave. What evolution has determined in the species turns out to be the freedom of the individual, which prevents the influence of the environment from becoming unremitting coercion.

Again, to avoid misunderstanding, I am not saying that experience and learning do not add to the freedom of action. They do. But they are not its origin; they are useful only because the basic faculties to choose and to decide are already there. They may be guides but are never governors.

All this we have learned by studying our cats, rather the cats have taught us, as R. F. Ewer once told me. What significance does it all have beyond the cat? As always, we must discern between what is typical of the organism under investigation and of any higher taxon it belongs to, in this case placental mammals. When we dissect a cat and remove its heart, the expert in comparative anatomy will still recognise the heart as the heart of a cat. However, it also possesses a number of features that are typical of all mammals. If we should discover a new species of mammal, we could predict without even the remotest chance of error that it would have a heart and circulatory system designed generally as in any other mammal. True, there are vast anatomical and functional differences between the hearts, say, of an elephant, a whale and a shrew. But still they are all immediately recognisable as the hearts of mammals. Thus, when we consider the motivational system of the cat we find many properties which are exclusively *cat*. However, the basic functional principles along which the system works are mammalian; all motivational systems of all mammals will be organised along these same principles, and that includes man.

The cat has taught us more about human freedom, its possibilities, its opportunities and its limits than we ever knew before. It has shown us why neither cat nor human can ever be entirely the products of their environment, and this is true also of the social and cultural environment. The cat walks by himself, under his own steam. We had better bear this in mind when we turn to investigating the cat's social systems.

The social life of domestic cats

Generally, all members of the cat family are believed to lead solitary lives. It is, of course, known that lions live in groups of up to 30 animals, and that cheetahs may occur in family and peer groups. But this does little to alter the overall impression.

I gave an account of what I believed then to be *the* social organisation of more or less free-roaming domestic cats (Leyhausen, 1965b). The picture presented could be summarised like this: cats, both males and females, occupy territories consisting of a home area of about 100 metres in diameter and a larger home range of 0.5 to 2 kilometres across, depending on population density and habitat structure. Neither part of the territory has clearly delineated boundaries, and home ranges may overlap considerably, especially with males, who tend to occupy larger home ranges than females. Females, however, defend their territories, particularly home areas, more fiercely than males. Fighting in males is for supremacy and rank rather than territory. Although territories overlap, there is not always mutual tolerance. The animals avoid encounters by sticking to more or less strict individual timetables when travelling through or staying in border areas. Control is by sight over some distance and by scenting conspicuous landmarks along the trail. Neighbours may come to tolerate each other at close quarters. At times, the neighbourhood seems to assemble at a place apparently considered by all as neutral ground for purely social purposes. Such social gatherings have since been observed by many people in many different places. Their precise role within the system is still not well understood. When there are several males of equal strength in a neighbourhood, they stop fighting after a while and may even form loose associations which I called brotherhoods. The most serious fighting between males occurs when a young male starts to fight his way into the brotherhood, as the novice will not readily acknowledge defeat and repeats his attacks over and over again. My conclusion was that the old notion that solitary animals had no kind of sociability and social organisation was wrong. I called that particular kind of organisation a neighbourhood system.

Since that time a great number of studies on the social behaviour and organisation of feral and semi-feral domestic cat populations have been published from many parts of the world (see Chapters 6 and 7). In no case was the social structure of one group exactly like that of another. Are methods and observers so incommensurable? Well, some variance in the results could perhaps be explained by these factors, but certainly not all of it. Females are strictly territorial in one case and mutually tolerant, even cooperative, in another. They may or may not tolerate dominant males within their territories. They may be fairly widely spaced or live in a crowd, share homes and dens or defend them, nurse and raise their young individually or in a kind of partnership. Males may share territories and females, or one superior male may terrorise all others and strive to exclude them, if not always successfully, from mating with any female within his 'jurisdiction'. Young may be tolerated and may take liberties with male and female alike, or they are cuffed and chased away by all except their mothers. When weaned, they may stay within the group, or they may be chased away. Can all this variability have been produced by domestication? Or is there no social order in the species and all is but a reflection of environmental differences and pressures? At least one investigator, Rosemarie Schär (1983) found that to some extent genetic differences between small populations were also responsible for their social diversity.

Unfortunately, we do not know anything of the

social behaviour and orgnisation of *Felis libyca*, the wild ancestor of the domestic cat, whose proper scientific name is not *Felis domestica* but *Felis libyca* forma *catus*. But let us shortly review what is known about the social systems of other felid species.

The social life of wild felids

The only wild cat similar in size to the domestic cat which has been observed extensively in its habitat is the Iriomote cat, *Prionailurus iriomotensis*, a close relative of the Leopard cat, *Prionailurus bengalensis*, and the Fishing cat, *Prionailurus viverrinus*. The genus *Prionailurus* is confined to South and East Asia and its extant species are not very closely related to the genus *Felis*, although *Prionailurus* is probably closest to the common ancestor of all modern cat species. The Iriomote cat has preserved many primitive traits and by and large may be considered the most primitive cat living. It is strictly territorial, the average size of a territory being two square kilometres. Only when they were mating could more than one animal be observed at a time. No observations were made of encounters in territorial border areas and the way territorial neighbours behave towards each other. The details of the social structure of the population are still obscure after three years of field study (Imaizumi, 1976, 1977; Yasuma, 1981).

The desert cats (*Felis nigripes*, *F. margarita* and *F. thinobia*) also seem to live widely spaced on established territories. Of *F. bieti*, the Gobi Grey cat, no field observation of any kind exists.

The European wild cat (*Felis silvestris*) follows the same pattern as the Iriomote cat. As far as details are known, we could assume that its social organisation comes fairly close to my original description of domestic cat sociality.

The same is true of the Bay lynx or bobcat (*Lynx rufus*). This species also seems able to form bonds between male and female of a more lasting nature than felids are usually credited with (Winegarner, 1985). Consort males join the female or female and young for periods ranging from a few hours to several days at intervals of days or weeks. In this context it may be mentioned that I observed some female domestic cats who remained 'faithful' to a particular male over many mating periods, although they did not associate with them in between. It is not quite clear yet whether the male bobcats also share in the task of providing for the young after weaning. The latter behaviour was

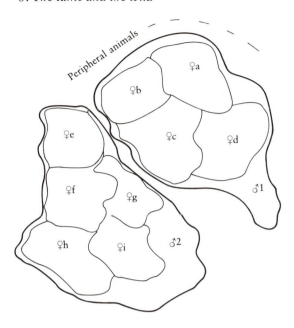

Fig. 5.2. Land tenure system as displayed by leopards in Sri Lanka and by tigers in Nepal and Central India.

Table 5.1. *Lion social structure in different habitats*

Habitat	Group size	Structure
Desert with dispersed waterholes N. and SW. Africa	1 male 1 female + cubs	Permanent
Semi-desert SW. Africa	1 male 2–3 females + cubs	?
Semi-desert with 1 regular rainy season Kalahari (Botswana)	1–3 males 2–6 females + cubs variable, nomadic	Form prides during rains. dry season
Savannah Zaire, Uganda	2–3 males 3–5 females + cubs	Form prides; pride males stay 6 years
Savannah East Africa from Kenya to Transvaal	2–5 males 5–20 females + cubs Nomads >50% of popul.	Form prides; pride males stay 2–3 years; variable groups
Bush with scattered grassland and forest Gir Sanctuary, India	2 males 3–4 females + cubs	Permanent?

observed in a captive family of Fishing cats (*Prionailurus viverrinus*) in Frankfurt Zoo and in a family of European wild cats in Magdeburg Zoo. In Samburu Park, Kenya, I observed a male leopard who joined a female and half-grown cub, played for a long time with the cub and then left, leading the two others away in single file.

Land tenure by the leopard (Muckenhirn & Eisenberg, 1973) is very similar to that of the tiger (Panwar, 1979; McDougal, 1981, 1982, 1983) in India and Nepal. Females own territories, several of which are contained within the territory of one male (Figure 5.2). Yet Schaller (1967) found that the territorial order is not so strict as to prevent all social contact outside the mating season and the rearing of a family. His summing up of tiger sociality: 'Solitary – yes, but not unsociable'.

Of all these and some other cat species such as the puma (*Profelis concolor*) we know very little about the variations their social system may show in different habitats, although some species like the bobcat, the leopard and the puma live in extremely diverse habitats. In the Amur area of Russia, tiger ranges extend over several hundred, even several thousands

of square kilometres. Under the circumstances it is impossible for a male to control more than two females, and territorial defence must of necessity be incomplete. However, more detailed knowledge is lacking, and we cannot yet know whether the social system of Amur tigers differs in other respects from that of their more southerly colleagues. Another extreme tiger habitat, though very different in nature from the Amur area, is the Sunderbans in Bengal. One might guess that the social system of the Sunderbans tigers should differ greatly from that displayed by the famous tigers of Kanha Park in Madyah Pradesh. But we have no certain knowledge of it.

The social and land tenure systems of felids reviewed above may present a fairly uniform picture. But we have seen that there is some flexibility and variation on the theme. The picture may also be deceptive, because we have inadequate data on all the species involved, too few and only incomplete studies from widely differing habitats and separated populations. The only species that has been studied in this way is the lion, and here we see a great variety of social structures which to some extent can be related to ecological factors (Table 5.1).

Best known is the social organisation of the lions in the Serengeti plains of Tanzania (Schaller, 1972; Bertram, 1975). The basic unit is a group of from four to twelve lionesses, which communally occupy and defend a piece of land as their territory. Such a group is called a pride. The pride is joined by two or more males, which are an even more closely knit group than what I described above as the brotherhood of male domestic cats. These pride males patrol the pride area and defend it and the females against any intruding males. Strange females are mostly driven away by the pride females. But only less than half the population is organised in prides and occupies clearly defined pride territories throughout the year. The majority live a vagrant life on the periphery of the pride lands, either by themselves or in small groups, unisexed or mixed. Male competition from outside groups is heavy and a pride male group succeeds only rarely in keeping the pride for more than three years. This, however, is not necessarily inherent to the system. In Uganda, for instance, males stay with a pride for six and more years (van Orsdol, 1982), that is, for all of their reproductive life. The pride females always recruit their ranks from their own offspring, so that they are all related to each other. Strange females are never allowed to join the pride. Nomad females may also breed, but are less successful in rearing the cubs than are pride members.

In striking contrast, the now extinct North African lion was reported as being monogamous, each pair occupying and dominating one of the rare waterholes or oases. Eloff (1973) states that this occurs also in some parts of the Southwest African Kalahari desert. Apart from this, the prides of lions in Southwest Africa are smaller than those in East Africa.

Whereas in most of the Southwest African Kalahari several years may elapse without rainfall, the Kalahari of Botswana regularly has one rainy season per year. But the greater part of the year is without any rain and water is so scarce that the lions' prey scatters widely and becomes extremely scarce and hard to get. The lions range extensively in search of food and behave socially much as do the Serengeti nomads. There is, however, little strife between them. At the beginning of the rainy season, prides are formed and territories occupied. The prides are not as exclusive as in the Serengeti, and the females often mate before pride formation and not always with the pride males. Females may join or leave the pride freely. Hence the pride females are not necessarily closely related (Owens & Owens, 1985).

This is but a sketchy outline of the wide potential of lion sociality. It will suffice, however, to show that a mammal's social system is not a cut and dried affair, but a range of social mechanisms which can be organised in many different ways and thus produce widely differing social orders and organisations, depending on factors like population density, age structure, ecological conditions, and maybe also genetic differences between populations. Schär in particular has found that social distance in the adolescent cat is determined partly by genetic factors, partly, however, by the degree of social tolerance and affection or repulsion it meets in the adults of its immediate social setting. Thus the form of social contact and structure the kitten will later help to create and maintain is dependent on what kind of 'social culture' it grows up with, in a kind of social tradition (see also Chapter 13).

The range of social adjustments displayed by different populations of feral and semi-feral cats reflects everything that we find in all the species within the cat family. That is probably much more than was expressed in their wild ancestors. How could we account for the possibility that the domestic form possesses a richer potential than the wild ancestral form?

Adolf Haas found that under conditions of stress or frustration a bumble bee of an 'advanced' species may fall back on behaviour patterns ordinarily shown only by a more 'primitive' species (Haas, 1962, 1965). He was, however, amazed to find that under extreme duress the 'primitive' species would also show behaviour patterns which are normally performed only by the 'advanced' species. Haas came to the conclusion that a species has in store the entire behavioural repertoire present in the genus and even in higher taxa to which the species belongs. He therefore called behavioural products of the species' potency to mobilise components that were not normally part of the repertoire 'generic behaviour'. It has long been acknowledged that generic behaviour is a common phenomenon not exclusively shown by bumble bees or even arthropods but observable in many taxa and probably common to them all.

The surprisingly wide range of social behaviour and societal structure displayed by domestic cat populations seems to be just another example of this. If so, it cannot be wondered at that this social variety exceeds what is shown by *Felis libyca*. Although this species ranges from Asia Minor to South Africa and in Africa from East to West, sparing only the extreme desert habitats, it has never met such an enormous diversity of ecological conditions as do feral domestic cat populations from Australia to industrial England, from rural Sweden to Galapagos, from Japanese islands to the ruins and parks of Rome. The fact that domestic cats show a greater social diversity than their wild ancestors does not necessarily mean that they possess a greater potential. They have simply been exposed to far more extreme, not to say diametrically opposed conditions.

The domestic cat's great social diversity does, however, raise a different problem. Other domestic animals when going feral do not present a similar social versatility. Feral horses, cattle, sheep, goats, pigs and dogs either fall back on social systems known from their wild ancestors, or they produce an impoverished version of these. So far, they never have shown enrichment.

Self-domestication

Lorenz (1940) described some similarities between civilised man and his domestic animals, both morphological and behavioural. As there was no other superior animal that could have domesticated man, Lorenz concluded that man must have domesticated himself. At the time, the notion of human self-domestication raised a great deal of controversy. Cultural anthropologists pointed out that there could be no comparison between the process by which man selected and bred his domestic animals and his own way of life. Any similarities could, therefore, only be superficial and in no way based on even partially identical processes. Culture provided Man, so runs the claim, with an entirely new 'adaptive dimension' that would automatically place all change in human behaviour, social behaviour in particular, on a level where all comparison with sub-human animals became meaningless.

Of course, there is the ticklish question what *is* culture? How do we define the dividing line between non-culture and culture? Or pre-culture and culture? And when we have found that line, how do we support the claim that it is now not only a mere quantitative, relative divide but an absolute, qualitative one? And how can we be so certain that the divide runs exactly between Man and all Other Animals? I think it is clear

by now to everybody that to meet the last condition it would need to be a very crooked line indeed!

This is where we return to Kipling's story. There is no evidence that at any time during its history the cat's way of life and its reception into human homesteads were purposely planned and directed by humans, as was the case with all other domestic animals at least from a very early stage of their association. The roughly one hundred and fifty years of Cat Fancy beginning early in the nineteenth century need not concern us here. In other words, there was no agent domesticating the cat besides the cat himself. The cat certainly did not create the domestic scene as man did for himself. But he grasped the opportunity when it was inadvertently offered. Like man, the cat was able to develop and adopt an increasing variety of communal organisation to meet the innumerable novel conditions which followed in the wake of new developments and the conquest of new and formerly uninhabitable parts of the earth. In every sense, the cat domesticated himself – if with some unimagined assistance from man. And as in man, the process of self-domestication developed a dimension not shared by intentionally domesticated and husbanded animals: the beginning of social culture and a seemingly infinite social diversity.

But is it all new? We already found that the social diversity displayed by different feral cat populations could be explained by the principle of generic behaviour. Does this not stir a suspicion that the seemingly unending variety of human social systems, when stripped of their more superficial cultural accessories, represents basically no more than the diversity of social organisations found in the order of primates? In primates, we find patriarchy and matriarchy, family groups and larger units, territorials and vagrants, neighbourliness and virtual tribal feuds, social hierarchies from simple single male tyranny to rule by a council of elders and even a kind of democratic equality. All the elements are there. Would it then really be so far-fetched to regard human social diversity as a special case of generic behaviour? And if it is so, are we not putting the cart before the horse when we traditionally regard adaptive social diversity as a product of culture? Is not the reverse true: that culture, social culture, could emerge only out of a social versatility and diversity which existed before all culture? Many exciting questions, indeed. Time is young yet, and much research is needed to answer them. But when looking at the panorama in the light of these questions, can we really doubt which way the answers lie?

Concluding remarks

For my part, I am convinced that cat behaviour is not only a fascinating subject to study, it is also a most promising way to probe more deeply into the evolution of mammalian behaviour in general and in so doing lift the veil from our own emergent existence. The mammalian heritage, far from being an ancient encumbrance to be shed as best we can, still provides the very core of our personal structure. The fundamentals of our motivational system, the functional principle on which the system is built, are still mammalian and will be forever. This does not turn cats into humans, nor humans into cats. But it can help us to understand that even our seemingly infinite resourcefulness carries with it its limits and shortcomings. With luck, knowing this may even help us to become more human.

6

Cat society and the consequences of colony size

G. Kerby and D. W. Macdonald

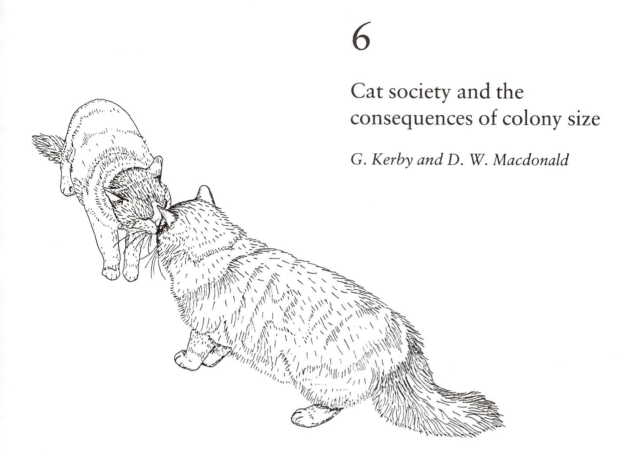

Introduction

Mammalian social behaviour is so complex that to describe adequately a social system requires analyses at several levels of resolution. Population structure and spatial organisation define a social system at one level, but at another the nature and flow of interactions between individuals are fundamental to understanding how a society functions. Evolutionary theory leads us to expect that individual members of a society will differ in their social relationships, and in the advantages, or otherwise, of group membership (Wilson, 1975). These costs and benefits of sociality may also vary along an additional dimension in so far as a species' social behaviour differs with circumstances. Domestic cats, *Felis silvestris catus*, are members of the Carnivora, an order in which intraspecific variation in social behaviour is commonplace. Explanations of this variation are generally sought in the contrasting ecological circumstances of different populations (Kruuk, 1976; Macdonald, 1983). One might expect the domestic cat's social system to

encompass great variation, since they live in habitats as diverse as sub-antarctic islands (van Aarde, 1978) and industrial cities (Rees, 1981), and at densities varying from less than one to more than 2000 per square kilometre (e.g. Langeveld & Niewold, 1985; Izawa, Doi & Ono, 1982). Domestic cats also differ in their dependence upon man; their degree of association with people ranges from nil on uninhabited islands to almost continual in crowded metropolises (Corbett, 1979; Natoli, 1985b). Cats vary intraspecifically in their feeding ecology (see Chapter 10), reproductive patterns (van Aarde, 1978) and genetic constitutions (Todd, 1978; O'Brien, 1980).

In this volume Liberg & Sandell (Chapter 7) have reviewed studies of the population densities and spatial organisation of domestic cats. They, along with others (e.g. Corbett, 1979; Macdonald *et al.*, 1987) conclude that, in general, cat populations can be divided into those in which females form groups and those in which they do not. The latter system, which often involves the smaller, non-overlapping ranges of females being encompassed by the substantially larger ranges of several males, is typical of undomesticated Felidae [e.g. leopards, *Panthera pardus*, (Hamilton, 1976); bobcat, *Lynx rufus* (Bailey, 1974); wild cat, *F. sylvestris* (Corbett, 1979)]. We suggest that these are two extremes of a continuum of social organisations, arising because of differences in patchiness and predictability of available resources (the principle is reviewed by Carr & Macdonald, 1986). Briefly, groups will be favoured where there is heterogeneity in the pattern of food availability. As an extreme, but appropriate example, the garbage 'skips' from which Dards' (1979) dockyard cats fed, constituted such rich patches that the minimum territory size required to support one cat also contained sufficient resources for several others. Since ecological factors underlying spatial organisation of cat societies are reviewed in the following chapter, we will confine ourselves to a finer level of resolution and review the consequences of individual relationships within and between social units. Our aim will be to shed light on the question: what, if any, are the advantages of sociality in domestic cats? Our material is drawn from studies of what are loosely termed feral cats (where feral means to have lapsed into a wild form from a domesticated condition). However, the nuances of cats' involvement with (and dependence upon) people are so complex that the single term feral cannot adequately describe them. The cats referred to here varied in many ways, including tameness and in the extent of their direct or indirect dependence on people for food or shelter. However, they share the quality that their everyday behaviour was not constrained by direct human interference.

We will first review the scant material available on the social behaviour of domestic cats living solitarily. Second, we will review social behaviour of group-living domestic cats, asking initially whether groups of cats are structureless and/or functionless aggregations around clumped resources. To answer this question we will turn to our own studies of the contrasts between three different sized colonies of farm cats.

Cat society
Solitary cats

In a paper memorably entitled 'The communal organisation of solitary mammals', Paul Leyhausen (1965b) drew attention to the apparently paradoxical fact that solitariness neither precludes social behaviour nor necessarily diminishes its complexity. Studies of mammalian social odours (reviewed in Brown & Macdonald, 1985) and vocalisations (e.g. Harrington, 1987) indicate the versatility of communication without visual contact. Amongst undomesticated felids both urine (e.g. Eaton, 1973) and faeces (e.g. Bailey, 1981) are thought to serve as social signals, and the lion's (*Panthera leo*) roar is an obvious example of very long range communication (Schaller, 1972). What evidence is there of social interaction amongst generally solitary domestic cats?

Encounters   Even cats which spend most of their time alone are seen occasionally in the company of other cats. The majority of such occasions involves an adult (presumably the mother) and kittens or subadults. For example, in SE Australia 71 per cent of Jones & Coman's (1982) sightings were of single cats, and 90 per cent of all adults sighted were on their own. When more than one adult was seen, the 'group' comprised a male and a female. Eighteen per cent of cats sighted were in groups of three or more, but these invariably involved subadults or one adult with kittens. Van Aarde (1978) presents similar data for cats on sub-antarctic Marion Island. There, 90 per cent of sightings were of single cats, 6 per cent of two cats, 2 per cent of three, 1 per cent of four and 1 per cent of five cats. Clearly the cats of Marion were generally seen alone, but van Aarde was able to identify some social groupings, and the mean size of these was 2.65. These groupings were not restricted to adult–kitten associations; 33 per cent involved adults only, 17.7 per cent juveniles only, and 7.6 per cent subadults only. Most groups consisted of a female and kittens. Konecny's (1983) study on the Galapagos led to similar conclusions. He noted 40 encounters between cats which were otherwise solitary. Eighty-five per cent were between males and 15 per cent between male and female; he never saw a meeting between two adult females. Corbett (1979) studied eight feral cats living at a population density of 3–4 per square kilometre on Heisker, an uninhabited island of the Monach group (Outer Hebrides). These cats fed largely on rabbits and were solitary. Encounters were rare but an adult female was seen to attack a young male who strayed near the den containing her dependent kittens.

Spacing   The weight of evidence is that the home ranges of cats which live solitarily generally overlap less than would be expected by chance (see Chapter 7). Such regularity implies an active spacing out or territoriality. Thus, the cats studied by Jones & Coman (1982) occupied intra-sexually exclusive home ranges (males 620 ha, females 170 ha) which overlapped minimally; a similar situation is described by Langeveld & Niewold (1985). However, the extent of exclusivity in the ranges of solitary females varies between populations. Greater overlap in ranges is associated with more patchy food resources. The cats in Konecny's (1983) Galapagos population were divided between two systems: where food was more uniformly dispersed overlap between home ranges was less than in an area where food was concentrated in richer patches. There, as on Dassen Island (Apps, 1983, 1986) several cats converged on the same area, but although their paths criss-crossed they appeared to avoid each other (see Social odours, below).

The dimensions of the home ranges in these studies varied amongst females from 11 to 270 hectares (Jones & Coman, 1982; Apps, 1983) and amongst males from 32 to 420 hectares (Apps, 1981; Langeveld & Niewold, 1985). Whether by spatial or temporal separation, or both, these studies have the common denominator that the cats lived solitarily and some avoided each other. As Leyhausen (1965b) pointed out, avoidance is not a passive phenomenon; clearly it can be an important aspect of cat social behaviour, and one that is likely to be moderated at least partly by scent marking.

Social odours   The sources of social odours in the domestic cat include their urine (Leyhausen, 1956a; Natoli, 1985b), faeces (and anal glands) (see e.g. Corbett, 1979; Panaman, 1981), perioral regions and feet (see e.g. Verberne & De Boer, 1976; Verberne & Leyhausen, 1976; cf. Rieger & Walzkoenig, 1979). The pattern in which scent marks are deployed, and possibly therefore their function, can vary intraspecifically (reviewed in Macdonald, 1985). Cats are among the species for which such variation has been recorded between both individuals and populations. Both sexes spray urinate, but males almost always do so at a higher rate [e.g. Apps (1981): maximum rates for males *vs* females = 62.6 *vs* 6.0 per hour]. Corbett (1979) provides the only detailed description of the pattern of scent marking by cats in populations where females are solitary. On Heisker, Corbett saw cats spray urinate (invariably on grassy tussocks) once

every 33 minutes. Of those faeces which were not covered, most were on elevated sites, and the great majority were on trails running through the best rabbit hunting habitat. Two or three faeces often accumulated at each site. In contrast, around the lair of a subordinate juvenile male he found a large accumulation of covered faeces. Corbett speculated that covering faeces may be a trait of subordinate cats (*vide* wolves, Peters & Mech, 1975).

Group living cats

Group membership does not necessarily entail travelling together or spending long periods in company. For example, Eurasian badgers, *Meles meles*, forage separately within their shared clan territory, and so when they are away from their setts, badgers are generally seen alone (Kruuk, 1978). Therefore we identify a social group as a number of adults whose interactions are generally tolerant and whose home ranges overlap more than would be expected by chance. In fact most studies of group-living cats concern rural populations, often around farms where, as a rule, cats are seen in close proximity when in the farmyard, but generally alone when in the fields.

Group size and structure   Two studies, Dards (1978, 1979) and Izawa *et al.* (1982) have concerned cats feeding on refuse dumps, the former in an English dockyard, the latter in a Japanese fishing village. In Dards' study the dockyard rubbish was localised into portable 'skips' which were emptied periodically. Some further food, also clumped but less abundant, was provided for the cats by dockers. The cats lived at a density of two per hectare in family groups of 2–11 (mode 4–5) adult females, at least some of which were relatives. In addition to 28 such family groups, Dards observed up to 31 solitary adult females. Mature males had large (mean 8.4 ha) freely overlapping home ranges whereas all other classes of male, and all females, shared group ranges (0.03–4.2 ha) which centred on skips. The behaviour of these cats, and the structure of their population, may have been influenced by the fact that the dockyard had been enclosed by a high wall since 1711. The food supply was also clumped in Izawa *et al.*'s study, where two village dumps were provisioned each day with waste from the local fisheries. The result was an overall density of 23.5 cats per hectare divided between two 'feeding groups' whose memberships were generally separate.

Each cat belonged to one or the other of these groups and typically occupied a home range which overlapped with those of other members of its own group but not with those of the other group. Adult males were, however, more mobile and occasionally switched sites. Furthermore, cats were seen feeding at many other sites and households in the neighbourhood, so the dispersion of food was highly variable and heterogeneous.

Cat food was also somewhat clumped in Natoli's (1985b) study of cats in Rome, where they lived at a population density equivalent to over 10 per hectare. A group of 24–39 adult females concentrated around food and shelter in the historic monuments and public gardens of Belvedere Tarpeo in Rome. Individuals of both sexes differed in their attendance records and in the particular sites they frequented. In Baltimore, Oppenheimer (1980) found cats at population densities of up to 7.4 per hectare, whereas Rees (1981) surveyed almost 300 colonies on industrial premises in England and found a modal size of 1–10, usually occupying less than one square kilometre. Only seven per cent of colonies Rees sampled consisted of more than 50 cats.

In more rural surroundings cats living under varying degrees of direct dependence upon people have been observed on farms by numerous researchers in recent years (see Chapter 7 and Macdonald *et al.* [1987]). In a survey of lowland farms in England, 82 per cent of farmers kept cats in numbers varying from one to 25. The modal colony size was 1–5, and the mean 4.0 (Macdonald *et al.*, 1987). These data indicated an overall cat density of 6.3 per square kilometre. Most farm cats confine their movements to the vicinity of the farmyard and the density around the farm was probably closer to 30 cats per square kilometre. The farmers in Macdonald *et al.*'s study estimated the proportion of their cats' food requirements which they provided; only a small minority provided their cats' total requirements, and two thirds provided less than 80 per cent. These conditions appear broadly typical of most studies of farm cats and those studies describe social organisations which share certain common factors: each farm is occupied by one or more (depending on the dispersion of food) groups of adult females and their young of both sexes. These groups can vary widely in size (2–7, Liberg [1981]; 15–20, Izawa *et al.* [1982]). The home ranges of group members overlap widely with each other, but little with those of neighbouring groups. These home ranges

encompass both farmyard and adjoining farmland and vary in size (e.g. 6 ha, Turner & Mertens [1986]; 50 ha, Liberg [1981]; 112 ha, Warner [1985]). Macdonald & Apps (1978) describe the widely overlapping ranges (mean size = 13.1 ha) of a kin group of three females which encompassed one farmyard and adjoining hedgerows; the single breeding male affiliated with them travelled a range of 83 hectares, which enveloped four farmyards. Several such group ranges (max = 9, Liberg [1980]) may be embraced by the larger, widely overlapping ranges of adult males. Groups of cats seem to be rather stable (e.g. < 15% of females emigrated from their natal group in Liberg's study and those that did invariably moved to a human dwelling without cats). It is generally concluded that the ranges of female farm cats encompass food and shelter, whereas those of males encompass groups of females (see Chapter 7).

Encounters and social dynamics   Whereas encounters between solitary cats are a rarity, group-living cats are in frequent social (and often physical) contact. Relations among females within each group generally appear amicable. Adult females may be in each others' company for periods of several hours, and frequently interact (e.g. pairs of individuals engaged in averages of 0.5–0.9 interactions per hour together in a group of four adults; Macdonald *et al.* [1987]). The behaviour of adult females toward both female and young male outsiders tends to be aggressive. Indeed, all the serious aggression observed by Macdonald & Apps (1978) was directed to outsiders. Natoli (1985b) also observed that females raising offspring attacked males which strayed into the colony's 'central area'.

The social relationships of the two sexes differ greatly. Dards (1979) found that adult males were never amicable but either avoided, tolerated or attacked one another, and actively persecuted younger males. The breeding males were not detectably affiliated with particular groups and maintained a hierarchy amongst themselves (again, the wall around the dockyard may have influenced the spatial organisation of these cats). In a detailed study of adult male farm cats Liberg (1980) identified four categories: Breeders (of which a single 'Central' male monopolised copulations at a given farm), Challengers (2–3 years old and involved increasingly in aggressive challenges of Breeders), Outcasts (young male emigrants, avoiding contacts with other cats) and Novices (yearling males remaining with their natal group and subject to increasing attack from older males). The ranges of Breeders overlapped widely, but their dominance relationships varied with location – each central male being dominant on the farm with which he was particularly affiliated.

Within female groups Izawa *et al.* (1982) found that feeding activity was synchronised and interactions between group members were generally amicable. Dards' (1978) data are similar: within the family group, individuals rested together, greeted and sometimes groomed one another. Females sometimes nursed kittens communally. Agonistic behaviour was rarely observed within the groups but interactions outside the group were usually aggressive. Natoli (1985b) never observed 'territorial behaviour' between the females of her colony and remarked on the amicable relations between females and independent daughters.

The mating system of cats is an enigma. Female cats are induced ovulators, i.e. they require multiple copulations to stimulate ovulation, and behave in ways which appear adapted to enhance competition between males: when in oestrus they call (Beadle, 1977) and during the first days of oestrus they are sexually attractive but not receptive (Scott, 1970). The result is that up to six adult males have been observed around an oestrous female. Dards (1979) recorded 93 occasions when males attended oestrous females, on 33 of which more than one male was present. However, whe never saw these males fight and could not confirm how many of them copulated.

Finally, our own studies have sought to describe farm cat society and to explore its adaptive significance by examining social interactions between group members and relating the results to reproductive success (Macdonald and Apps, 1978; Macdonald *et al.*, 1987; Kerby, 1987). We will review our findings in the second part of this chapter.

Social odours   Leyhausen & Wolff (1959) proposed that some cats might time-share their joint occupation of an area. They proposed that these comings and goings might be controlled by urine marks and drew an analogy between the age of the scent marks and the changing colour of traffic signals. Although several authors have thought this traffic signal system applicable to wild felids (e.g. Hornocker, 1969; Eaton, 1970), neither the mechanism nor the notion of time-

sharing has been tested quantitatively for the domestic cat. However, the idea of avoidance through scent is compatible with Corbett's (1979) and Konecny's (1983) observations of several cats hunting the same area at different times.

Adult male cats spray frequently, especially while travelling. Liberg (1981) reported non-breeding males averaging 12.9 urinations per hour of travel, whereas breeders averaged 22.0 per hour. Panaman (1981) observed that females sprayed most when hunting (1 per 16.7 min or 70 m). Corbett's (1979) cats on the island of N Uist left most sprays in the entrances of rabbit burrows. These cats sprayed on average once per 5.4 minutes as they travelled, with dominant cats (and those with the largest ranges) spraying most frequently. Just over half of the sprays made by one adult male followed in the study by Macdonald *et al.* (1987) were in the farmyard, while the remainder were left while travelling. Of this male's sprays, 14.8 per cent followed agonistic encounters, and in this context the tendency to cheek rub on or near the urine trebled. Both Panaman (1981) and Macdonald *et al.* noted that females tend to bury urine and faeces around the farmyard, but to leave them exposed elsewhere. This difference might reduce the olfactory conspicuousness of the lair to predators. (It might also be a tendency subject to selection during domestication.) Natoli (1985a) demonstrated that adult cats of both sexes could distinguish the urine of strange males from that of familiar males, and that males investigated urine odours for longer than did females (see also De Boer [1977]).

Cats allomark (mark each other) by rubbing the cheek and perioral regions against each other. The initiator of such a rubbing interaction may thereby deposit scent on the recipient (and/or pick it up). The odours may come from the interactants' dermal glands and saliva or from urine on which they have rubbed previously. In Macdonald *et al.* (1987) it is suggested that this allomarking is an important clue to cat social relationships. It is also noteworthy that some greetings involve rubbing the dorsal surface of the tail down the cheek and under the chin of the recipient.

Laboratory studies   Laboratory studies of cat society have focused on the question of whether they form dominance hierarchies. Although experimental designs have varied they all involved ranking cats through their success at gaining access to food. The results vary; for example, Winslow (1938) found that one male invariably dominated all other cats in a group, irrespective of their sex. Cole & Shaffer (1966) found that reliable dominance hierarchies involving up to eight cats were stable, and unperturbed by differential levels of hunger. None of these studies shed light on the workings of a hierarchy in the cat's natural history, and none has reported the subtle behavioural cues one might expect to signal the *status quo*, outside direct competitive situations in a mammalian society. They focus instead on instances of overt aggression and threat. Winslow (1938) concluded that the dominant cat expressed its status by pseudo-copulating with males and females, but neither Baron, Stewart & Warren (1957) nor Cole & Shaffer (1966) ever observed this behaviour.

Variation

The studies reviewed here show great variation in the social circumstances of domestic cats. Within populations the behaviour of male, female, old, young, dominant and subordinate all differ. Population densities vary from 0.9 to 2350 per square kilometre (see above). Colony sizes vary from one to 52 (e.g. Rees, 1981; Jones & Coman, 1982), patterns of scent marking vary, and spatial organisation embraces many shades of variation. Females' home ranges vary from 0.03 to 170 hectares (Dards, 1978; Jones & Coman, 1982) and adult males' from 0.8 to 380 hectares (Dards, 1978; Liberg, 1984). This variation prompts the question: are some behavioural traits characteristic of local populations (reflecting underlying genetic differences) or can individuals swap between different social *modi vivendi*? Corbett's (1979) study shows that the latter was the case for the cats living in the crofting communities of N Uist (Hebrides). These free-ranging domestic cats were associated with a particular croft; females were self-supporting, hunting rabbits on overlapping home ranges in summer but returning to crofts where they were subsidised in winter. Females took their kittens in to the croft when about eight weeks old. Males remained in the fields throughout the year (expanding their ranges in winter). Breeding females maintained exclusive breeding territories adjacent to their croft while rearing young. They lived at a population density of 19 cats per square kilometre in a population where 56 per cent of cats were adult and there was

annual recruitment of young. The degree of overlap and priority of access to rabbit warrens differed with respect to age, sex and social status of the cats. Male, adult and dominant cats had larger ranges than female, young and subordinate cats. Corbett's findings emphasise not only that the ecology of the two sexes was different, but also that individuals switched between contrasting spatial and social arrangements on a seasonal basis as resource dispersion and availability altered.

Farm cat society

The concentrations of cats on farms around the world tend to be dismissed as aggregations rather than social structures. For example, Laundré (1977) concluded that their social order was poorly formed and that little group bonding behaviour existed. He speculated that farm cats fluctuated between solitary and social circumstances and therefore never fully developed the 'refined intricacies of social or solitary living' (Laundré, 1977, p. 997). To investigate whether groups of farm cats are structureless and/or functionless aggregations around clumped resources, we have studied three such colonies, selected because of their different sizes. By selecting colonies which varied in size we hoped to uncover (a) generalisations about farm cat society and (b) differences associated with colony size. Furthermore, certain questions can be most appropriately studied in colonies of a certain size. For example, it was practical to explore the detailed dynamics of social interactions among the adults of our 'Small' colony, whereas it was impractical to do so for all 70 cats (and nearly 5000 possible cat dyads) studied over three years at our 'Large' colony. On the other hand, it was realistic to seek generalisations about the behaviour of age–sex classes at the large colony, but not at the small one. A brief description of the three sites is given below:

1. *Small:* Church Farm, Bradford, Devon. Between four and nine adult cats were observed between 1977 and 1981. Their circumstances have been detailed by Macdonald & Apps (1978) and Macdonald *et al.* (1987). The colony was founded in 1977 by a pair and their two adult daughters (transferred as a complete group from another farm). The cats were provisioned with milk daily, but otherwise left undisturbed by the farmer. They foraged extensively for themselves, hunting the hedgerows and outlying buildings (principally for rodents) and scavenging chicken food. Their

movements centred on a barn filled with bales of straw. In 1979 for logistical reasons the whole colony was translocated to Oxfordshire where observations were continued sporadically until May 1981. At both sites shelter and nest sites were abundant. In total approximately 900 hours of direct observation were recorded.

2. *Medium:* Church Farm, Elsfield, Oxfordshire. Between 5 and 15 cats were observed at this pig farrowing unit between 1980 and 1982. They spent most of their time around the farmyard and nearby buildings, but also ventured into the surrounding pasture and arable fields, gardens and woods. The cats were provisioned daily with household scraps and were able to scavenge farmyard casualties and after-births. Individuals differed in the extent to which they hunted away from the farmyard. Shelter and nest sites were abundant around the farm buildings. Annually or biannually the cats were culled by the farmer to reduce their numbers to 10 or less. In total approximately 1200 hours of observation were recorded.

3. *Large:* Horspath Piggery, Oxfordshire. Between 25 and 30 cats were observed at this pig fattening unit between 1980 and 1987. The pigs were fed swill whose preparation generated abundant scavengable food. This was supplemented with erratic provisioning by the farmer, who supplied copious high quality food (e.g. joints of cooked meat, entire cooked piglets). The cats spent the majority of their time around the farmyard area in order to exploit this food. Some cats occasionally caught rats or birds. Shelter and nest sites were abundant around the farm buildings. Between 1980 and 1982 approximately 1400 hours of intensive observation were recorded, with a further 500 or so hours accumulated during weekly visits thereafter.

Using data drawn from these three colonies we will answer briefly a series of questions; some of these analyses can be found in Kerby (1987) and Macdonald *et al.* (1987), others will be published in full elsewhere.

Were the cats avoiding or attracting each other in the timing of their visits to the farm?

At the Small colony all four cats spent much of their time (male: 31%; females: 65–85%) in the vicinity of a straw-filled barn. Radio tracking revealed that the remainder of their time was spent foraging around the farmyard or in the surrounding countryside. During

484 hours of observation, the identities of all cats present at the barn were noted every five minutes. These data were used to generate an expected probability that each pair of cats would coincide at the barn. The four adult cats provided six pairwise comparisons, and in none of these did the observed frequency of coincidence at the barn differ significantly from the random expectation (nor did it do so in any one of five months analysed individually, nor when the exercise was repeated after the group had been translocated to Oxfordshire). Therefore, we conclude that each cat's attendance at the barn was independent of the attendance of each of the other cats: that is to say, members of the colony were neither seeking nor avoiding meetings at the barn more than expected by chance.

Once in the farmyard were the cats actively sociable?

If a colony was only a structureless aggregation its members would none the less meet, and presumably interact, occasionally. Therefore, observation of interactions is evidence neither of social structure nor of active sociality. A rudimentary proof of the existence of social forces would be departure from randomness in the spacing (with respect to resources) of cats around the farm. Even a brief acquaintance with our three colonies would make it obvious that in each of them some cats actively sought out others. In none of the colonies was there any restriction of space or sites that might have forced the cats into close proximity.

In the Small colony, on average when a cat was present in the barn it had another cat at less than one metre away on 20 per cent of our scan samples (male: 18%; females: mean 21.5%, SD = 6.0). This level of proximity was not due solely to adults sitting with kittens: on average, each adult female was within one metre of another adult cat (and often touching) on 14 per cent of the scans. All three females sought to position themselves close to the adult male, who had at least one female within a metre of him for 15.7 per cent of the scans for which he was in the barn. The frequency with which given cats positioned themselves close together was not simply a reflection of the probability of finding themselves in the barn simultaneously. On the contrary, each cat differed in the individuals to which it tended to be close.

In the Small colony adults spent about half their time in the barn asleep and adult females were in bodily contact with one or more other cats for more than half the time they were asleep. Each adult differed in the tendency to sleep in bodily contact with others and showed different preferences for sleeping partners.

In the Medium colony the cats congregated in one area of the farmyard. When in this area, members of both sexes spent about 40 per cent of their time within one metre of another cat, but adult females were found touching another individual twice as often as adult males (13%, SD = 9.1 vs 6.5%, SD = 3.5). At the Large colony, when in the farmyard, members of both sexes spent almost 40 per cent of their time within one metre of another cat, and adult females spent slightly more time actually in bodily contact than did adult males (9.4%, SD = 7.7 vs 7.6%, SD = 7.7).

We conclude, on the evidence of the close proximity between them, that the cats were actively sociable, and that this sociality was spatially structured in that individuals differed in the cats with which they chose to associate.

Were interactions between cats socially structured?

In a structureless grouping one might expect interactions between given pairs of cats to occur at frequencies proportional to their likelihood of meeting. In the Small colony the scan samples indicated when each pair of cats was together, and 6544 documented interactions revealed that there was no correlation between the time that two cats spent in each other's company (as defined by being in the barn simultaneously) and either the frequency or rate of interactions between them (Table 6.1). The identity of the cats affected the frequency of their interactions, and these frequencies were positively correlated with the tendency to maintain close proximity. That is, individuals interacted most with the cats whose close company they sought. These results demonstrate that the cats' interactions were socially structured.

The average hourly rate of interaction between adults was lowest in the Small colony (Small = 1.1, Medium = 1.45, Large = 1.34). However, the numbers of adults differed between the colonies, and was inversely related to the average hourly rate of dyadic interactions (Small = 0.4, Medium = 0.18, Large = 0.064). Thus, the average adult in the Large colony interacted less with each other adult, but interacted more in total, than its counterpart in the Small colony (see Table 6.2). These rates are affected not only by the

Table 6.1. *Hourly rates of interaction when together in the farmyard for each focal animal at the Small colony. The four bottom rows show the interaction rate when in each other's company for each pair of cats. These data are from April to December 1978 when the colony consisted of one adult male, TM, three adult females, SM, DO and PI, and one male kitten, LU (the kitten is only represented in the data for 487 of the 789 h of observation of the adults). SM was mother, and TM very probably father, to DO, PI and LU (data from Macdonald et al., 1987)*

		TM	SM	DO	PI	LU
Hours present of 789		253.3	520.7	670.7	603.6	(409.2)
Adult interaction per hour present		3.5	1.4	1.7	1.4	4.2
Interaction with ♀ per hour present		3.5	0.78	0.93	1.12	4.15
Interaction with ♂ per hour present		—	0.62	0.77	0.28	0.05
Interaction with kitten per hour present		0.3	3.6	1.8	0.38	—
Interaction per hour in company	SM	0.98	—	—	—	—
	DO	2.67	0.54	—	—	—
	PI	0.76	0.86	0.65	—	—
	LU	0.34	4.0	2.0	0.42	—

numbers of cats in each colony, but also by the pattern of their attendance in the farmyard. The rates would obviously be increased if we considered only time during which cats were present in the farmyard simultaneously, and therefore available for interaction. In the case of the Small colony, for example, such a correction for cat availability increases the hourly rate of interaction between two adult cats by a factor of about 2.7.

Are relationships between colony members qualitatively different?

The nature of interactions between two cats can be summarised by their type, total number and prevailing direction from initiator to recipient (asymmetry).

All three of these measures are shown in Figure 6.1

Table 6.2. *Hourly rates of interaction observed between pairs of average representatives of each adult sex (e.g. at the Large colony each adult male interacted with each adult female on average once every ten hours or 0.1 times per hour). The calculation and interpretation of rates of interaction amongst cats is greatly complicated by the differential availabilities for interaction of given cats, depending on the pattern of their attendance in the farmyard. This is not taken into account in the figures given in the table but has the effect of increasing the rate of interaction between average pairs of cats. For example, at the Small colony the male and each female interacted at an average rate of 1.47 times per hour during periods when they were in the farmyard simultaneously; pairs of females interacted 0.68 times per hour when in each other's company. In brief, these differences arise because the male was rarely present, but interacted at a high rate with females when the opportunity arose.*

	Small	Medium	Large
Male–female	0.37	0.228	0.100
Female–female	0.39	0.114	0.046
Male–male	—	0.178	0.057

for the frequencies of each of three types of interaction for all four adult cats present in the Small colony from April to December 1978. Of these 1547 interactions, 64.7 per cent were licking, 27.8 per cent rubbing and 7.5 per cent aggression, but the numbers and proportions of different types of interaction varied between pairs of cats. For example, female DO initiated 377 interactions with male TM of which 42.2 per cent were licking and 57.8 per cent rubbing, whereas female PI initiated 100 interactions with TM of which 26.0 per cent were licking and 74.0 per cent rubbing. Neither female was ever seen to be aggressive to TM although he was aggressive to them. Furthermore, the magnitude of asymmetry in the direction of interactions differed not only between cats, but between behavioural categories for given pairs of cats. It is clear from Figure 6.1 that relationships between adults in the Small colony differed in type, frequency and prevailing direction. Overall the Small colony was generally amicable (approximately half of the inter-

actions involved licking) and rarely agonistic (< 5% of interactions involved even mild aggression). Individuals differed in the number of interactions that they initiated, allowing some to be classified as net initiators of interactions and others as net recipients.

From these analyses it is clear that farm cat colonies are highly structured in terms of the nature of individual relationships. That the existence of this structure has not been more widely appreciated is doubtless due to the low frequency and inconspicuousness of some important behavioural patterns [Macdonald *et al.* (1987) point out that they saw only 1 rubbing interaction between adult females per 46.5 h of observation.]

Can individual relationships be organised according to consistent age–sex class distinctions?

Figure 6.2 shows a simplified representation of the interactions between selected age–sex classes in each colony. In small colonies there will inevitably be few members of most age–sex classes, and none of some. This makes it difficult to distinguish individual variation in social behaviour from variation which is characteristic of a given age–sex class. Figure 6.1(*b*) displays equivalent age–sex class data for the Small colony, broken down into three types of behaviour. Even with this simple catalogue of behaviour, it is clear that the quality of relationships differed between the male, females and kitten. In summary, kittens were initiators to adults, females to the adult male, and some adult females were initiators to others.

To search for such generalisations in the Medium and Large colonies we assigned each cat, each month, to one of six classes: (a) adult (breeding) male, (b) adult (breeding) female, (c) juvenile male (> 6 months but not yet breeding), (d) juvenile female (> 6 months but not yet breeding), (e) male kitten (< 6 months), and (f) female kitten (< 6 months). We calculated the hourly rate of each type of behaviour that an average initiator cat of a particular age–sex class manifested towards an average recipient cat of a particular age–sex class (correcting for variation in cat availability, numbers of animals in each age–sex class per month, and hours observed per month). A rank order of recipient age–sex classes was drawn up for each initiator class, and these were tested for significance between the rank positions. The results indicated that interactions initiated by adults were not distributed among the other age–sex classes in

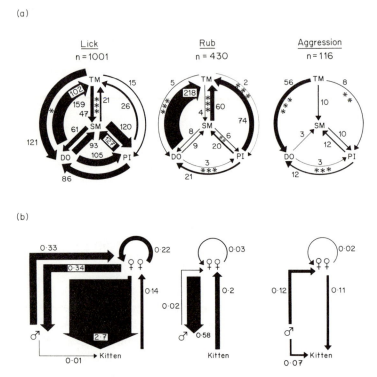

(a)

(b)

Fig. 6.1 (*a*) Sociograms of the relationships between adult cats at the Small colony from April to December 1978, when the colony members were an adult male, TM, an adult female, SM, and her two adult daughters, PI and DO. Three behaviours are illustrated, and initiators are distinguished from recipients. The thickness of the arrows is proportional to the percentage of interactions of that category between the cats in question. The asterisks indicate the statistical significance of the asymmetry of flow between each pair (* $p < 0.05$; ** $p < 0.01$; *** $p < 0.001$). The numbers on each arrow indicate the numbers of interactions observed between the cats in question. (*b*) Sociograms for the same three behaviours illustrating the hourly rates of interaction between each age and sex class in the Small colony during the period when a male kitten was growing (June–December 1978). The numbers on each arrow indicate the average hourly rate of interaction between average individuals of each age–sex class (e.g. the average adult female initiated 0.22 licking interactions per hour with another adult female during each hour that they were simultaneously present in the farmyard). (Details of methodology in Kerby, 1987).

proportion to the availability of those classes (either in terms of their numbers in the colony, or their immediate presence in the farmyard). However, there were differences between the Medium and Large colonies.

Figure 6.3 shows, for average pairs of interactants, which age–sex classes were interacted with preferentially. For example, at the Large colony adult males interacted with kittens at a significantly lower rate than that at which they interacted with any other age–sex class, whereas at the Medium colony adult males interacted preferentially with juvenile males and juvenile females. These results emphasise the over-riding preference for juvenile male recipients at the Medium colony, contrasting with the lack of any clear preference for given classes of recipient at the Large colony. The results summarised in Figure 6.3 concern all behaviour patterns. Different preferences emerge when different categories of behaviour are selected. For example, 'parental' behaviour was defined to include behaviour patterns such as suckle, retrieve kitten, bring food, and groom another individual.

Analysis of the recipient age–sex classes for 'parental' behaviour revealed, not surprisingly, that adult females directed such behaviour at a significantly higher rate towards kittens than towards any other class. Similarly, analysis of 'aggressive' behaviour showed that adult males at the Large colony interacted at a significantly higher rate with other adult males, while at the Medium colony adult males interacted at a significantly higher rate with both adult and juvenile males.

These analyses will be presented in full elsewhere (Kerby, 1987); here they lead us to conclude that there are characteristic differences in the behaviour profiles of given age–sex classes, but that these may vary with circumstances between colonies.

Can social categories be identified within age–sex classes?

In our studies a detailed social profile was drawn up for each cat on the basis of four criteria: (a) presence (the amount of time spent at the resource centre), (b) proximity (of the time present, the proportion

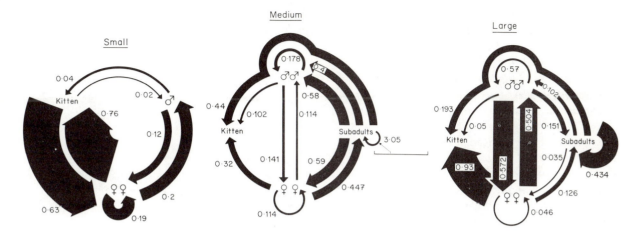

Fig. 6.2. A comparison of the hourly rates of interaction observed between representatives of selected age–sex classes in three colonies. The thickness of the arrows is proportional to the percentage of the total hourly interactions that was exchanged between average individuals representing given classes of cat. The data are expressed as the average number of interactions observed per hour between one average member of one class and an average member of the other. These averages are written alongside the appropriate arrows. For example, in the Large colony each adult male initiated an interaction to each other adult male 0.057 times per hour. The overall pattern would be different if we considered the proportion of observed inter- actions between age–sex classes as a whole. The data presented here have been corrected for the variation in the numbers of representatives in each class thus making the three colonies directly comparable (see Kerby, 1987).

LARGE

Significantly preferred recipient class

		A♂	A♀	J♂	J♀	K♂	K♀
INITIATOR AGE/SEX CLASS	A♂	✓	✓	✓	✓		
	A♀	No	significant		preference		
	J♂	✓	✓	✓	✓		✓
	J♀	✓	✓	✓	✓		

MEDIUM

Significantly preferred recipient class

		A♂	A♀	J♂	J♀	K♂	K♀
INITIATOR AGE/SEX CLASS	A♂			✓	✓		
	A♀			✓		✓	
	J♂			✓			
	J♀			✓			

significance level *p = 0.01*

A♂ = adult male
J♂ = juvenile male
K♀ = kitten female
etc.

Fig. 6.3. Results of an analysis of discrimination between recipient age–sex classes for all behaviour categories by adult and juvenile initiator age/sex classes. A tick indicates that a given age–sex class of recipient was significantly preferred (in terms of rate of initiations) by a given class of initiator at *p* < 0.01 (Mann-Whitney U-tests). (Full details in Kerby, 1987.)

Table 6.3. *A summary of the qualities that distinguished Breeding and Non-Breeding males, and Central and Peripheral females in each of the three colonies. The measures are (a) Presence: the proportion of scans of the farmyard in which eact cat was present; (b) Proximity: the proportion of scans in which each cat was within 1 m of its nearest neighbour and (c) Interactivity: the number of interactions in which each cat was engaged per hour of observation. The judgements 'High' and 'Low' indicate whether the scores, on a given measure, of cats in a particular class, fell predominantly in the high or low half of the distribution of scores for members of their sex in their colony on that measure*

		Presence	Proximity	Interactivity
Adult male	Breeders	Low	Low	High
	Non-Breeders	High	High	Low
Adult female	Central	High	High	High
	Peripheral	Low	Low	Low

Table 6.4. *Indicators of reproductive success of adult males at each of the three colonies*

	Small	Medium	Large
Number of Breeders: number of Non-Breeders	1:1	3:4	7:5
% Intromissions by Breeders	100	60	78
Proportion Breeders seen to intromit	100	67	42
Proportion Non-Breeders seen to intromit	0	50	20
Proportion ♂♂ who attempted to mate and who succeeded	66.6	57.1	57.1
Number of mate attempts that were observed	?	124	113

spent at given distances from a nearest neighbour), (c) interactivity (hourly rate of interaction when present) and (d) behavioural profile (the proportion of interactive behaviour assigned to each of several behaviour categories). Within and between colonies these social profiles revealed great individual variation. None the less, across all three colonies it was possible to identify adults which for each sex fell into one of two distinct classes. Their qualities are summarised in Table 6.3. We label these classes Breeder and Non-Breeder males; Central and Peripheral females.

At the Medium and Large colonies, where comparison between adult males was possible, Breeder males were characterised by low presence scores, avoiding close proximity to other cats, and by interacting at a higher rate than Non-Breeding males when present. Breeders were more 'alert' than Non-Breeders, more overtly aggressive, and mate-called and scent-marked more. Non-Breeders had high presence scores, maintained close proximity to other cats, but interacted at a lower rate than Breeders (although they were present for a greater proportion of the time), and in particular had low scores on scent-marking. Non-Breeders tended to be defensive rather than aggressive.

All adult females bred, but at all three colonies some spent more time than others in the vicinity of the resource centre, and on this basis we draw a distinction between Central and Peripheral females. At both Medium and Large colonies, Central females were more frequently present, and had high proximity scores and interaction rates. In general, Central females were more alert and aggressive than Peripheral females.

We conclude that despite great individual variation, it is useful to distinguish at least four social classes of adult cats within colonies.

Does social class affect reproductive success?

The observational difficulties of inferring paternity increased with colony size. Only one breeding male at a time was affiliated with the Small colony (being present about 25% of the time) and although other adult males passed through, only the affiliated male was seen to mate. Two successive breeding males were observed mating with all the adult females, whereas neither strangers nor younger male members of the group were seen to succeed in this despite occasional attempts. In such a reproductive monopoly the second male left more offspring because his tenure spanned a period when there were more reproductive females in the Small colony.

In the Medium and Large colonies no single male could monopolise matings. We recorded both attempted copulations and successful intromissions. Mating is a rare event and our data-gathering protocol

Table 6.5. *Indicators of reproductive success of adult females at each of the three colonies. Females are categorised as explained in Table 6.3*

	Overall			Central			Peripheral		
	Small	Medium	Large	Small	Medium	Large	Small	Medium	Large
Kittens per ♀ per year	1.00	1.25	0.97	0.90	1.40	1.56	1.20	1.14	0.42
Proportion of litter failing (%)	44	57	68	50	50	53	30	62.5	82

was not designed to facilitate such observations. None the less our observations sufficed to show that as colony size increased the proportion of those males attempting to copulate that succeeded in intromission decreased. When males were classified as Breeders and Non-Breeders, Breeders secured 60–100 per cent of matings (Table 6.4). Many of the mounts by Non-Breeders were on inappropriate recipients (young females, kittens or occasionally other males – see Winslow [1938]). In the Medium colony Non-Breeders, collectively and on average individually, were seen mounting slightly more often than were Breeding males, but the latter achieved on average 50 per cent more intromissions. Similarly, in the Large colony, although Non-Breeders were responsible for 39 per cent of the observed mount attempts, they secured only 22 per cent of the observed intromissions, and individually averaged only 40 per cent of the average Breeder's number of intromissions. In all three colonies, Breeder males were at a reproductive advantage; but as colony size increased each Breeder could expect, on average, a smaller proportion of the intromissions (see also Natoli & De Vito, Chapter 8). Our data are insufficient to show (a) the extent to which this loss was compensated by the increased number of potential mates available as colony size increased, or (b) consistent differences in mating success between individual Breeders, or (c) any variation in the ratio of Breeder to Non-Breeder intromissions at different stages of a female's oestrus.

In the Medium and Large colonies females termed Central and Peripheral were distinguished by the location of their kitten nest sites (i.e. whether they reared their kittens near the resource centre, or towards the periphery of the farmyard). The central nest sites were characterised by higher kitten survival than peripheral nest sites, where kittens frequently

died before weaning (see Table 6.5). At the Medium colony one successful breeding female bred peripherally, but at this colony the practice of culling may have affected the female's choice of nest site.

Although all adult females bore kittens, many litters died in all three colonies due to disease, accident or apparent maternal neglect. We measured reproductive success on the basis of the number of kittens surviving to post weaning per female per year. Individual female's reproductive success varied from zero to five kittens per year, and considerable individual variation occurred amongst both Central and Peripheral females (Central, 0–5.0; Peripheral, 0–0.67). Table 6.5 presents the average female reproductive success for Central and Peripheral classes at the three colonies. At both the Medium and Large colonies the Central females enjoyed the highest reproductive success on average. The proportion of litters failing completely increased with colony size, but the burden of this increasing loss was carried by the Peripheral females (see Table 6.5). In the Small colony small numbers of cats and high kitten mortality confound any generalisations about females' social roles and their reproductive success.

In the Large colony it was possible to see an interaction between the effects of lineage and centrality. Table 6.5 shows that 82 per cent of litters born to Peripheral lineages failed completely, whereas 53 per cent of those born to Central lineages failed. If the data are analysed in terms of litters failing in peripheral versus central nest sites the figures are 52 per cent versus 15 per cent. The difference between these two sets of figures arises because some members of the Central lineage bred in peripheral nest sites and suffered higher litter losses. These results beg the question of what underlay female centrality. We suggest that the answer lies in social affiliations based upon kinship. Of the three colonies there was inevitably the greatest scope for genealogies to diverge in the Large one. Spatial status seemed to be determined primarily by kinship. During the study period, two Central and six Peripheral lineages were identified. Four of these Peripheral lineages were probably side branches of the two Central lineages, while two derived from immigrant females.

Averaging reproductive success of members of the lineage revealed that kitten survival in each of the two Central lineages exceeded that in all the Peripheral lineages. Reproduction was so poor among Peripheral females that their lineages became progressively more fragmented. After seven years of observation, some old Peripheral females still lacked any descendants. With time, the Peripheral lineages would be expected to die out, and the central ones to split, pushing low status females to peripheral positions and low productivity. Not surprisingly, the effect of kinship ties was much less apparent in observations of the Peripheral cats than of the Central cats.

This effect was less marked at the Medium colony, probably partly because the annual or biannual cull of about one third of the cats reduced competition, fragmented lineages and destabilised social structure. Furthermore, the higher overall reproductive success of the Medium colony (see Table 6.5) may arise because a major mortality factor there was unconnected with food supply or social dynamics.

What selective pressures affect sociality in farm cats?

As mentioned at the outset, we conclude from the literature that the pattern of food availability largely determines whether or not cats live in groups. Within that ecological framework other, sociological selective pressures may affect group size or the fitness of colonial cats.

At all three colonies we observed communal denning and allomaternal behaviour (including nursing and providing food). The frequency of nursing coalitions was highest in the Small colony (> 80% of possible cases were observed). With the larger number of females in the Medium and Large colonies the numbers of possible combinations of potential cooperators was large. However, observations of alloparental behaviour did not increase proportionally. At the Medium colony we documented one case of two females nursing their litters communally, and another case of a nursing female adopting an orphan. In

neither case were the genetic relationships known. At the Large colony communal nursing was more common and 10 communal dens were observed over three years, all of which were occupied by mother–daughter nursing coalitions. Overall it appears that alloparental behaviour is generally (but not exclusively) confined within lineages.

A case of infanticide by an unfamiliar adult male was observed at the Small colony, and circumstantial evidence of cats killing kittens was gathered at both the other colonies. In the light of the observed case at the Small colony, where females combined forces against the infanticidal male, it may be beneficial to have several mothers in attendance at a den. In addition to their greater strength of numbers, larger coalitions will reduce the time during which the nest is unguarded.

Entire combined litters succumbed to contagious disease at all three colonies. It is possible that communal denning increases the risk of disease transmission. On the other hand, it might reduce the risk if kittens susceptible to cat flu were nursed by an alloparent who was immune (Csiza *et al.*, 1971; Johnson, Margolis & Kilham, 1967).

Discussion

We have discussed variation in cat social behaviour at three levels. Firstly, the distinction between populations in which adult females are generally solitary and those where they are gregarious. Secondly, the variation in group sizes and consequently in social structure. Thirdly, individual variation within and between age and sex classes in terms of the nature of social relationships. It has been convenient to distinguish these levels of variation, although they are only different magnifications of the same image; all three stem from differences in the behaviour of individual cats. At all levels it is clear that the frequent assertion that lions are the only sociable felids is unfounded (e.g. Kleiman & Eisenberg, 1973; Fox, 1975). It also seems unwarranted to dismiss domestic cat sociality as a creation of selection by cat fanciers (e.g. Packer, 1986).

Reviewing our findings and those of others, we conclude that one social unit is fundamental to the organisation of all groups of cats, irrespective of their sizes, compositions and superficial differences. That unit is the social matriline – the long-term affiliation between a female and successive generations of her direct descendents. The expression of matrilineal organisation varies with resource dispersion, such that it is most clear cut where food is highly clumped and abundant and where adult mortality is low – in other words, under the circumstances of our Large colony.

Initially the females in our Small colony were all so closely related that there was no scope to interpret their social affiliations in terms of differential relatedness. The same situation probably prevails in many small colonies: all the females are related as daughters, grand-daughters or nieces. Such groups tend to be amicable, cooperative and spatially tightly knit. Each matriline in the Large colony was roughly analogous to the entire Small colony in composition. Members of each lineage were amicable amongst themselves, but members of the central matriline were at a social and spatial advantage over peripheral cats. Doubtless, all the matrilines in the Large colony were genetically related through the paternal lines (and at least distantly through the maternal line too) but the large number of cats at the farmyard and consequent reduction of the average coefficient of relatedness, allowed greater distance in kinship to be reflected in polarised social affiliations. At the Large colony the rich food supply consisted of one large clump. Therefore, aside from emigration, there was no possibility of further spatial separation between the matrilines. If the resources had been divisible we would predict that the Large colony would have split along the matrilineal rifts. Such splits might underlie the circumstances described by Dards (1978) where closely neighbouring groups of females were each associated with their own clumped food supply (in that case rubbish skips). One might speculate that the heterogeneity in resource dispersion in Dards' study area, and in those of Izawa *et al.* (1982) and Natoli (1985b), was reflected in a heterogeneity in the populations' genetic constitutions, with patches of closer kinship coinciding with patches of food resources.

Might such a matrilineal organisation be preserved in populations where cats are solitary? Corbett (1979) describes a solitary dominant female cat whose summer home range encompassed that of a subordinate female. The latter was forced to forage in suboptimal habitat, but the two cats, and others from neighbouring home ranges, shared the same household when food was clumped there in winter (see above). We wonder whether the social structure that might force a young female towards the periphery of a farmyard (under circumstances where resources were clumped), could also force her into less favoured corners of the maternal territory, or even out of it altogether (under circumstances where food was more uniformly dispersed). The result might be clusters of related females in overlapping or adjoining ranges.

The situation of males in different populations varies more in degree than in kind. It seems that the ranges of Breeding males are structures to encompass several ranges of females, whether each of these ranges contains a solitary female or a group of them. Amongst the Carnivora there are close parallels between the spatial arrangements of male domestic cats and those of many male mustelids. Our division of males into Breeders and Non-Breeders is compatible with Liberg's (1980) finer level of classification. Other details of the mating system remain obscure (see Chapters 7 and 8).

Concluding remarks

Previously the detailed social dynamics within groups of cats have been studied only at the crude level of laboratory experiments contrived to provoke clashes over food. It seems likely that such experiments will inevitably reveal a hierarchy, irrespective of whether such ranking has any relevance to social behaviour 'in the wild'. Macdonald & Apps (1978) and Macdonald *et al.* (1987) argue that there are distinct differences in the relationships between cats in a colony. In this chapter we propose that cat colonies comprise a network of social relationships within and between matrilineal subunits. We believe that the largest colonies of 50 or more cats are not social units in any functional sense, but rather populations of social units. The social relationships between cats are reflected in the juxtaposition of the cats with respect to each other and resources such as food and shelter, and in the interchange of behaviour.

Acknowledgements

We are grateful to Dr L. Corbett and P. Apps, who made helpful comments on the manuscript, and to the Editors for their forbearance. Our research was supported by grants from the Natural Environment Research Council and National Geographic Society.

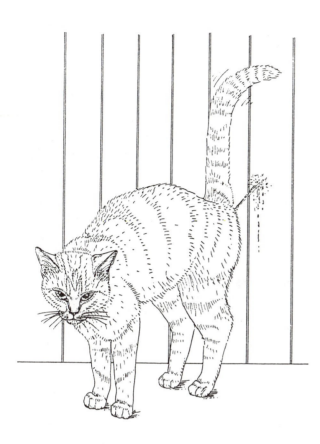

7

Spatial organisation and reproductive tactics in the domestic cat and other felids

Olof Liberg and Mikael Sandell

Introduction

As its vernacular name implies, the domestic cat has a long history of coexistence with man; but as we all know, it is still capable of reverting back to the feral state. The cat enjoys a very special status as a domestic animal. There has been little artificial selection by man in cats, and many cats are allowed complete freedom of movement. In many respects the cats' way of life more closely resembles that of certain 'wild' symbionts of man, like the rat or the house sparrow, than that of a true domestic, such as the dog. It is therefore probable that many, if not most factors influencing the social behaviour of wild felids are also operative in the domestic cat.

Wild felids are difficult to study. They are shy and rare, and they often live in remote or inaccessible areas. Domestic cats are at least in the non-feral state tame; they occur at high densities all over the world and are available for study just outside the gates of universities. Besides being interesting study objects themselves, domestic cats are also excellent 'model

animals' for studies on how different ecological factors shape social organisation, including spacing, more generally in the Felidae. The intermediate position of the domestic cat between a solitary way of life, which is typical for most wild felids, and more well developed group-living, resembling that of the lion, *Panthera leo*, might also shed light on factors favouring social life.

For clarity's sake, when we speak of the domestic cat, we mean all categories of *Felis silvestris catus* L. With house cat, or house-based cat, we are referring to cats that live in close connection with a household, which assumes some responsibility for feeding the cats. When we speak of a farm cat we mean a house cat that lives on an agricultural farm. Finally, with feral cat we mean a domestic cat that is not attached to a particular household. This does not mean that it cannot live close to humans on a more anonymous basis. A feral cat can subsist either entirely on its own, hunting and scavenging like any wild carnivore, or by being fed anonymously by humans at the garbage depot or by direct hand-outs from 'cat lovers'. The latter source seems to be especially common in larger cities (Tabor, 1983).

Scientific literature on the behaviour and ecology of free-roaming domestic cats has increased rapidly in the last decade from less than a dozen articles in 1975, to more than one hundred in 1986. Since these studies also cover cat populations at the extreme ends of such ecological gradients as food abundance and distribution, we are in a position to test hypotheses on the influence of these factors on spacing and other social behaviour.

This review is based primarily on published studies or material 'in press'. Results from a few unpublished dissertations are also included. Methods and results have been critically examined, and problems connected with the evaluation and synthesis of results are discussed. We will also question some traditional ways of thinking about felid spatial organisation. Our main purpose has been to assess whether a pattern exists in the spatial organisation of the domestic cat. We assume that spacing pattern is an effect of the reproductive tactics chosen by the individuals in the population. Since the cat is a polygynous (or rather, promiscuous) species, we expect that males compete primarily for access to receptive females, while females compete over food and other environmental resources to improve their production and rearing of offspring (Trivers, 1972; Clutton-Brock & Harvey, 1978). These hypotheses can be tested with the data available on domestic cats. A comparison with other felids is included to assess the generality of the patterns, and to reveal possible effects of domestication.

Density

We begin with a section on cat population density. This is important for our later discussion of spatial organisation for two reasons: density is a potential causative factor, and a population variable that might be affected by spacing behaviour.

Population densities reported in the various cat studies show tremendous variation, from about one cat per square kilometre to around 2000 cats per square kilometre (Table 7.1). This certainly calls for an explanation. Our basic hypothesis is that density of both free-ranging house and feral cats is determined by absolute food abundance.

One problem when testing this hypothesis is that many different methods are used to determine densities (see Table 7.1). Thus, one has to keep in mind

that there is a large variation in accuracy between studies.

Another problem is the almost universal lack of quantitative data on food abundance. All authors report the type of food available to their cats and, in most cases, some estimate of relative abundance. But this is insufficient for a normal regression analysis of density over food abundance. Instead we have had to group the studies into three broad density classes, and relate these to a rough estimate of the food situation (Table 7.2).

Densities above 50 cats per square kilometre were only found in urban areas where cats fed on rich supplies of garbage or were fed by large numbers of 'cat lovers', i.e. people not owning the cats, but who frequently gave them food at traditional places. Intermediate densities (5–50 cats per sq km) were found in farm cat populations where the cats were supplied with all, or at least part, of their food requirements by owners, and in rural feral populations subsisting on very rich, often clumped natural prey such as colonies of ground-nesting seabirds. Densities below five cats per square kilometre were only found in rural feral populations subsisting on widely dispersed prey, mainly rabbits and rodents.

This is certainly not a satisfactory test of our food hypothesis, but it does indicate that absolute food abundance is at least roughly related to density. A second factor that might seriously affect densities is human control. It is interesting to note that two rural populations where the cats were based mainly at non-farming households (Liberg, 1980; Warner, 1985), and where one might expect a lower tolerance of large cat groups, also had lower densities than two populations where the cats lived on dairy farms (Panaman, 1981; Turner & Mertens, 1986). Direct control operations are also common, both in urban feral populations (Natoli, 1985a) and in rural populations (e.g. Hubbs, 1951; Pascal, 1980).

The only comparable density figures for wild small felids is one Scottish population of European wild cat, *Felis s. silvestris*, which exhibited a density of three animals per square kilometre (Corbett, 1979). This agrees well with figures for Australian and New Zealand feral cats of one to two cats per square kilometre (Jones & Coman, 1982; Fitzgerald & Karl, 1986). The main prey for all three populations was rabbits occurring at roughly the same densities. This is an indication that the same factors may determine the densities of wild felids and feral cats living in similar habitats.

Home range size

Two basic methods have been used to determine home range size: ratio-tracking and sightings of identified individuals. Radio-tracking naturally gives a less biased result, since locating the subjects is not dependent on habitat visibility. Also the risk of missing less frequented parts of the home range is higher when range size is based only on sightings. We therefore expect that the sighting method will yield smaller home range estimates than radio-tracking, which is supported by data from Izawa, Doi & Ono (1982). With very large samples, as in the study by Dards (1978), the sighting method will also yield reliable results, especially if the study is conducted in a confined area and all parts are evenly searched by the observer. From our review we noted that home range sizes based on only sightings were either from urban studies, or studies of single farm cat groups. All others (multiple farm cat groups, rural feral populations) have used radio-tracking.

Due to differences in sampling methods, length of tracking periods, sample size and, especially, the methods used to calculate range size, there is great variation in the data on home range size. As far as possible we have used values resulting from the 'convex polygon method' (Mohr & Stumpf, 1966).

Some authors have split up their tracking data into subperiods. We find that monthly ranges are rather meaningless, since there is no biological reason to expect monthly differences. But seasonal ranges based on various biological criteria can be useful for answering certain questions. For cats the most relevant division probably would be into mating and non-mating seasons. For female cats litter rearing periods might also be meaningfully considered separately (e.g. Corbett, 1979; Fitzgerald & Karl, 1986).

Female home range size

As with density, there is a 1000-fold variation in mean home range size given in the different studies. Female ranges span from 0.1–1.8 hectares in a Japanese fishing village (Izawa *et al.*, 1982) to 170 hectares in the Australian bush (Jones & Coman, 1982). Our primary hypothesis is that female range size is determined by food abundance and distribution. If these are the only factors influencing range size, females are expected to include just enough space to give them access to the food needed to get them through the year. Unfortunately the lack of data on food abundance again prevents a direct test of this prediction. It is obvious, however, that food has just as strong an influence on female home range size as on cat density. In fact we found a significant negative correlation between female home range size and density (Figure 7.1). We believe the reason for this correlation is that density and female home range size each are correlated to a third factor, namely food abundance. The smallest female ranges were found in those urban feral populations that subsist on rich clumped food resources; intermediate ranges were found in farm cats; and the largest ranges were shown by feral cats living on dispersed natural prey (Table 7.3). The wide scatter of points around the regression line in Figure 7.1 is caused by the farm and house cats, which get food from their owners, independent of their range size. If only feral cats are considered the correlation is even higher ($r = -0.97$, $n = 7$, $t = 8.62$, $p < 0.001$).

Harder to test than the influence of food abundance is that of food *distribution*. Konecny (1983) found that when food occurred in patches, the feral cats in his study moved over larger areas than when it was evenly distributed, in spite of a higher overall food abundance in the former case. Farm cats and others subsisting on a concentrated food source, rich and stable enough to support them throughout the year, obviously move over larger areas than are needed to fulfil their food requirements. But other needs may explain this. For example, some of the female cats living on fish dumps in Japan with relatively small home ranges, still moved far away from the food source itself, obviously in search of appropriate resting places (Izawa *et al.*, 1982). Many female farm cats, which could stay near the farm buildings for their entire life as far as food acquisition is concerned, still move considerable distances away, usually to hunt natural prey in the surrounding fields.

Male home range size

The variation in range size between different areas is just as large for males as for females (see Table 7.3). When plotted over density, the male range regression line has an almost identical slope with that of females in Figure 7.1, but lies at a higher level. On the average, male ranges are 3.5 times larger than those of females. Energetically this increase in range size corresponds to

Table 7.1. *Characteristics of the studies from which quantitative data were taken for analysis of spacing behaviour in cats. Studies are arranged in order of population density*

Study no.	Place, country	Duration of study (yr)	Study area size (sq km)	Method[a]	Habitat	Food Type	Relative abundance	Distribution	Cat status	Group/ Sol.[b]	Population density (n/sq km)	References
1.	Ainoshima, Japan	1.5	0.1	R, S	Fisher village	Fish dumps	Rich	Clumped	Feral	G	2350	Izawa, 1984, Izawa et al., 1982
2.	Rome, Italy	1.5	0.02	S	City park	Anon. hand-outs	Rich	Mod. clump.	Feral	G	1000–2000	Natoli, 1985a
3.	Portsmouth, England	4	1.0	S	Dockyard	Anon. hand-outs	Rich	Mod. clump.	Feral	G	200	Dards, 1978, 1983
4.	Oxford, England	5	1.0	S, R	Pig farm	Regular feeding	Rich	Clumped	Farm cats	G	High	Kerby & Macdonald, this volume
5.	Cornwall, England	0.5	0.16	S	Dairy farm	Milk, some prey	Mod.	Clumped	Farm cats	G	30	Panaman, 1981
6.	Lorraine, France	0.2	0.75	R	Dairy farm	Milk, wastes	Mod.	Clumped	Farm cats	G	?	Pericard, 1986
7.	Wisconsin, USA	0.5	One farm	S	Dairy farm	Milk, some prey	Mod.	Clumped	Farm cats	G	?	Laundré, 1977
8.	Dassen Island, South Africa	1.3	2.2	R, S	Sub-tropical scrub	Rabbits, bird carcasses	Mod.	Dispersed	Feral	S	20–50	Apps, 1983, 1986
9.	Hebrides, Scotland	2	1.0	S	Sand dunes	Rabbits, food scraps	Mod.	Mixed	Semi-feral	G/S	19	Corbett, 1979
10.	Hirzel, Switzerland	1	1.3	R, S, I	Agricul. land	House feeding, rodents	Mod.	Clumped	Farm cats	G	14	Turner & Mertens, 1986
11.	Kerguelen, S Ind. Ocean	2	600	S	Sub-antarctic heath	Rabbits, sea birds	Mod.	Mixed	Feral	S	10–15	Derenne, 1976, Pascal, 1980

No.	Location			Method[a]	Habitat	Food		Dispersion	Cat type	Group[b]	Group size	Reference
12.	Marion Island, South Africa	1.5	33	S	Sub-antarctic heath	Seabirds	Mod.	Clumped	Feral	S	5–14	van Aarde, 1978, 1979
13.	Illinois, USA	5	52	R, I	Agricul. land	Farm feeding, rodents	Mod.	Clumped	House cats	G	6.3	Warner, 1985
14.	Devon, England	0.5	0.6	R	Dairy farm	Milk, some prey	Mod.	Clumped	Farm cats	G	6	Macdonald & Apps, 1978
15.	Macquarie Island, New Zealand	?	120	T, S	Sub-antarctic heath	Rabbits, seabirds	Mod.	Mixed	Feral	S	2–7	Jones, 1977
16.	Revinge, Sweden	8	20	R, S, I	Farms, pastures, woods	House feeding, rabbits	Mod.	Clumped	Mixed	G/S	3–7	Liberg, 1980, 1981, 1983, 1984
17.	Monach Island, Scotland	2	2.4	R	Dunes, heath	Rabbits, birds	Poor	Dispersed	Feral	S	3.7	Corbett, 1979
18.	Galapagos The Pacific	1	10 + 15	R, S	Tropical scrub	Rodents, birds, lizards	Poor	Dispersed	Feral	S	2–3	Konecny, 1983
19.	Victoria, Australia	4	190	R	Subtropical grassland	Rabbits	Mod.	Dispersed	Feral	S	1–2	Jones & Coman, 1982
20.	Schiermonnikoog, Netherlands	1	40	R	Rural open land	Rabbits, rodents, birds	Poor	Dispersed	Feral	S	0.9	Langeveld & Niewold, 1985
21.	Orongorongo, New Zealand	2	15	R	River valley bottom grass slopes woods	Rats, rabbits	Poor	Dispersed	Feral	S	1	Fitzgerald & Karl, 1986

[a] R = radio-tracking; S = sightings; I = interviews with owners; T = trapping and shooting.
[b] Group = most females and some males live in groups; Sol. = solitary cats.

Table 7.2. *General food situation in three density categories of cat populations. For identification of populations refer to Table 7.1.*

Density category	More than 100 cats / sq km	5–50 cats /sq km	Less than 5 cats sq/km
Identity of populations within category	1, 2, 3	5, 8, 9, 10, 11, 12, 13, 14, 15, 16	17, 18, 19, 20, 21
General characteristics of food situation in category	Rich clumps (garbage, fish dumps, provisioning by cat lovers)	Thinner clumps (farms and other households, bird colonies on oceanic islands) or Rich dispersed prey	Scarce dispersed prey; might occur in patches, but no rich concentrations of food

a body weight 5.3 times that of females. As males rarely are more than 1.5 times as heavy as females (Liberg, 1981), we interpret this as a clear indication that food is not determining range size for males, at least not directly.

According to our basic assumption, males compete for access to females. From that we predict that the primary factor determining male range size is female density and distribution. We expect males to maximise access to females, and this means that male ranges generally will be larger than those of females. We will return to this point, but first two other aspects supporting our original hypothesis have to be considered.

The first concerns dominance categories in males. In most polygynous species both dominant breeding males and subordinate males that are partly or totally excluded from breeding occur. When such a situation exists in a cat population, we would expect breeding males to have larger ranges than non-breeding males, if they are living under otherwise similar conditions. Unfortunately most authors have not distinguished between these categories. Liberg (1981, 1984) recognised six categories of adult males, based on dominance and ecological status (house-based or feral). In house-based cats breeding males had ranges of 350–380 hectares; ranges of subordinate, non-breeding males were around 80 hectares, or not much larger than those of females. Turner & Mertens (1986) also found that the male they presumed to be the 'breeder' of their small population had the largest male range in the study. We believe the reason subordinate males generally have smaller ranges than dominants is that they gain little by travelling widely in search of females

(see below). However, under certain circumstances they can have even larger ranges. In the Swedish study some subordinate males were driven out of their primary homes by dominant rivals and assumed a feral status. These males had larger ranges than breeders, partly because they were no longer fed by humans and had to subsist on hunting, and partly because they were 'pushed around' by dominant males during the breeding season. To a certain extent these males corresponded to the male lion category that Schaller (1972) named 'nomads'.

The second aspect concerns seasonality. If breeding is seasonal we would expect female density and dispersion to be important for male range extension only during the mating season. At other times of the year breeder male ranges might be determined by the same factors as those of females and subordinate males. As mentioned earlier, there are few studies that have presented data on differences in range size between mating and non-mating seasons. But Corbett (1979) showed graphically that male ranges in his Hebrides study were largest in early spring, when presumably mating activities were at their highest, and then declined as the year proceeded. He did not present separate data for breeding vs. non-breeding males. Nor did Izawa *et al.* (1982), who also showed that male ranges were larger during the mating season than during the rest of the year. In a previously unpublished study we found that in the Revinge area of southern Sweden, breeding males had significantly larger ranges during the mating season than in the autumn when females were anoestrous (Table 7.4). We also found that breeding males had larger ranges than non-breeding males during the mating season, but

Table 7.3. *Range characteristics of male and female domestic cats. References are found in Table 7.1*

| Place of study | Density (n sq km) | Female ranges | | | | Overlap/Exclusive | | Male ranges | | | |
		Mean size (ha)	Range	n		Within groups	Between groups	Mean size (ha)	Range	n	O/E
Group-living females											
Japan[a]	>2000	0.51	0.06–1.8	6		O	E	0.72	0.31–1.7	6	O
Portsmouth	200	0.84	0.03–4.24	68		O	E	8.4	0.08–24.0	32	O
Switzerland	14	6.0	1.2–17.8	6		O(55%)	E(4%)	7.2	0.8–16.0	3	O
Illinois[a]	6	112	4.8–185	7		O	—	228	109–528	4	O
Sweden	3–7	50		15		O	E	370	84–990	18	O
Solitary females											
Dassen Island	30	19	11–32	3		O		44	32–63	5	O
Monach Island[a]	4	42	24–60	2		—		—	—	—	—
Galapagos	2–3	82	21–210	4		O		304	35–760	10	O
Victoria	1–2	170	70–270	2		—		620	330–290	2	O
New Zealand	1.1	80	20–170	5		O		140	50–130	4	O
Holland[a]	0.9	113	50–180	3		E		367	320–420	3	O

[a]Not annual ranges.

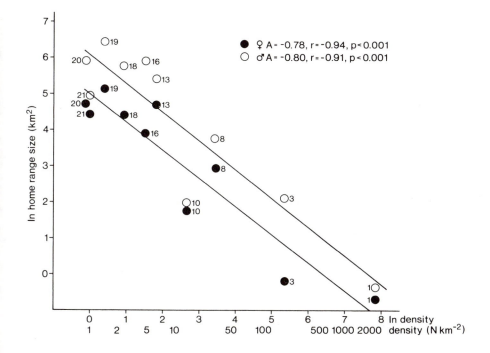

Fig. 7.1. Relationship between density and home range size in male and female cats. Figures refer to study number in Table 7.1. Lines are regression lines.

Table 7.4. *Seasonal changes in range size for dominant and subordinate males in the Revinge area, Sweden, 1984*

	Range size (sq km)					
	Mating season			Non-mating season		
	$\bar{x}$	Range	n	$\bar{x}$	Range	n
Dominant males	2.18	1.58–3.26	4[a]	0.44	0.21–0.63	3
Subordinate males	0.10	0.01–0.18	2	0.85	0.02–1.69	2

[a] $p < 0.05$ Mann-Whitney U-test.

similar-sized ranges during autumn, although these latter findings could not be confirmed statistically.

The range size ratio males:females

Even if male ranges generally are larger than those of females, the male:female range size ratio from the different studies varies from almost 1:1 to 10:1. We believe this reflects the variation in female distribution, but then it is surprising that both the lowest and the highest ratios are found in populations where females live in groups and intermediate values are from populations with solitary females. We must therefore ask more specifically under what conditions we would expect a low, respectively a high range size ratio.

Again we start with the assumption that males strive for access to as many females as possible. We further assume that males visiting many different female groups or 'clumps' will have larger ranges relative to females, than those visiting one or just a few groups. When female groups are large and widely dispersed it may not pay for a male to include more than one such group in his range, in which case he would not need a larger home range than any of the females living in that group. This seems to be the situation in the Swiss study, where the lowest male:female range size ratio of all was found. There, no less than eight females lived on four closely situated farms, which is in effect just one clump. The dominant male visited all four farms, and therefore did not have to cover more ground than the most mobile of the females (Turner & Mertens, 1986). Thus, the first condition, many females in the 'group', was met. The second condition, of widely spaced clumps, was, however, not met, since

the next female 'clump' was just 500 metres away (Turner, personal communication). This condition may, however be less important than the first. In the Japanese study where females lived in very large groups of up to 20 adult females, the groups were also closely spaced, and still males did not have much larger ranges than the females. They usually stayed at one group. Only a few visited two (Izawa *et al.*, 1982).

The conditions favouring a high male:female range size ratio are just the opposite of those favouring a low ratio, namely small female groups that are evenly distributed and not too far apart. This was the situation in the Portsmouth dockyard, and here the highest ratio of all was found (Dards, 1978). Although a few males stayed with only one female group, most males wandered widely and incorporated many smaller groups in their ranges (Dards, 1983). In the Revinge area in Sweden female groups were also small, but here they were more widely spaced (Liberg, 1980). Breeding males incorporated on the average five female groups in their ranges, with a maximum of nine. The range size ratio here was still fairly high at about 7:1. This again indicates that female group size might be more important than distance between groups in determining how many groups a breeding male will visit.

In populations with solitary females the ratio would increase the more exclusive, and therefore dispersed, the female ranges are.

Liberg (1984) showed that variation in range size was much higher than variation in number of female cats included in those ranges for breeding males; the opposite was true for subordinate males, where range size was more constant than number of females in the ranges. It is plausible that breeding males simply visit and check as many females as they have time to, and that this figure is rather constant for all males in a given area; heterogeneity in female distribution would then cause a larger variation in the area covered while performing these visits.

Group living

Many studies report that female cats live in groups which sometimes include adult males (Table 7.5). Since felids generally are known to be extremely solitary, with the lion and possibly the cheetah, as the notable exceptions, one may ask what factors favour group living in the domestic cat. We hypothesise that it is the occurrence of a concentrated and stable food

Table 7.5. *Characteristics of cat groups in the different studies*

Study no.	Characteristics of the central area of the group	Group size (ad. fem.)	Number of groups studied	Group structure
1. Japan	Fish dumps at fisher village	15–20	2 (5)	Stable membership. Kinship unknown. Several adult males in each group
2. Rome	Daily provision in city park by cat lovers	15	1	Stable membership of females. Males occurring irregularly. Kinship unknown
3. Portsmouth	Garbage and provisioning by cat lovers	2–9	20	Female kin groups. Sometimes one adult male attached to a group
4. Oxford	Pig farm with *ad lib.* provision of pig food	Large	1	Female kin group with two kin lines. Adult males coming and going
5. Cornwall	Dairy farm with regular provision of milk	5	1	Female kin group. Adult males loosely attached
6. France	Dairy farm with regular provision of milk	2	1	Female kin group. Adult males loosely attached
7. Wisconsin	Dairy farm with regular provision of milk	6	1	Female kin group. Adult males loosely attached
10. Switzerland	Four closely located farms, fed daily	2	4	Female kin groups. Also some kinship between cats of different farms. Only one dominant male in the area
13. Illinois	Various rural households with regular feeding of cats	No data	Many	No data
14. Devon	Dairy farm, milk provided	3	1	Experimentally started group with 3 related females introduced to new farm
16. Sweden	Rural, non-farming households with regular feeding of cats	1–7	Around 20	Female kin groups. Males usually leaving groups when 1–2 years old

resource large enough to support more than one individual (but see also Kerby & Macdonald, Chapter 6). All cases of group-living cats reported include this condition. There are two categories of group-living cats: farm cats in the countryside and feral cats subsisting on food concentrations such as garbage dumps in urban areas. Group living has never been clearly documented in cat populations living on natural prey. Van Aarde (1978) claimed that at least some adult cats lived in small groups in his feral population on subantarctic Marion Island, and that one reason for this might be heat preservation when several cats curl up together to rest. But this interpretation was based on just a few sightings and further documentation is required before any firm conclusions can be drawn.

Thus, since cats living on natural prey do not form groups, we assume that behavioural advantages such as communal care and cooperative defence of kittens are not responsible for the appearance of group living in the domestic cat, as has sometimes been proposed (e.g. Macdonald & Apps, 1978; see also Chapter 8). Such behavioural patterns are secondary benefits of living in groups, once these groups have arisen as an effect of food distribution.

But are these true social groups or are they mere aggregations around food concentrations? Most data point to the former. All studies that have any relevant data at all report that female membership in the group is stable over time. In most cases it has also been documented that female membership is based on kin relationship, which is an effect of philopatry and internal recruitment of female offspring coupled with hostility towards strange females (e.g. Liberg, 1980; Turner & Mertens, 1986). There is also some evidence that individual bonds develop between different cats within groups, and persistent hostility (although usually on a low level) occurs towards others (see Chapter 6). As mentioned earlier, female group members also interact cordially when rearing offspring (Macdonald & Moehlman, 1982).

Males usually have a much looser attachment to groups. In several studies the majority of males dispersed from their natal groups after attaining sexual maturity (see e.g. Liberg, 1980; Warner, 1985; Pericard, 1986), and only a few ever reach breeder status there (Liberg, 1981). In the large groups at fish dumps in Japan no female transfer between groups was observed, but an occasional male transfer (Izawa *et al.*, 1982). Males obviously manage to enter strange groups much more easily than females. The reason for this will be discussed below.

Spatial distribution

Degree of range overlap or exclusiveness tells something about how animals in a population distribute resources among themselves. A low degree of range overlap can either be the result of mutual avoidance and an equal sharing of resources and space at low population densities, or of animals defending their ranges from which they exclude conspecifics, at least of their own sex. The latter case is called territoriality and we adhere to the more restricted definition of this, requiring active defence of the range.

There is a large asymmetry between the data needed to show range overlap and exclusive ranges. Data on two adult individuals of the same sex can be enough to show range overlap, whereas the documentation of exclusive ranges requires either a high degree of confidence that all animals within the study area are monitored, or that a number of animals with adjacent ranges are followed simultaneously. Since it is often uncertain that all individuals in an area are monitored, the latter alternative is advantageous for demonstrating the presence of exclusiveness. We consider three or four adjacent ranges showing a mean of less than 10 per cent overlap (measured on 'convex polygons') as a convincing indication of exclusive ranges.

Range overlap in females

Throughout this review we have assumed that food is the most critical resource for female cats. Group-living females utilise a food source that is predictable in time and clumped in rich, concentrated patches. Predictability is considered an important condition for defendability, whereas a clumped distribution generally is not, at least not when the clumps are very rich (Davies & Houston, 1984). The latter is true, however, only when the defender is a single individual and the clump contains more food than this individual can utilise by itself. A stable and rich clump can be defended by a group of individuals, and this is what we think the group-living female cats do. Within groups home ranges overlap extensively, especially at the primary feeding place, be it a farm, a garbage dump or the corner of a city park where 'cat lovers' regularly place food (Figure 7.2). Between groups there is little range overlap (see Table 7.3). This was very nicely illustrated by Izawa and colleagues (1982, 1984) in their work with feral cat groups subsisting on fish waste dumps. And in their small Swiss farmer village Turner & Mertens (1986) measured degree of range overlap quantitatively within and between groups and found it to be, on average, 55 and four per cent respectively.

There is no published evidence of active defence of ranges or core areas by group living females, but the complete lack of female transfer between groups (Liberg, 1980; Izawa, 1984; Natoli, 1985a), while male cats obviously move between groups, does point to some kind of repulsion of strange females. There could be many reasons why strange males are accepted in female groups, e.g. greater physical strength (although females can unite to drive away a strange male when they have small kittens [Macdonald & Moehlman, 1982; Liberg, 1983]), sexual relationships, or simply because males pose a lower competitive threat than strange females, making it less worthwhile for females to exclude them. An invading female would not only compete herself for food, den sites, etc., but might also start a new matriarchal line in the group. This would pose a much more serious threat to the future reproduction of the established females than an invading male would. The situation directly parallels pride-living lions, where strange females are kept away by the pride females, but males are not; but male lions are certainly more capable of parasitising

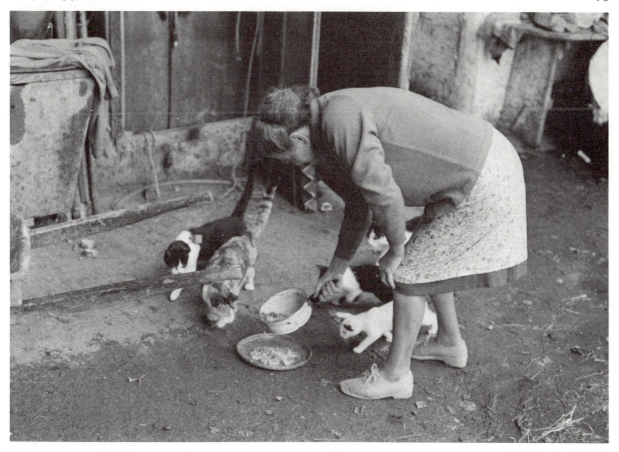

Fig. 7.2. Food resources for many cats are rich and clumped today, affecting population density and home range overlap. (Photo: D. Turner.)

the pride females than male cats are (Schaller, 1972; Bertram, 1978).

The discussion above about territoriality of course also applies to solitary-based females, which have easily defendable, predictable food patches too: their primary homes. The situation for solitary feral females which subsist on natural prey, is different. Their food is usually more dispersed and less predictable than that of house-based and other group-living cats.

Generally we expect exclusive ranges when the food resource is stable and evenly distributed, whereas variations in space and time give rise to a system of overlapping ranges (for a detailed discussion, see Waser & Wiley, 1979). Food distribution is notoriously difficult to record, and most workers do not

even mention the characteristics of the food resource; therefore the following analysis will have to be a very rough one.

Fitzgerald & Karl (1986) worked with a low density population (one cat per sq km) that subsisted on a patchily distributed food source, and they recorded large overlap between female ranges. A high density population (30 cats per sq km) was studied by Apps (1986). These cats lived partly on a rich and patchy food resource (ocean bird colonies), and the females had overlapping ranges. Thus, density *per se* does not have much influence on range overlap. Langeveld & Nievold (1985) reported exclusive female ranges in a population with a low density of about one cat per square kilometre. Since they radio-tracked three adjacent females simultaneously and were also able to record the replacement of one of these females by another, still with exclusive ranges, they seem to have good indications of exclusiveness. Unfortunately, the food distribution in their study area was not reported, but we predict an even prey distribution.

Range overlap in males

When discussing the spatial organisation of male ranges, we again have to be aware that the pattern may differ between seasons and that different categories of males may show different patterns. In our unpublished study referred to above, the dominant males showed almost complete overlap during the mating season (Figure 7.3), whereas their smaller ranges during the non-mating season were completely separated. The ranges of subordinate males were covered by those of the dominant males all year round. Once again this demonstrates that one has to know the social status of the subjects investigated, and the influence of seasonality in the area, to understand the data obtained in a study of spatial patterns.

The reasons we get these differences in male range *overlap* between seasons and social categories are the same as those discussed in the section on male range *size*. During the non-mating season food is the most important resource for both males and females, and a similar spacing pattern can be expected for both sexes. During the breeding season food is still the most important resource for females and no change in their spatial organisation is expected or found. For breeding males the most important resource is receptive females, and if that resource has different spatial and temporal characteristics than food, then a different tactic has to be used to exploit it and this will give rise to a different spatial organisation (cf. Erlinge & Sandell, 1986).

The male spacing pattern during the mating season will be determined by the tactic used by the dominant males to achieve matings. There are two alternatives for a male: to stay in a relatively small area and try to defend and monopolise a number of females during the breeding period, or to roam over a large area and compete for receptive females as they are encountered, i.e. to stay or to roam. We suspect that the former system is only possible when it is in the interest of all dominant males in the population. It is then maintained through a mutual interest in exclusivity. It is probably impossible to defend a territory against

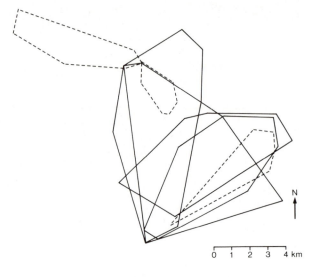

Fig. 7.3. Spatial organisation of dominant males during the mating season (solid lines, $n = 4$) and during the non-mating season (dashed lines, $n = 3$) in 1984 in the Revinge area (cf. Table 7.4).

other dominant males if they are not also interested in having exclusive areas. As soon as a roaming tactic is more rewarding for *some* dominant males, the whole system of exclusivity might break down.

If females are clumped, it may pay for a male to stay with one female group if it is very large; but then it will probably be impossible for him to monopolise the whole group, since the females are not always close together. If groups are smaller, it would probably be more rewarding for a dominant male to check several groups (thereby increasing the potential number of matings) than to defend one group, again resulting in a roaming tactic.

The only case where we expect exclusive areas in males is when females are dense and evenly distributed.

Given these predictions, there are very few populations of domestic cats where we would expect exclusive ranges in dominant males. Female domestic cats are seldom evenly distributed (see above), and if they are the population densities are low. As shown in Table 7.3 all studies with data on male spatial organisation have reported overlapping male ranges. Dards (1983) reported one case where a dominant male

Table 7.6. *Differences in dispersal between house-based males that are protected from harassment by conspecifics and non-protected males in the Revinge area (Liberg, 1981 and in preparation)*

	Protected	Non-protected
Dispersed 2nd or 3rd year	7	16
Dispersed later or stayed	12	3
	$\chi^2 = 7.05$	$p < 0.01$

stayed and monopolised one group, but other dominant males visited several groups. In a situation with evenly distributed females (but low density) in Australia, the ranges of two adjacent males did not overlap (Jones & Coman, 1982). These two were the only males tracked, however, and other adult cats were seen within the ranges of the instrumented cats, so the situation is not clear. Thus, overlapping ranges is the general pattern found among male domestic cats. This pattern is not one of mutual tolerance, but one of continuous strife. All males try to keep other males away, but since roaming is the best tactic for dominant males, it is impossible to accomplish this.

Liberg (1981) studied these relations in detail. In his area females occurred alone or in small groups at well spaced households. Dominant male ranges overlapped completely, but relative dominance varied between different places, so that at each farm there was only one male holding the 'breeder status'. Other males also visited the farms regularly, presumably in search of unattended females, and occasionally also to test the 'breeder'. The system was very dynamic with frequent changes in the dominance order.

For subadults it is a situation of continuous harassment, and many are forced out of their natal homes by aggression from older males. That inter-male aggression is the factor causing dispersal is shown by the significantly lower dispersal rate of young house cats that could find protection indoors (Table 7.6).

In a population of dominant roamers a subdominant has poor prospects. Roaming would be useless, as he would not be able to take over any of the receptive females he encounters, and during his movements he would be more susceptible to harassment from dominants. Therefore the best tactic for a subordinate

male is to stay at home, where he might be able to mate with receptive females in his group when no dominant males are present. Thus, if roaming is the tactic employed by the dominant males, staying will be the best tactic for subordinate males. Liberg (1981) showed that in this case, subordinate males do indeed employ a staying tactic until they are old and strong enough to establish themselves as dominants. When staying is the dominant male tactic, roaming will be the best alternative for subordinates. Their only chance to achieve matings in this situation is to encounter females with no dominant male present.

Mating tactics

Individual variation in mating behaviour has hardly been studied at all in the domestic cat, although this species provides an excellent opportunity to do so. In this section we will demonstrate some possible approaches to this topic together with some scattered observations that are available.

Do females choose their mates? The available data indicate that there is no active mate choice in female cats; females are mated with the most dominant male present (Liberg, 1981, 1983; Liberg & Sandell, personal observations). There are, however, other more subtle ways in which the female may influence the paternity of her offspring. Some behavioural patterns of female oestrus can be interpreted as ways of inducing competition between the courting males. The receptive female sometimes makes quick rushes, which may force the most dominant male to re-establish his position close to her (Liberg, 1983). Other patterns that attract more males to the receptive female, e.g. increased scent-marking activity, will increase male competition, and thereby decrease the probability that she mates with an inferior male (cf. Janetos, 1980; see also Chapter 8).

Another aspect of mate choice concerns avoidance of inbreeding. The detrimental effects of inbreeding in domestic cats are not known, but close kin matings are not uncommon; six out of 17 matings in our study area were with related females from the males' natal group (personal observations). There was, however, a tendency for females with males in their groups to leave home more often during oestrus than females without males in their groups (Liberg, 1983). This is possibly a behaviour selected to avoid inbreeding. Unfortunately, these as well as most other aspects of female reproductive tactics remain unexplored.

Besides the different movement patterns shown by males, other behaviour also indicates that males have many 'decisions' to make when trying to maximise their mating success. A dominant male can take over almost all receptive females he encounters. During the peak mating season several females will be in heat at the same time, and he will find himself in a conflict situation: to stay with one and be sure of paternity, or to mate with many but reduce his probability of paternity in each litter (see Chapter 8).

During the mating season 1984, the dominant male in our study area (male A) showed varying behaviour towards receptive females as the breeding season progressed. Early on he guarded one female during two days, and none of the other males in the area showed any interest in her before or after that. During the peak of the mating season, the top male stayed less than one day with a receptive female, and that same female was courted by male C (third in the hierarchy) before, and male B (second in the hierarchy) after male A took her over. Thus, the dominant male showed dynamic behaviour as the mating season progressed. The other categories of males also showed changes in behaviour: when male A guarded during the whole oestrus, the other males didn't bother to stay around; but when he just took over the female for a while, they stayed close. Therefore, the alternatives open to subordinate males would also be interesting to analyse. These variations in behaviour between individuals, and in the same individual over time, can be relatively easily studied in the domestic cat, and detailed predictions can also be made.

Spatial organisation in other felids

All of the above-mentioned difficulties in studying free-roaming domestic cats apply to an even greater extent for studies of wild felids, and in many cases it is just as difficult to interpret the data on their spatial organisation. Most wild felids live in rough terrain and are very hard to spot, so radio-telemetry is the only reliable method of securing data on spatial patterns. Again, data on at least two adult individuals of the same sex is the absolute minimum for studying spacing patterns, which means we have a rather small number of studies on only a handful of the 37 wild species (Table 7.7).

The negative correlation between density and home range size found in the domestic cat is also present in wild felids, both for all species combined ($r = -0.942$, $n = 12$, $t = 8.88$, $p < 001$) and separately for the mountain lion ($r = -0.961$, $n = 5$, $t = 6.02$, $p < 0.01$, data from Hemker, Lindzey & Ackerman, 1984) and bobcat ($r = -0.98$, $n = 5$, $t = 7.60$, $p < 0.005$, data from McCord & Cardoza, 1982). As discussed above we think both of these variables are influenced by prey biomass (the total weight of prey in the area). For lions a correlation was indeed found between range size and lean-season prey biomass, and between the latter and measures of density (Van Orsdol, Hanby & Bygott, 1985). A negative correlation between home range size and prey density has been reported for the bobcat (Litvaitis, Sherburne & Bissonette, 1986). A change in range size with changes in prey density was recorded for lynx in Yukon, where ranges increased with decreasing density of snowshoe hares (Ward & Krebs, 1985). Density of lynx was also influenced by changes in hare density (Brand, Keith & Fischer, 1976; Ward & Krebs, 1985). Thus, both density and home range size in wild felids are strongly influenced by prey biomass, and this explains the correlation between the two variables.

For the same reasons as discussed above for domestic cats, female spacing patterns should be determined by the characteristics of the food resource. Exclusive ranges are expected when food is evenly distributed and stable, while in all other situations, we expect overlap. Reliable data from wild felids are so scarce that these predictions cannot be properly tested. Female tigers in Royal Chitawan National Park, Nepal had a stable and evenly distributed food source, and they had exclusive ranges (Sunquist, 1981). In the Idaho wilderness ungulates show seasonal migrations between high and low elevations. Female mountain lions there had almost totally overlapping ranges in winter when the ungulates were concentrated at lower elevations (Seidensticker *et al.*, 1973). During summer, when prey were more evenly spread out, the ranges were larger, but overlap was greatly reduced. In a habitat with patches of variable prey density, female lynx had overlapping ranges and several animals utilised the same high density patch (Ward & Krebs, 1985). With evenly distributed prey female bobcats also had exclusive ranges (Bailey, 1974).

Whereas female spacing patterns are determined by a single resource, food, males have two decisive resources: food and receptive females. Outside the mating season, there should not be any notable dif-

Table 7.7. *Range characteristics of wild solitary felids*

Species	Place of study	Density (*n*/100 sq km)	Female ranges $\bar{x}$ (sq km)	Female ranges Range	*n*	Overlap/ Exclusive	Male ranges $\bar{x}$ (sq km)	Male ranges Range	*n*	O/E	Reference
Lynx	Minnesota	—		51–122	?	O		145–243	?	E?	Mech, 1980
	Alaska	0.9	70	51–89	2	—	783		1	—	Bailey *et al.*, 1986
Bobcat	Idaho	5	19.3	9.1–45.3	8	E	42.1	6.5–107.9	4	E	Bailey, 1974
	Minnesota	4–5	38	15–92	6	E	62	13–201	16	O	Berg, 1979
	California	5	43	26–59	4	O	73	39–95	3	O	Zezulak & Schwab, 1979
	Tennessee	—	25.9		3	O	76.8		?	O	Kitchings & Story, 1984
	Alabama	77–116	1.1		6	E	2.6		6	E	Miller & Speake, 1979
Mountain lion	Idaho	1.4	268	173–373	4	O	453		1	—	Seidensticker *et al.*, 1973
	Utah	0.3–0.5	685	396–1454	4	O	826		1	—	Hemker *et al.*, 1984
	California	3.5–4.4	94	54–119	3	O	178	78–277	5	O	Sitton *et al.*, 1976
	California	1.5–3.3	66	57–74	2	—	152	109–238	4	O	Kutilek *et al.*, 1980, cited in Hemker *et al.*, 1984
Jaguar	Brazil	4–8	29.5	25–34	2	(O)					Schaller & Crawshaw, 1980
Tiger	Nepal	2.8	16.9	16.4–17.7	3	E	66	60–72	2	(E)	Sunquist, 1981

ferences in male and female spatial organisation. Some supporting evidence was found during a snowshoe hare decline in Yukon, where both male and female lynxes showed the same response to the declining food resource (Ward & Krebs, 1985). In the European wild cat males and females had about the same monthly range sizes during winter, but when the mating season started, the males moved away (Corbett, 1979).

In situations where males have exclusive breeding areas they might have to maintain them throughout the year. Unfortunately there are no data to test this; data on range sizes analysed separately for breeding and non-breeding seasons are badly needed. In species where breeding occurs at any time of the year the males will of course employ their breeding tactic throughout the year.

In wild felids there might also be different categories of males, including roamers. Even if the authors in many studies mention non-resident males (e.g Seidensticker *et al.*, 1973; Bailey, 1974), they usually discard them as 'transients', assuming that only the resident males take active part in breeding. From studies of other carnivores, there are indications that wide-ranging, 'transient' males perform most of the matings (e.g. Mills, 1982; Sandell, 1986). Thus, there is reason to believe that 'transient' males also in many felid species may play an important role in the breeding of the population.

As predicted for domestic cats, wild males should also have exclusive ranges when females are dense and evenly distributed; a patchy distribution and low female densities would favour a roaming male tactic.

Indeed we find exclusive ranges in males when females are evenly spaced and have ranges of less than about 20 square kilometres, i.e. when density is rather high (see Table 7.7, Bailey, 1974; Miller & Speake, 1979; Sunquist, 1981); but larger female ranges seem to cause overlap among the males, even if the females are evenly spaced (see Table 7.7; Berg, 1979). When female ranges overlap, we need to know whether there are patches of high female density with low density areas in between, or if there is an even distribution. The former situation would resemble the female group pattern in domestic cats (see above), resulting in overlapping male ranges, independent of density. An even distribution of overlapping female ranges would be equivalent to the situation with exclusive female ranges, and should give rise to exclusive male ranges at high densities and overlapping male ranges at low densities. In this case we would expect to find a threshold density at which the system changes from exclusive to overlapping male ranges. This value will of course differ between species, but we think the change would take place in a rather narrow density interval. The data in wild felids needed to test these predictions are unfortunately lacking.

We conclude that there are no great discrepancies between domestic cats and wild felids regarding the principles of their spatial systems and the factors influencing these. We therefore believe that future studies on domestic cats have great potential, not only for increasing our understanding of that species in itself, but also to gain further insight into felid behavioural ecology generally.

Concluding remarks

We have seen that domestic cat population density varies by three orders of magnitude, from less than one cat, to more than 2000 cats per square kilometre. Density level is determined by food abundance. Home range size also varies by three orders of magnitude; in females from 0.1 to almost 200 hectares, in males up to almost 1000 hectares. Female range size is determined by food abundance and distribution. Males have ranges that are on average three times larger than those of the females. Male ranges are larger during the mating season, and dominant males have larger ranges than subordinates. The size of dominant male ranges is determined by female density, and even more so, by female distribution.

Group living in cats depends on human subsidies, and is an effect of rich food concentrations. The groups are stable and consist of female kin, with males usually being loosely attached. Most young males disperse from their natal groups, while young females are philopatric. The home ranges of group-living females overlap very little with those of females from other groups. Solitary females show range overlap when living on patchily distributed prey. Male home ranges overlap extensively, especially during the mating season. This pattern of spatial organisation in the domestic cat is also found in various wild felids, making the former a handy 'model' species for studies of general patterns in felid behavioural ecology.

Acknowledgements

We want to thank Ulrika Göransson and Isabella Levay for help with radio-tracking, J.-Å. Nilsson and H. Smith for comments on the manuscript, and Dennis Turner for all the work he has put into this manuscript. Our field study was supported by a grant from Løvens Chemical Industries, Copenhagen.

8

The mating system of feral cats living in a group

Eugenia Natoli and Emanuele De Vito

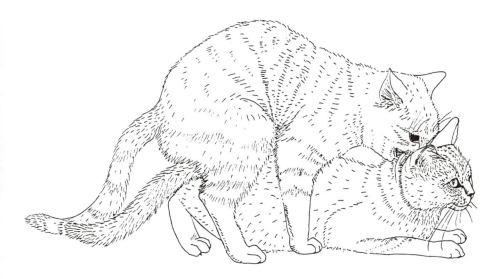

Introduction

Mating behaviour of the domestic cat has attracted the attention of scientists for a long time and several laboratory studies have focused on sexual behaviour of both males and females (Michael, 1958, 1961; Rosenblatt & Aronson, 1958; Whalen, 1963; Prescott, 1973; Leyhausen, 1979). However, few observations have been carried out on cat mating behaviour in a natural setting. Probably this imbalance between laboratory and field studies was due to the fact that the domestic cat was traditionally an animal chosen for physiological studies (see e.g. Liche, 1939; Maes, 1939; Wildt, Guthrie & Seager, 1978) and consequently, readily available for studying behaviour in captivity. Interest in cats' lives outside the laboratory developed later on.

Even though during the last ten years the interest in free-ranging cat behaviour has increased sharply and cats have been examined in many different environments, surprisingly few scientists have focused their attention on cat mating behaviour and on their mating

system in natural situations. The few studies on this topic (Liberg, 1981, 1983; Dards, 1983) have provided a basis for further analysis of the problem, rather than clearing it. This is even more surprising given the interest in sociobiological problems in recent years and the fact that many of those studies have concentrated on less available species of felines (e.g. Bygott, Bertram & Handy, 1979; Packer & Pusey, 1983).

Liberg & Sandell (Chapter 7) have discussed the scant information available on cat reproductive tactics within the context of spatial organisation. Mostly they consider mating tactics within populations of fairly well dispersed animals or small groups of animals. But some cats live in large groups at high densities and a study of their mating system might provide an interesting comparison. We have conducted one such study and report our results here; but we caution the reader against generalising our findings until more studies on cat mating systems at different densities have been conducted. We include a fairly detailed description of our methods, which is not only required to enable

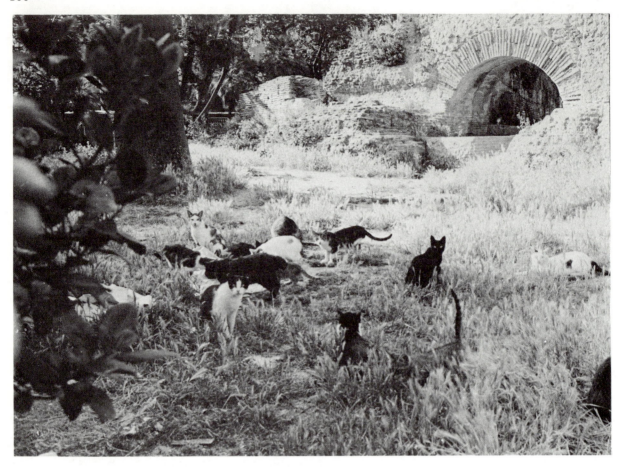

Fig. 8.1. A group of feral cats in front of the historical ruins
in Rome. (Photo: courtesy of E. Natoli.)

future comparisons, but also illustrates to the non-scientist how such a study is conducted.

The study area

We conducted our study in a market square (Piazza Vittorio Emanuele) in Rome, located in the centre of the city near the main train station. This square is the largest in Rome (6.54 ha) and it has several concentric rings, each ring with a different function. The outer and largest ring is occupied by shops, all under arcades that surround the square; the second is represented by a street with heavy traffic; the third, by the market-stalls with diverse consumer goods (food, animals, clothes, flowers, etc.); and the last area is a public garden in the centre with green areas, some offices, a car park, a merry-go-round, and historical ruins (Trofei di Mario). The latter are surrounded by a high wire fence prohibiting admittance to the public.

But the fenced area around the ruins (measuring 2570 sq m) is available to a cat group, which has colonised the ruins and established its 'core area' within the enclosure (Figure 8.1). There were also other smaller, but discrete groups of cats in the square, whose members sometimes had contact with the cats belonging to the group under study.

The cat population

The cat group living in the study area was similar to that described in a previous study of a cat colony living in another part of Rome (Natoli, 1985a). It had no constraints placed on breeding or movements (by human owners) and very few individuals were tame enough to be handled. Still, they were completely dependent on food provided by people (either from direct feeding or from refuse found around the market-stalls). The cats were fed by people at least two to three times a day (we counted up to seven visits by cat lovers bringing food for cats during seven hours of observation); thus, they were so well fed that a lot of food was wasted. Death of adult and young cats was never due to starvation but to other causes such as respiratory diseases, or violent acts by humans.

During our study the group consisted of 81 'residential' cats and a number of 'transients'. To determine which cats regularly frequented the study area, we calculated a 'presence percentage' by dividing the number of days each cat was observed in the area by the total number of observation days. The 81 cats showing a regular presence of more than 10 per cent were defined as 'residential': 37 adult females, 4 sub-adult females, 32 adult males and 8 sub-adult males. Of the adults, 33 females and 29 males showed clear signs of sexual maturity; the rest were too ill or old for such activities and some died during the study.

Eight adult male, and five adult female 'transients' (< 10% presence) belonging to other groups living in the square were occasionally spotted near the ruins; and during our four-month study over 40 cats were abandoned at the site by humans. Most of these were found dead shortly thereafter, or disappeared. When the study began there were no kittens in the group.

Observational methods

We observed the cat group during 315 hours on 112 days, between 8 January and 30 April 1986. Out of 315 hours, 172 were devoted to data collection on mating behaviour; during the remaining time general observations were made.

Data on occurrence and length of oestrus (heat) of females belonging to the group were collected. When a female came into oestrus, she advertised it with all features typical of the oestrus state described e.g. by Beaver (1977) and Michael (1961). Vocalisations, rubbing of the head, chin and neck on vertical objects, rolling on the floor and crouching were frequent, but the real onset of oestrus was characterised by the complete acceptance of the males' efforts to copulate. During the oestrus period an observer followed the female for four hours a day, for a total of four days (or

for the duration of oestrus when it lasted less than four days), in order to collect data on copulatory behaviour and on male spatial distribution while courting the female and within five metres of her. The frequency and duration of two kinds of mount were scored: those with pelvic thrusting and intromission, and those with pelvic thrusting, but no intromission. These are termed mounts with intromission (M) (true or successful mounts), and mounts without intromission (MW) (false mounts) respectively. Mounts without intromission could be easily distinguished from those with intromission because of the strong reaction of the female to the latter. When intromission occurred, the female emitted a sharp cry, showed an aggressive reaction by turning toward the male and threatening him, and usually rolled on the ground vigorously afterwards.

The number of males that courted and copulated with the same female during a single oestrus period was recorded. Since males courting a female arrived and left the courtship area irregularly throughout the oestrus, observation time on females was divided up into 81 'sessions' of observation. Each 'session' represented a time period during which the female was continuously observed and the number of males that courted and copulated with her during that session was also recorded.

We were particularly interested in analysing the spacing pattern of males around the female courted. To this aim, we imagined a circle of five metres radius around the female and divided it into three concentric rings: the first was from 0 to 1 metre around her; the second from 1 to 3 metres; and the third from 3 to 5 metres from her. The position of each male in the three rings was recorded every 60 seconds (Instantaneous Sampling Method, Lehner, 1979). From these data, we wanted to assess whether there was any kind of spatial-position dominance that might be correlated with a higher number of mounts, as suggested by Liberg (1983).

The main results
Synchrony of oestrus period

The literature on social felids suggests that in colonies females tend to synchronise their oestrus (Bertram, 1975; Liberg, 1983); in this study, considering the great number of sexually mature female cats belonging to the group, oestrus periods were less aggregated than one might have expected (Table 8.1). The

Table 8.1. *Test of breeding synchrony. From 12 January to 21 March = 69 days; mean oestrus length = 4.39 days. The probability of a female being in oestrus on a given day is therefore 0.06 with 18 females present during the period (oestruses of unknown length were excluded)*

	Number of females in oestrus per day				
	0	1	2	3	4
Observed numbers	19	28	16	5	1
Observed frequency	0.28	0.41	0.23	0.07	0.01
Predicted frequency (Poisson)	0.34	0.37	0.20	0.07	0.02

$\chi^2 = 0.025$ $df = 4$ NS
Tendency for *asynchrony*

maximum number of females in oestrus on the same day was 5 as deduced from Figure 8.2.

On the average, the first oestrus of the year occurred in mid-January and lasted 4.39 days (SD = 1.46); this figure is based on 18 females observed from the beginning to the end of heat.

In April 7 females came into their second heat of the year. They either had aborted or lost their kittens during the previous months. The mean duration of this second oestrus was less than half of the first ($\bar{x} = 2.17$ days, SD = 1.34).

Number of courting males

During a single oestrus period the number of adult males courting a particular female ranged from eight to 20 ($\bar{x} = 13.80$, SD = 3.72), whereas during a single session (mean duration of a session = 2 h) it ranged from 1 to 16 ($\bar{x} = 6.07$, SD = 3.20) (Figure 8.3).

Spacing pattern of courting males

Nineteen adult males out of 29 that showed clear signs of sexual maturity (courtship activity and marking behaviour) were seen mounting a female of the group. The analysis of spatial distribution of males around females in heat was therefore restricted to these. Recall that we wanted to find out if certain males more consistently occupied a central position than others and whether this position represented an advantage in terms of mounts performed.

The highest frequency for male presence was scored for the ring nearest the female (analysis of variance: $F_{2,36} = 21.42$, $p < 0.01$) (Figure 8.4). Generally males tried to remain as close as possible to the female courted. But there were hardly any individual differences in their presence within the rings around the female: scores for the time spent within one metre of the female did not differ significantly between males ($\chi^2 = 19.16$, $df = 18$); nor did they differ for the second ring ($\chi^2 = 17.78$, $df = 18$). However, there were significant individual differences between males on their presence in the outer ring ($\chi^2 = 51.59$, $df = 18$, $p < 0.01$) (see Figure 8.5). Percentage of time spent in the first ring by an individual was not correlated with percentage of successful mounts ($r_s = -0.112$, NS).

Copulatory behaviour

The general sequence of copulation-related behaviour closely resembled that described elsewhere (Michael, 1961; Whalen, 1963). All males displayed 'pattern number 11' in Dewsbury's (1972) classification system: no copulatory lock, extra-vaginal thrusting, ejaculation on single insertion, and multiple ejaculations.

Fewer mounts with, than without intromission were observed (68 *vs* 187). Mean duration was 2.08 minutes (SD = 1.54) and 1.40 minutes (SD = 1.72) respectively. On the average, we observed one copulation without intromission per 51 minutes, or 29 per 24 hours, and one copulation with intromission per 140 minutes, or 11 per 24 hours. Considering both types of mount, this yields one copulation per 38 minutes, or 39 per 24 hours.

Copulations were performed by all males courting females under direct observation. Two out of 19 males performed only mounts with intromission, and another two males performed only mounts without intromission (see Figure 8.5). There were significant differences between the individuals' scores for mounts without intromission ($\chi^2 = 165.57$, $df = 18$, $p < 0.01$), mounts with intromission ($\chi^2 = 77.23$, $df = 18$, $p < 0.01$) and all mounts taken together ($\chi^2 = 85.17$, $df = 18$, $p < 0.01$). Each male differed in individual number of females mounted, and the difference, expressed as percentage of females mounted out of the total number of females under direct observation, was statistically significant ($\chi^2 = 46.48$, $df = 18$, $p < 0.01$) (see Figure 8.5).

Two main strategies could be recognised: some

Days of the month:

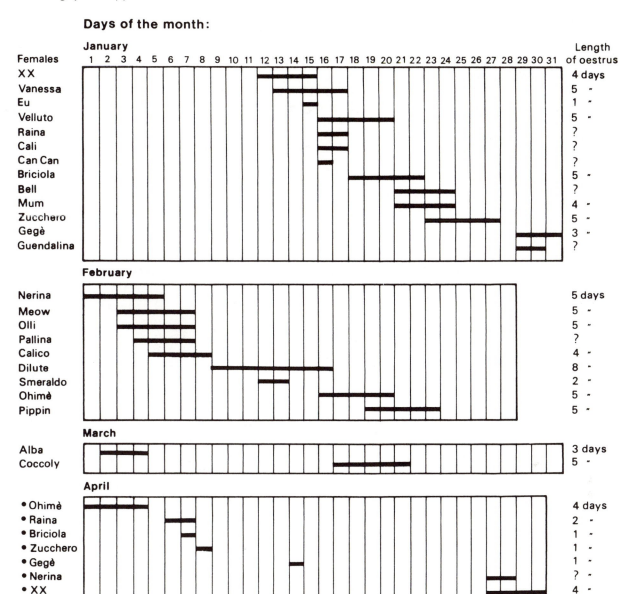

Fig. 8.2. Monthly distribution of oestrus periods in the cat population studied, from January to April 1986.

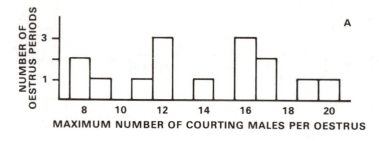

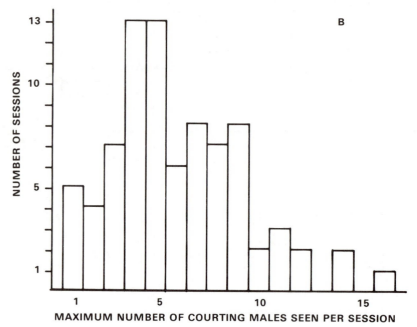

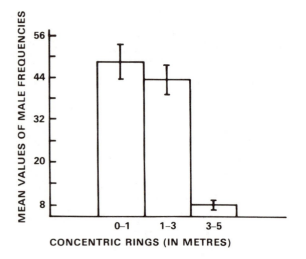

Fig. 8.3. Frequency distribution of the maximum number of male cats observed courting a particular female during an oestrus period (A), and at the same time (± 2 h) during a session (B).

Fig. 8.4. Mean values over all males of male frequency in three concentric rings (from 0 to 1 metre, from 1 to 3 metres, from 3 to 5 metres) around the female courted.

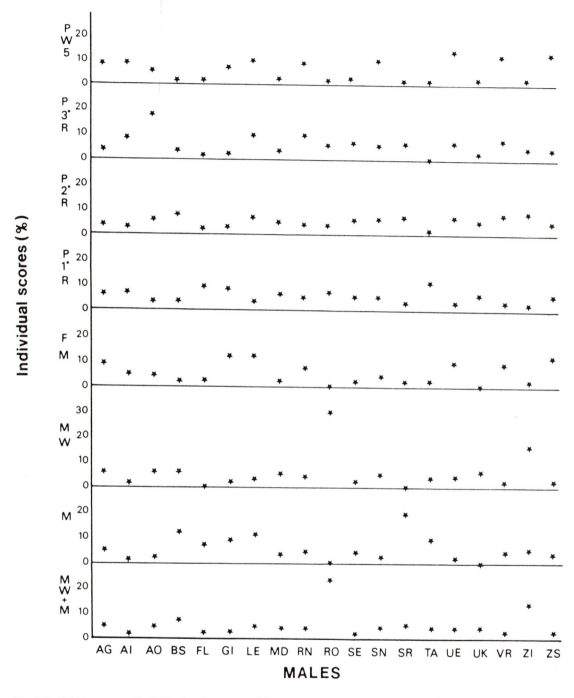

Fig. 8.5. Relative scores of individual males corrected for differences in observation time and presented here as percentages. From *top* to *bottom*: Presence within 5 metres (PW5); presence in the third, second, and first ring around a female (P3°R, P2°R, P1°R respectively); proportion of females mounted (FM); mounts without intromission (MW); true mounts (M, with intromission); total mounts (MW + M).

Table 8.2. *Number of oestrus periods and sessions during which females mated with none, one, or more than one male. Symbols: MW = Mount without intromission; M = Mount with intromission*

Oestrus periods

Number of males	Number of oestrus MW + M	Mean number of males present	Number of oestrus MW	Mean number of males present	Number of oestrus M	Mean number of males present
0 males mating	0		1	16	2	9.5
1 male mating	2	12	2	8	2	14
2 males mating	2	10	4	14.25	4	13
3 males mating	1	11	2	11.5		
4 males mating	3	12.67	2	15	4	14.5
5 males mating	3	17	1	16	1	19
6 males mating	1	14	2	14.5	1	14
7 males mating					1	17
8 males mating	2	16	1	20		
10 males mating	1	17				

Single sessions

Number of males	Number of sessions MW + M	Mean number of males present	Number of sessions MW	Mean number of males present	Number of sessions M	Mean number of males present
0 males mating	32	5.93	42	6.11	45	5.88
1 male mating	22	5.72	22	5.27	26	6.11
2 males mating	18	5.72	11	5.36	9	6.00
3 males mating	6	6.33	3	8.33	1	14
4 males mating	2	10.5	2	10.5	0	0
6 males mating	1	14	1	14	0	0

males were seen courting a female for only a short time, whereas other males spent a considerable amount of time following a single female (see 'presence within 5 metres' in Figure 8.5). Males who followed the first strategy might have been more successful: although not statistically significant, the correlation between presence and proportion of true mounts was negative ($r_s = -0.332$, NS; $p < 0.05 = 0.399$).

Female behaviour

Most of the females copulated with more than one male during a single oestrus and usually even during a single observation session. In 27 out of 81 sessions females mated with more than one male, in 22, with one male, and in 32 with none. In order to assess whether the number of males courting a female influenced the number of males that succeeded in copulating with the female, an analysis of variance compared the mean number of males courting during sessions in which females mated with one male, with more than one male, or with none. (Sessions with four and six males copulating were too rare to be included in the analysis.) The differences were not significant, either when mounts without and with intromission were considered separately (MW: $F_{3,74} = 1.77$; M: $F_{2,77} = 0.22$), or when considered together (MW + M: $F_{3,74} = 0.11$). Thus the number of males courting a female did not influence the outcome of copulations (Table 8.2).

Discussion

There appears to be no information in the literature about groups of cats as large as the one observed in this study. The existence of such a situation was probably made possible by the great amount of clumped resources available in that environment (see Chapters 6 and 7). The context was even more interesting since male and female cats regularly visited the study area and formed a stable group, at least in terms of daily spatial interactions. Such a situation provided a unique opportunity to study the mating system of cats under extreme density.

Timing of oestrus

One important factor shaping an animal mating system is the timing of the females' oestrus. Synchrony of oestrus in female cats might act to lower competition among males, while the spacing out of oestrus probably would increase it. Females might have benefits from asynchronous oestrus if their multiple matings with different males and the high copulation frequency found in this study (11 per day) and others (10–20 per day, Eaton, 1978; 15 per day, Liberg, 1983) serve to assess the males' vigour, as Eaton has hypothesised. On the other hand, females might benefit from synchronising their oestrus, and consequently time of deliveries, since this would facilitate communal care and communal defence of small kittens (Liberg, 1983).

Felids living in a group are said to be able to time their oestrus in response to social factors, although the exact physiological basis for this is unknown (Bertram, 1975). Bertram showed that in pride-living lions there was an oestrus synchrony within prides but not between them. The same has been shown for other domestic cats (Liberg, 1983). Timing of oestrus found in this study suggests that synchrony of oestrus in domestic cats may be due to other environmental factors than simply a large number of sexually active females in the group.

Given the general difference in duration of the first and the second oestrus of the year, it would have been interesting to note whether the second oestrus resulted in fewer kittens (fewer successfully induced ovulations). Unfortunately, we were unable to collect the appropriate data to answer this question.

Male behaviour

Several males courted the same female during a single oestrus period and simultaneously. Courting males drew close to the female, and their interest seemed focused more on her than on the other males. No one male was always clearly closer to the female and we therefore could not identify a 'Central Male' and other 'Peripheral Males', as suggested by Liberg (1983). Nor does the difference we found for presence in the third ring support the idea of 'Peripheral Males'. The statistical difference was due to just one male who spent more time between 3 and 5 metres of the female

relative to other males (see Figure 8.5), but whose highest presence was actually shown in the second ring. Furthermore, since no correlation was found between time spent close to the female and percentage of successful mounts, it can be concluded that holding a central position does not necessarily lead to a higher number of copulations. Besides, all 19 males were seen copulating (with or without intromission) with a female of the group and there was no dominance hierarchy among them with respect to their spatial distribution around females. We cannot conclusively say why our population behaved differently from Liberg's Swedish one, but both density and group structure differed between the areas.

Concerning the difference between true mounts and mounts without intromission, it is possible that the latter might be related to either preparing the female for the true mount (induced ovulation) or a demonstration of rank. These hypotheses need further testing.

Whatever the meaning of mounts without intromission is, it is important to distinguish them from true mounts when evaluating dominance hierarchy among male cats based on copulatory behaviour. Male RO in our study (see Figure 8.5) shows how important this can be: he scored the highest percentage of mounts when both false and true mounts are considered together. But if considered separately, it is clear that he performed the highest percentage of mounts without intromission and not one mount with intromission. In other words he completely failed in terms of reproductive success, at least concerning the females we observed. The same was true for male UK, whereas the opposite held for males FL and SR. Thus, the statistically significant differences found between individuals on mounts with and without intromission, considered separately as well as combined, cannot be used to determine dominance relationships among males of the group.

On the other hand, it was quite clear that males followed two different courting strategies, some of them remaining longer near the same female, others not. Since a greater amount of time spent courting a single female did not correspond to a greater number of mounts with that female, this strategy might be less than optimal. But why, then, didn't all males follow the 'short time' strategy? Perhaps this strategy has its disadvantages too. The fact that some males were able to copulate after being present only a short time may indicate that they utilised their time very well; but it does not necessarily mean that they fertilised a larger number of females. In any event the fact that the 'mobile' males in some way managed to bypass the queue did not seem to be dependent on open conflict or aggressive behaviour among courting males (Natoli, unpublished).

Female behaviour

In this study females mated with up to seven males (considering only mounts *with* intromission) during a single oestrus period. Also during a single session, females mated with more than one male, but the number of courting males did not seem to influence the number of males they mated with.

We suggest four reasons why a female should copulate with more than one male: firstly, if multiple matings with different males can produce a single litter sired by several males, the resulting increased genetic diversity of the offspring might be advantageous (Williams, 1975). Secondly, the quality of the paternal genetic contribution might be improved by means of sperm competition (Parker, 1970). Thirdly, by increasing paternal uncertainty, the females might succeed in reducing male aggressiveness toward their offspring (Hrdy, 1977). And finally, females might have been selected to increase the *average* degree of relatedness of their offspring (Davies & Boersma, 1984) through multiple paternity.

Any one or a combination of these hypotheses might explain the female cat behaviour observed in our study. Especially the last two deserve more consideration: even though infanticide in domestic feral cats has not been reported to occur frequently, it nevertheless occurs (Macdonald *et al.*, 1987). At the high density found in this study, the probability that a tomcat will meet up with very small kittens is particularly high. It would be extremely adaptive for a female living in such an environment to increase paternal uncertainty. And lastly, *if* it is true that the domestic cat living in rural and urban environments is evolving toward a higher form of sociality, as has been implied by several authors (Fagen, 1978; Corbett, 1979; Liberg, 1981; Panaman, 1981; Dards, 1983; Natoli, 1985a, b; Macdonald *et al.*, 1987), then increasing relatedness of offspring would facilitate kin selection, an important precursor for the evolution of many cooperative social systems (Hamilton, 1964; Holmes & Sherman, 1983).

Concluding remarks

We have presented data on matings within a large group of cats at an extremely high density. Some of our findings will probably hold true for cats under other conditions; others may not. But one aspect, that of multiple matings by several males with the same female, certainly deserves more attention than in the past, since it has often been noted at various densities and has important consequences for the biological 'fitness' (genetic contribution to the next generation) of each male involved.

Acknowledgements

Financial support for this research was provided by the Association for the Study of Animal Behaviour. We thank Prof. Giovanni Costa, Drs Francesca D'Amato and Alfonso Troisi for support and valuable discussions through all stages of this research. We also would like to thank the Archaeologic Superintendence of Rome for allowing us to carry out the study on the cat population that colonised the historical ruins.

IV

Predatory behaviour

9

Hunting behaviour of the domestic cat

Dennis C. Turner and Othmar Meister

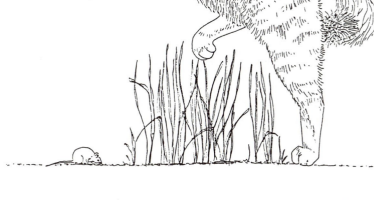

Introduction

Domesitic cats fulfil two very different roles in today's civilisation: they are kept as pets and/or for their propensity to hunt and kill agricultural pest species. This review concerns the latter aspect of their behaviour and we will describe the 'how, when and where' of hunting by cats on the following pages. Since many pet cats with outdoor access hunt, we hope to summarise available information of interest to the cat owner. But we are also interested in comparing the relative success of different hunting strategies and their application e.g. by male and female cats, for different prey types and in different habitats. Such questions are asked by the behavioural ecologist, and their answers also have practical consequences for those who keep cats for their pest-killing abilities, i.e. many farmers.

Two very important aspects of the cat's predatory behaviour are covered in other chapters of this volume: as part of their general treatment of behavioural development in cats, Martin & Bateson (Chapter 2) include the development of predatory

skills in kittens, the role that mother cats and siblings play in that, and the role mothers play in the development of prey preferences of their offspring. And Fitzgerald (Chapter 10) discusses prey selection from an ecological viewpoint, including the impact domestic cats have on their prey populations.

Given the domestic cat's notoriety as an excellent hunter, it is surprising that very few studies have concentrated on its actual *hunting* behaviour. Most investigations on prey-related behaviour have dealt with the cat's activities after a prey item has been detected (or presented in an experimental situation), and many have concentrated on the acts of grasping, killing, handling and/or consuming the prey (see e.g. Caro, 1980a, b; Leyhausen, 1956c, 1965a, 1979). Although these are certainly important aspects of predation by cats, 'hunting' begins with the search for potential prey, and includes all behaviour leading to the successful capture of that prey and/or a renewed search for other prey items. Essentially, we agree with and will use Panaman's (1981) definition of hunting as (a) making a roving search of the environment, i.e.

111

travelling alertly, stopping every few metres and appearing to look and listen intently; or (b) being stationary, attentive and oriented towards a locus, often between bouts of roving searches; and (c) including pouncing (onto the prey) during (a) or (b).

We begin our review with a general composite description of the hunting methods cats use, which leads to a discussion of potential hunting strategies applied by the individuals in a population. General hunting success and factors affecting that are discussed in the next section. Activity patterns and budgets (particularly for hunting) are then covered, followed by a section on 'where' the cats hunt. We conclude with a short summary of what is known on prey-handling once prey has been caught (see references above).

Hunting methods or 'how' cats hunt

Cats have evolved specialised hunting techniques which require crypticity for success (Kleimann & Eisenberg, 1973). According to Leyhausen (1956c), all cats show both the sit-and-wait hunt as well as the stalking hunt, exploiting local cover during the latter.

We have often observed and can describe the typical hunting excursion over pastures and fields (and thereby, tailored to hunting burrowing rodents) as follows:

When the cat departs for a hunt, it often appears to head for a particular area that is somehow different from the surrounding land, e.g. a freshly mown pasture, and it utilises streets, roads and paths that more or less directly lead to that area. When it has arrived there, it begins its search by moving more slowly and looking towards the ground nearby. Occasionally, it will stand still and look up, as if to check what is going on in its extended surroundings, before continuing its search. A particular field can be either searched while crossing over it, or more thoroughly in a zig-zag pattern of movement. Experienced cats can reportedly follow urine-stained mouse trails to the burrow entrances (Leyhausen 1956c); since even humans can smell these, this is probably true, though no hard evidence exists.

When the cat has found a potentially productive spot, e.g. the entrance to a mouse burrow, it carefully approaches this – slowly, quietly, always staring at the point of maximum interest and usually low to the ground. There, it continues to stare at the locus while standing, sitting or crouching. For our discussion later

on, we call this behaviour 'interest for a locus' and we can speak of the 'duration of (that) interest'. When a mouse appears, the cat usually 'waits' until it has moved some distance from the burrow entrance. The tension building up in the cat increases to its highest level just as the cat makes its pounce at the prey item, which is reflected in its subtly changing body posture. By our definition, interest disappears with a successful pounce, or when the cat moves away from that locus (> 0.5 m in our study). If a rodent is captured it is either eaten shortly thereafter near the place of capture or carried home; if the prey is an invertebrate, it is usually devoured on the spot.

After an unproductive 'interest' (no prey appeared) or an unsuccessful pounce, the cat usually looks around for a few seconds before moving on to another potentially attractive locus. The behavioural pattern is then repeated. Since pounces only occur in the presence of prey, 'interests' are often shown without ending in a pounce. The cat may hunt for a while on a particular field, and the loci of its 'interests' can be spatially clumped, often within a radius of some 20 metres or so. When the cat changes fields, it rarely shows interest along the way until it reaches another potentially good place. After a while and with or without success, the cat will depart for home once again moving faster and directly along the various transit routes (personal observations).

Hunting for birds requires stalking, since many species of birds have an up to 360° field of view and can detect a cat coming up on them from behind (Tabor, 1983). The cat must very carefully gear its moves to the bird's behaviour and local cover. During the stalk, head and body are kept low and to be successful the approach must be either extremely slow, or extremely fast when the bird is preoccupied or has moved out of sight behind leaves. Then the cat sprints forward to where it resights the bird and 'freezes'. This procedure is repeated until the hunter is within pouncing range of the prey; but by then, it is often too late – the bird has already flown away or to another branch.

The 'wait' just before the pounce is a characteristic element of the cat's hunting behaviour and many birds also fly away during this 'wait' without ever having noticed the cat. But because of these failures, many cats soon give up bird hunting altogether. The predominance of the 'wait' prior to a pounce is one indication of specialisation in cat hunting behaviour for capturing small burrowing rodents; another is the fact that cats are generally attracted to crevices and holes in the ground (ethologists say they have an 'appetite' for these [Leyhausen, 1956c, 1979)].

The importance of acoustic cues, once the cat has begun its search, cannot be overemphasised. Cats have better acoustical discrimination abilities and respond physiologically to higher-pitched sounds than either dogs or men; over twenty muscles control their pinnae (external ears) allowing independent swivelling to locate sounds (see Tabor, 1983). Scratching noises and high-pitched mouse calls act upon an innate releasing mechanism which directs a kitten's attention soon after birth to the source of the sound; with experience, adult cats are capable of locating the prey at close range by sound alone (Leyhausen, 1956c). It has even been suggested (though not proven) that they can learn to distinguish between mice and shrews by the sounds they emit (Kirk, 1967).

Nor can vision be forgotten when considering prey detection and recognition. After the cat's attention has been gained by an appropriate sound, movement towards the 'prey' is elicited by any moving (or moved) object within the cat's field of vision that is neither too large, nor too fast and is moving more or less along a straight path (Leyhausen, 1956c). Once again, experienced cats are capable of recognising and attacking immobile prey. But there is no unitary 'schema' in the cat's central nervous system which would identify an object as 'prey', nor is there a releasing mechanism, which would innately identify any particular species as prey (Leyhausen, 1979). Learning through experience is again of great importance.

With few exceptions, hunting methods for prey *within* a major animal class do not appear to be *species*-specific. Most small mammals are caught using the sit-and-wait technique after a roving search of the area, the notable exception being moles, which cats often scratch out (but infrequently eat) while the mole is digging up to the surface. Rabbits and large tunnel-living birds, e.g. Antarctic prions and petrels on some islands, are either ambushed by a cat waiting at the burrow entrance (Corbett, 1979; Liberg, 1981) or actively sought out by entering the burrow if it is large enough (Jones, 1977; van Aarde, 1980).

Small songbirds are of course more mobile (faster and in three dimensions) and less predictable when they move than rodents, which might try to rush back to the burrow entrance upon attack in two-dimensional space. The longer approach by the cat over the branches is added to the behavioural repertoire for hunting birds (but again, is not *species*-specific); as mentioned above, both this and the wait just before the pounce (for both mammals and birds) do not favour success at bird hunting.

Even if hunting methods are not particularly prey species-specific, cats can reportedly become 'specialists' for particular prey *types*, e.g. birds. Prey specialists are mentioned by numerous authors (e.g. Heidemann & Vauk, 1970; Lüps, 1972; Tabor, 1983), but we are unaware of any *field data* demonstrating their existence. Two routes would lead us to conclude specialisation: (a) an individual cat might only (be able to) apply one hunting method, which is particularly suited for capturing one prey type, resulting in a high proportion of that type in the diet, and (b), an individual might prefer a particular prey type and only apply the hunting method best suited to that type. A number of experimental studies on captive cats indicate that early experience with a particular prey type (capture techniques) or diet (food preferences) influences later behaviour and/or preferences (Caro, 1979a, 1980a; Baerends-van Roon & Baerends, 1979; Kuo, 1930, 1967), and we might expect some specialists to exist in the field depending on their own experiences or the prey that their mothers brought back to them as kittens.

We might also expect to find a correlation between the following hunting methods and prey types: roving search, then 'sit-and-wait' – for small mammals; sight, then stalk – for song birds; sight and pounce or observe, then pounce – for insects; and either 'sit-and-wait' or enter large burrows – for rabbits and tunnel-living birds. Of course each of these methods might also represent a hunting 'strategy' depending on the circumstances.

Hunting strategies

We may speak of hunting strategies whenever a number of individuals in a population use the same method, or one or more individuals use the same method for one prey type and other methods for other prey types. There is a host of studies indicating that many cats are opportunistic predators, taking the various prey randomly or in proportion to their availability, and/or scavengers, feeding from carrion or human refuse (e.g. Hochstrasser, 1970; Tabor, 1981,

1983; Dards, 1978, 1981; see also Chapter 10). We can therefore either speak of an *opportunistic/ scavenging hunting strategy* or include this under what has more generally been called the 'mobile' or 'M-hunting strategy'.

Cats are said to be following the mobile hunting strategy whenever they are moving e.g. between two farms and pause when attracted by a potential prey (Macdonald & Apps, 1978) or whenever moving around within an area and seeking out prey visually (Corbett, 1979). It is quite clear that opportunism plays a role in both situations though more so during the former, and that scavenging could occur during either situation.

The counterpart of the M-strategy is the 'stationary, sit-and-wait- or S-strategy' which also covers lie-and-wait and ambushing, terms used by other authors. Strictly speaking, this can only be applied by the cats after they have arrived at, or found an area or locus of interest, whereas the M-strategy can be applied within potentially good prey areas or between any two locations. In the future and to enable better comparisons between studies, researchers should carefully describe whether they are referring to the hunting behaviour shown once the cat has reached a potentially productive area, along the way to such an area, or between any two places not necessarily used for hunting. Probably most of the hunting methods mentioned in the last section could then be assigned to the S- or M-strategy at the population level. Only Corbett (1979) has compared the application of both the mobile- and stationary-strategies while hunting the same prey type, rabbits; domestic cats were more successful using the M-strategy at that study site.

Cats are apparently capable of less-than-random searches for prey, but quantitative field data are sparse. Jones (1977) observed cats 'methodically' entering and inspecting rabbit burrows on Macquarie Island; and Leyhausen (1956c) reported the qualitative observation that cats often return to the precise place of an earlier capture, days or weeks later. We have already mentioned the numerous observations of cats using streets, roads and paths for their transit routes to and from places where they hunt; but whether they systematically visit various hunting areas within their home ranges is unknown (see below).

Systematic searching patterns have, however, been demonstrated in laboratory cats (Lundberg, 1980). In an artificial, hidden-prey distribution, the animals spontaneously showed individual, direction-stable search strategies. For example, some animals always searched the hides from left to right, others from right to left. Using rewards, Lundberg was able to induce a change in search direction preference, which occurred suddenly after a phase of seven to eight days of non-adaptive search orientations. He also found that cats tend to show a maximising strategy when solving probability-learning problems, i.e. binary discrimination. It would be most interesting to assess whether free-ranging farm cats apply direction-stable search strategies and/or a maximising strategy, when they 'decide' where to hunt.

Success rates

Generally cats are considered to be successful hunters. Spittler (1978) found that 63 per cent of 300 cats shot while straying had at least some prey in their stomachs; numbers of prey per stomach ranged from one (31 cats) to 12 (one cat). Lüps (1976) determined that 41 per cent ($n = 416$), and Goldschmidt-Rothschild & Lüps (1976) found that 44 per cent ($n = 259$) of their strays had recently caught prey. But percentage of cats with prey in their stomachs is only a weak measure of success, since we do not know how long the animals took to find and capture that prey.

Hunting success can legitimately be measured by any number of parameters, e.g. number of prey captured per hour, per hour-hunting, per pounce, etc. That not every pounce results in a successful capture is illustrated in Table 9.1 summarising values reported in the literature. For comparative purposes, it is important that researchers pay more attention than in the past to reporting details of how they calculate success rates (particularly when based on 'observation' time). Still, we do have some evidence that one or more of the measures of success are influenced by a number of factors which we will consider in this section.

Prey size and predator defence mechanisms

Although morphologically and behaviourally best-adapted to catching small, burrowing rodents, cats are probably capable of catching any animal not larger than themselves; but they generally don't try to capture anything larger than rats, pigeons (Leyhausen, 1979) or young rabbits (Corbett, 1979). Most domestic cats aren't strong enough to take healthy, full-grown rabbits, but will take young or weak (myxoma-

Table 9.1. *The number of pounces required to capture a prey item*

No.	Pounces per prey type	Source
3.6	Pounces/vertebrate prey[a]	Panaman (1981)
ca. 2	Pounces/rodent	Liberg (1982a)
5	Pounces/rabbit	
ca. 2	Pounces/mouse	Leyhausen & Wolff (1959)
4.4	Pounces/rodent	Meister & Turner (in prep.)
3.0	Pounces/invertebrate	

[a] 16 rodents and 1 bird.

Table 9.2. *Time spent per captured rodent*

Hours	Conditions	Source
3.0	—	Panaman (1981)
0.95	January–April	Liberg (1982a)
1.22	May–August	
0.63	September–December	
11.2	Non-mothers (both sexes)	Meister & Turner (unpublished)
1.6	Mother cats	

tosis) ones (Jones, 1977; Corbett, 1979). As deduced from Table 9.1, the highest number of pounces (attempts) per successfully captured prey item has been reported for rabbits.

Leyhausen (1956c) proposed that preferred prey size might be imprinted on kittens when their mothers bring back prey to them, since kittens whose mothers only carry in mice, rarely become rat-killers. Caro (1980a) found that none of his cats had benefited from prior experience of prey on their ability to deal with rats, and suggested that the cats might simply be fearful of these larger prey.

Success rates are indeed affected by the predator defence mechanisms of the prey. In an experimental study, Biben (1979) found that the probability of a kill decreased when prey was large or difficult. On the other hand, cats will capture and feed to satiation on smaller, defenceless prey, e.g. a swarm of grasshoppers (Hochstrasser, 1970). Shrews are easily located and captured, since they are rather noisy when moving about in search of food and active day and night (Tabor, 1983). Many species on islands have not co-evolved with mammalian predators and do not, therefore, show defensive behaviour against introduced cats; according to Fitzgerald (Chapter 10), this has often spelled their doom.

Prey availability

The amount of time a cat takes to successfully capture a prey animal is certainly influenced by prey availability. Three studies, which are summarised in Table 9.2, present data on time spent per captured prey. Seasonal differences in this parameter were related to seasonal differences in prey abundance by Liberg

(1982a). When rodents were at their highest density in autumn, the cats took only an average 40 minutes for a successful capture; at lowest rodent density in early summer, they took 70 minutes. But prey availability may be indirectly affected by the cats' social organisation: Corbett (1979) showed that dominant cats excluded subordinates from good rabbit areas, which certainly reduced success rates of the latter animals.

Individual and sex–class differences

Every farmer and observant cat owner knows that some cats are better (more successful or more active) mouse hunters than others. While the majority of cats in Spittler's (1978) study had captured one or two mice just prior to their death, one individual had twelve mice in its stomach! Since all of these cats had caught mice, we doubt that such differences are due to variation in the cats' *ability* to capture and kill the prey (Baerends-van Roon & Baerends, 1979; Caro, 1979a); rather, the explanation may be sought in motivational differences between individuals, or classes of individuals, which in turn, affect their hunting behaviour.

From the most extensive study of cat hunting behaviour to date, Liberg (1982a) found that feral males, i.e. males not attached to households, were somewhat more efficient rodent hunters than domestic females, especially during the spring (based on minutes of hunting per prey taken). He suggested that the communally-living, house-attached females might deplete their hunting grounds more than the feral males do.

At Liberg's study site, the cats hunted primarily voles (*Microtus* and *Arvicola*) and/or young rabbits. Rabbit kittens and juveniles weighed on average 300 g, or about ten times more than the average rodent; but per rabbit, they took only about five times more time to catch than a rodent. Therefore, rabbit hunting provided double the rewards of rodent hunting – at least during the summer. Still, Liberg found that his female cats spent more time hunting rodents than hunting rabbits. The author interprets this inconsistency as follows: firstly, the females he observed were fed at home and therefore less dependent upon their catch; there was little pressure to optimise their behaviour. Secondly, the activity periods of the females away from home were relatively short (less than two hours), due to the presence of kittens at home. If they were not hunting to fulfil their energy requirements, but to satisfy their motivation to hunt (see Leyhausen, 1956c), it would indeed be more rewarding to hunt rodents, since their short activity periods would rarely be long enough to capture a rabbit. On the other hand, the feral males were not hampered by having to care for kittens at home, but were indeed dependent upon their catch for food. For them, rabbit hunting would be the optimal strategy and indeed, they spent more time hunting rabbits than hunting rodents.

However, we found that females with kittens at home tended to be more efficient hunters than cats in other classes when (a) all cats were fed similarly and (b) rodents alone were the main prey available (Meister & Turner, unpublished). We recorded the behaviour of 23 farm cats during 143 hunting excursions over one summer. The sex–class of each animal was determined after completing the observations so as not to bias the recordings. Unfortunately, we had too few individuals in some classes and had to pool all of the non-mother animals (male and females) into one class to compare their hunting behaviour with that of mothers. Additionally, some individuals yielded more data (more excursions) than others, which probably adversely affected our statistical tests. In the following, we shall therefore only speak of trends toward differences between mothers and non-mothers.

The six mothers captured more rodents than the 17 non-mothers did (23 of 26 successful captures) and spent an average 1.6 hours per successful capture, as opposed to 11.2 hours per capture by the non-mothers (see Table 9.2). The average duration of hunting excursions by both mothers and non-mothers was the same, namely, *c.* 30 minutes. However, their behaviour during those excursions was quite different. Mothers travelled faster than the other cats

(8.4 *vs* 4.0 m/min). They showed almost twice as many 'interests' for loci per minute than the non-mothers (0.13 *vs* 0.07), but the duration of those interests was much shorter (median for 291 interests = 75 sec *vs* median for 162 interests = 168 sec). In other words mothers don't sit as long as non-mothers do at a mouse burrow, before moving on; and after an unsuccessful pounce, we found that they leave the present burrow faster than the non-mothers, presumably for a new locus of interest.

Most of the animals we observed were fed about the same, i.e. milk with pieces of bread and table scraps. But in our study as opposed to Liberg's, the mothers were probably more dependent on their catches than the non-mothers due to higher costs for lactation and bringing prey back from the field to older kittens. They were also the more efficient (minutes hunting per prey taken) and successful (pounces per prey, see below) hunters. It would appear that *both* sexes are capable of adjusting their hunting behaviour to maximise efficiency, if necessary.

Whether the hunting activity (time spent hunting) or efficiency (when hunting) of females drops when they are not caring for young is still an open question. They are reported to catch considerably more prey when they have young and it is assumed that the kittens themselves provide the stimuli that promote carrying prey home (Leyhausen, 1979). But it is possible that the mothers simply bring home a greater proportion of their prey (to their offspring) than they do at other times, giving the (false?) impression that their hunting activity increases when they have young. Since it is known that folliculin increases the readiness of female cats to catch prey in the laboratory, while other sex hormones inhibit it (Inselman & Flynn, 1973), it is still likely that their hunting activity, and possibly efficiency, increase when caring for young at home. We did find that mothers require fewer pounces to capture a rodent than the non-mothers pooled (3.4 *vs* 12.3 pounces). This might more clearly indicate a higher motivation to capture prey (with resulting higher efficiency) than the amount of time needed to capture a rodent shown in Table 9.2, but again data showing changes in this measure within the same individual over time still need to be collected (Meister & Turner, unpublished).

This raises the question of the effects of castration on the hunting behaviour of both males and females. At this point, we can only say that castrated animals *do* catch and eat or bring home prey (Borkenhagen, 1978; George, 1974, 1978). No field study has compared the hunting activities of cats of either sex before and after castration, and only Borkenhagen presents data on the number of prey *brought home* by castrated and intact animals of the same sex (males): 2.2 prey per castrated male ($n = 6$) *vs* 1.7 prey per intact male ($n = 19$). [His intact females ($n = 28$, many with young) carried in an average 9.5 prey per female, but he had only one castrated female in his sample.]

Supplemental feeding

Feeding a cat might conceivably reduce its motivation to hunt, which could affect the amount of time it spends hunting and/or its hunting intensity when in the field. Farmers have historically believed that keeping cats somewhat undernourished will make them better rodent catchers, and many have been poorly fed for this reason (Tabor, 1983). This is unfortunate for at least three reasons: (a) there is no conclusive proof that under-fed cats are more avid rodent hunters; (b) poorly fed cats are more susceptible to disease and parasites and tend to raise small offspring; (c) ill-fed cats are more likely to stray and be less attached to the farm (buildings and people).

The evidence, which is currently available on this, is somewhat contradictory. Liberg (1984) found that females fed at home spent just over half as much time hunting as feral (non-fed) females did, on an annual basis. But they still hunted and it is important to compare how intensively they did when in the field and what proportions of the captured prey were actually eaten. Most studies on the stomach contents of cats shot while straying indicate that a fairly large proportion of those ($\bar{x} = 21.3\%$) not only had been fed at home, but had also fed on field prey; and many of those with only field prey in their digestive tracts had also been fed regularly at home, as indicated by dental plaque (Lüps, 1972, 1976; Spittler, 1978; Goldschmidt-Rothschild & Lüps, 1976). A number of studies have reported on the hunting activities of cats that were well fed at home (e.g. Laundré, 1977; Panaman, 1981; Turner & Mertens, 1986), but again, it's a question of how intensively they hunted, and comparisons are difficult.

Still, it should not surprise us if supplemental feeding has little effect on the cats' hunting behaviour, given Leyhausen's (1956c, 1979) findings that prey capture, killing and consumption are relatively inde-

pendent of each other and the former two activities, independent of hunger. In most carnivores, hunger triggers the initial stage – searching – of predatory behaviour (Kruuk, 1972); but we have frequently observed domestic cats depart to hunt immediately after a full meal containing meat! This may be related to the fact that the cat has evolved while hunting small rodents on an opportunistic basis, i.e. to hunt frequently for relatively small meals. Indeed, colony studies show that when cats are offered unlimited food over the entire day, they adopt a 'nibbling' pattern of food intake, eating many (8–16) discrete meals over a 24 hour period (see e.g. Mugford & Thorne, 1980; Thorne, 1985).

Activity patterns and budgets, or 'when' cats hunt

Given the fact that colony cats spread out their feeding bouts (and most probably, activity) over the entire 24 hour period, it is somewhat surprising that domestic cats are generally thought to be crepuscular or nocturnal animals. That today's cats are not particularly nocturnal (see below) may either be an effect of the domestication process and/or simply a behavioural adaptation to life with diurnal humans. The assumed ancestor of our house cats, the African wildcat (*Felis silvestris libyca*) is predominantly nocturnal (Guggisberg, 1975; see Serpell, Chapter 11). In laboratory cats maintained under stable environmental conditions, behavioural and brain activity do show two peaks during the night, but are also registered during the day (Sterman *et al.*, 1965). Only two field studies on semi-dependent cats report the amount of activity during different phases of the 24 hour day, and both give the impression of a shift towards more diurnal activity in modern cats: George (1974) observed three castrated cats over four years for periods of various duration covering 8500 daylight and 7300 crepuscular-nocturnal hours, and found that 49.8 per cent of their prey were caught during the day, 20.1 per cent at dawn or dusk and (only) 30.1 per cent during the night. Although not necessarily, hunting behaviour is probably correlated with general activity level. Panaman (1981) observed five females during 360 hours and additionally, each of those during 48 consecutive hours. He found that 62.6 per cent of their 'active' behaviour occurred between dawn and dusk and that 82.1 per cent of their sleep fell between dusk and dawn.

The amount of time a cat spends hunting per day varies from individual to individual (Panaman, 1981); between the sexes, with supplemental feeding, and with social status (Liberg, 1984); and between seasons (George, 1974; Fennell, 1975). Values range from zero to 46 per cent of the 24 hour day over all studies. For the five females in Panaman's study, an average 14.8 per cent of the day was used for hunting, whereas one cat only hunted 2.5 per cent and another, 33.7 per cent of the day (his minimum and maximum values based on 24 h observations).

Liberg (1984) observed 18 female and 19 male cats during over 4000 hours and found that (a) house-attached females spent 26 per cent, feral females 46 per cent of the day hunting; (b) under similar conditions, males spent generally less time hunting than females did; (c) males in the different social (reproductive) status classes spent different amounts of time on hunting, ranging from 5 per cent (for domestic 'breeders') to 34 per cent of the day (for 'outcasts' and feral 'breeders'). But again, hunting intensity was not directly compared.

Cats are generally more active and active for longer periods during spring and summer than during autumn and winter (Fennell, 1975). Within their active phases, they possibly shift their hunting times too, as George (1974) qualitatively found for his three, castrated cats (2 females, 1 male). During the winter, they hunted mainly over the six mid-day hours, longer on clear, bright days and little at night or when very cold. They caught prey during and after snow storms. During spring, there was a slight shift towards dawn and dusk, but they still avoided the night for hunting. They hunted often during light rains and immediately after heavy rains. And over summer and fall, they avoided the hot mid-day to hunt mainly in the crepuscular and nocturnal hours.

Whether the duration of single hunting excursions changes seasonally is unknown. Our average duration of just under 30 min (for both mothers and non-mothers; range of 5 to 133 min) was determined during the summer and early autumn (Meister & Turner, unpublished). The duration of interests at loci in the field might also change seasonally; we can only say that it will probably be much shorter than the incorrect impression of cats patiently waiting for 'hours' at a particular mouse burrow (Leyhausen, 1956c).

Hunting areas, or 'where' cats hunt

Apparently cats have an excellent memory for locality and often return to the precise place of an earlier capture to 'look for more' (Leyhausen, 1979). Several field researchers have spoken of hunting 'areas' or hunting 'grounds' which the cats regularly utilise within their home ranges, implying at least some degree of temporal permanency (Leyhausen & Wolff, 1959; Laundré, 1977; Liberg, 1980; Panaman, 1981). Unfortunately, none of these authors presents data demonstrating the differential use of, or delineating, areas within the home range for hunting. On the contrary, one quantitative analysis of home range utilisation patterns among eleven adult cats yielded no concentrations of sightings away from the primary home, which would have been indicative of such areas (Turner & Mertens, 1986). One might argue that the authors pooled sighting-data over too long a period, to allow the appearance of successively used neighbouring areas. But the first author, upon a qualitative re-examination of those data, found no hint to support this.

Nevertheless, the attractiveness of a particular field or clearing, which is in some way different from the surrounding habitat, is frequently mentioned; this may be a freshly mown pasture, a recently harvested grain field or a new forest clearing, where one might expect increased chances of finding prey due to lack of cover (Leyhausen, 1979; Schär & Tschanz, 1982). The cats appear to travel more or less directly to such places, as mentioned earlier, but the decision-rules they use to select or combine the places they visit for hunting have not yet been examined.

Few data are available on the effective distances cats travel during single hunting excursions. For complete excursions, i.e. beginning and ending at the primary home, we found a median distance travelled of 211 metres ($n = 15$, $\bar{x} = 371$ m) and a maximum of 1578 metres (Meister & Turner, unpublished). Panaman (1981) reported values per individual for the 24 hour day (and therefore, probably for more than one excursion) ranging from 30 to 1770 metres ($n = 5$ females, $\bar{x} = 519$ m/d). The distances travelled on such hunting trips are certainly affected by home range shape and size, and the distribution and abundance of prey, which in turn are related to the different habitat types within the range.

The cats at Liberg's (1982a) study site in Sweden hunted most often in wet meadows or bogs and grass fields, rarely in forests (deciduous or coniferous). This does not mean they avoided the forest totally. Indeed, in one study from the Swiss midlands, the highest proportion of cats shot while straying (46.8%, *n* = 109) was found for the woods; but these animals rarely had forest-living prey (e.g. *Clethrionomys*, *Apodemus*) in their digestive tracts, indicating that they had not been hunting or had had little success there (Lüps, 1972). Male cats tend to be found more often in the woods than females (Goldschmidt-Rothschild & Lüps, 1976; Lüps, 1976, 1984), which might be related to their larger home ranges (see Chapter 7) and the location of primary homes, generally away from forest edges. Heidemann (1973) reported that 68 per cent (*n* = 156) of the stray cats shot, captured or run over at his site in northern West Germany were on fields, and many studies on the stomach contents of cats indicate hunting exclusively field- (or bog-) living prey species, at least in northern latitudes (see also Chapter 10).

The presence of conspecifics can also influence where a particular cat hunts. Rosenblatt & Schneirla (1962) reported that kittens follow their mothers when they depart from the nest area and are present *when they hunt*. This is certainly not that common, as we are unaware of corroborating observations from field researchers. Cats generally hunt alone, and a dominant animal may even forcibly exclude subordinate cats from a particularly good area (at least for rabbits; Corbett, 1979). But this is usually not necessary, since domestic cats avoid contact outside their primary homes, especially while hunting (Leyhausen, 1979). Prey size neither requires, nor allows, a cooperative hunt by several individuals. Cats from the same home coordinate their hunting excursions in time and space, usually to avoid (Leyhausen, 1965b), occasionally to promote (Turner & Mertens, 1986) contact with conspecifics. This is accomplished visually and/or olfactorily with urine marks (Natoli, 1985b; Matter & Turner, unpublished). Only one study (Turner & Mertens, 1986) has demonstrated a significant positive coordination of hunting trips, but that was between an adult brother and sister. Still, other studies have reported cats hunting in the field within sight of each other (usually within 50 m distance or closer), with few agonistic interactions, and

for no apparent reason, e.g. because of prey distribution (Leyhausen, 1965b; Laundré, 1977; Liberg, 1980; Panaman, 1981). Although Liberg's cats apparently did not take notice of each other, we frequently observed quick glances between the cats, and suggest that they might be checking on their neighbour's success. Probably most of the cats which have been observed hunting near each other were related and based (fed) at the same primary home, two predominant factors affecting cat sociality according to Kerby & Macdonald (Chapter 6). And although cats are basically solitary hunters, positive coordination of hunting excursions has been added to the growing list of phenomena which Fagen (1978) calls 'facultative sociality' in the cat, and makes this species a fascinating subject for studies in behavioural ecology and social ethology.

Prey-handling, or what the cat does after a successful capture

Essentially, the cat has three choices of what to do with a successfully captured prey item: it may kill and consume the prey immediately, at or near the place of capture; it may carry the prey (dead or alive) back to the primary home; or it may first 'play' with the prey before killing and consuming it (in the field), or allowing it to be killed and consumed (at home).

Adult cats are extremely efficient at dispatching their prey. The constriction between the head and body of the prey acts upon an innate releasing mechanism to direct the cat's bite to the back of the neck; with their strong jaws, they sever the spinal cord (or destroy it with pressure) causing immediate death (Leyhausen, 1956c). Small mammals are usually consumed entirely, being careful to ingest the prey with, as opposed to against the grain of the prey's hair, birds are defeathered before consumption (Leyhausen, 1956c).

As mentioned earlier in this chapter and covered in more detail by Martin & Bateson in Chapter 2, adult cats often carry prey home. Females, and most probably those with kittens at home, do this more often than either intact or castrated males (Borkenhagen, 1978), but this behaviour is shown by members of both sexes to varying degrees. Leyhausen (1979) mentions this 'bring hypertrophy' in castrated males, implying that the phenomenon in males has something to do with the lack of male hormones; but since intact males also carry prey home, another explanation must be sought. He also suggests that the human to which the prey is often brought may be serving as a 'deputy kitten', but we should not forget that male cats have nothing to do with raising their offspring. Perhaps the cat without kittens brings home prey that it usually doesn't eat but doesn't know what to do with, i.e. when the cat finds itself in a conflict situation. This phenomenon might also conceivably be related to the early domestication of cats and their being used to retrieve game hunted by their domesticators (see Chapter 11).

Mothers first bring kittens prey which they have killed themselves; later, when the kittens are at least four weeks old, live prey which they release in their presence. The competitive races and play with live prey by the mother and her offspring may seem cruel, but they help the kittens reach the motivational threshold required to apply the killing bite (Leyhausen, 1979).

But playing with live prey also occurs in other contexts. Whenever hunger and prey size place the cat in a conflict situation, e.g. when a hungry cat is confronted with a large or difficult prey item, adult cats tend to play with the prey before, after or instead of killing it (Biben, 1979). It is probable that this also tires the prey and reduces its ability to defend itself. Leyhausen (1979, pp. 118–27) has described the various ways cats play with prey and believes this to be a natural consequence of the different endogenous rhythms for each of the predatory activities (e.g. stalking, seizing, biting, consuming). In 'overflow play', which is most common after killing mice, the tension accumulating in the cat up to the kill suddenly 'overflows' with relief.

Whenever a cat brings prey home and releases it from its mouth, it risks 'losing' that prey to another conspecific. Mothers promote the transfer of prey to their young by calling them upon their return. Leyhausen (1979) reported that cats will readily snatch up another's prey once it has been put down, but rarely attempt to steal it from the captor's mouth; we can confirm this from numerous observations in the field. George (1978) observed 'piracy' of prey at a high cat density, but it is unclear whether this occurred before, or after the prey had been put down in his 'delivery area', and whether the captor was even present. We should not forget that many of the conspecifics present at the primary home are probably related (and not just kittens of the captor) and *prey-sharing* might be more common than previously thought. Macdonald & Apps (1978) have observed the adult daughter of a female with another five-week-old kitten repeatedly bring in and share prey with her mother. Indeed, the domestic cat might be just as interesting to study for the modern sociobiologist as for the behavioural ecologist!

Concluding remarks

In closing, we are now in a position to summarise what is known about the hunting behaviour of domestic cats. The general hunting methods used by cats, including the sensory systems involved, have been adequately described. Domestic cats are opportunistic hunters and scavengers. They employ two basic hunting strategies: the 'mobile' and/or the 'stationary/sit-and-wait' strategy. Although generally considered successful hunters, their success rates depend upon (a) prey size and defence capabilities; (b) prey availability (which is seasonal); (c) the individual and its sex–class. Both males and females are capable of adjusting their hunting behaviour to maximise efficiency.

Supplemental feeding reduces the amount of time spent hunting, but does not eliminate it. How it affects hunting intensity and/or efficiency is unclear. Domestic cats have shifted more of their activity (including hunting) into the daylight and crepuscular hours than their wild ancestors. They spend between zero and 46 per cent of the 24 hour day hunting, depending upon the individual, its sex, whether it is fed, its social status, and the season.

Cats are attracted to freshly cut fields or clearings for hunting, but since these change in space over time, one should not speak of hunting 'grounds' within their ranges. In northern latitudes, they hunt mostly on fields (including wet meadows and bogs), but are also found in forests (where they rarely hunt). Cats usually avoid hunting near other conspecifics, but not always.

Once prey has been caught, it is either killed and consumed or carried back to the primary home. Play with prey (dead or alive) has also been examined and its causes fairly well explained. But more work is required to predict what a particular cat will do with a specific prey item once it has been caught.

And lastly, for a number of reasons mentioned above, it appears that the domestic cat is an ideal subject for studies in behavioural ecology and social ethology.

Acknowledgements

The studies by Meister and Turner, and Turner and Mertens were financed by the Swiss National Science Foundation (Grant Nrs. 3.338.83 and 3.247.85 to Turner); Effems Beratung für Kleintierhaltung, Zürich, provided additional support for Turner's projects. We are grateful to Tim Caro and Claudia Mertens for their comments and criticisms.

10

Diet of domestic cats and their impact on prey populations

B. M. Fitzgerald

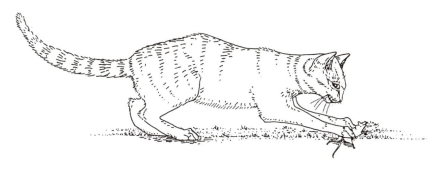

Introduction

House cats have long been associated with humans and have travelled with them to most parts of the world, including many remote islands. Although domesticated for several millennia they readily revert to the feral or wild state and feral populations of cats persist on islands in many parts of the world after human settlements have been abandoned. Near human habitations though, the distinction between feral and house cats is less clear; even well fed house cats hunt for prey, and feral cats will feed from garbage.

Many myths and misconceptions about the predatory habits and diet of cats are present in the literature; they can be corrected only by detailed studies of the feeding habits of cats, and by experiments on the effects of cats on prey populations. In this review the various methods used to study and report on the diet of cats are examined and those diets are analysed, particularly for variations in relation to the cats' dependence on man, to habitat, latitude, sex, age,

season and prey size and availability. Then the effects of cats in determining the numbers of prey, including rodents, rabbits, game species, songbirds and island faunas, are examined.

Diet of cats
Methods of study

Many methods have been used for studying the diet of cats and to try to draw conclusions from the diverse material (see Appendix 10.1) I have had to seek a common denominator. This requires some discussion of the methods, each of which has advantages in different circumstances.

Quantitative studies of the food of cats are based mostly on gut samples from cats killed whilst straying, or from feral cats. Other methods include scat (faecal) analysis, records of prey brought home by house cats, and the uneaten remains of prey found in the field. This last method has been used mostly on islands where cats are the sole mammalian predators and remains of their prey are readily distinguished from those of avian predators. Gut analyses are usually of

Table 10.1. *Results for studies given only as per cent volumes (McMurray & Sperry, 1941, Gibb et al., 1978), converted to per cent occurrences, using correction factors derived from studies that presented results by both methods. Correction factors for McMurray & Sperry (1941) are calculated from data in Nilsson (1940), Hubbs (1951) and Eberhard (field cats) (1954) and for Gibb, Ward & Ward (1978) from Gibb, Ward & Ward (1969). Trace amounts have been given figures of 0.5%*

	McMurray & Sperry (1941)			Gibb, Ward & Ward (1978)		
	% volume	Correction factor	Estimated % occurrence	% volume	Correction factor	Estimated % occurrence
Mammals, chiefly rodents	55	1.37	75.3			
Hedgehog				Trace	1.0	Trace
Rabbit				77	1.37	100
Rats				Trace	2.5	1.25
Mice				2	2.67	5.34
Stoat				Trace	1.0	Trace
Sheep				Trace	1.0	Trace
Birds	4	2.86	11.4	4	2.41	9.64
Reptiles	2	3.20	6.4	Trace	10	5
Insects	12.5	10.25	100	9	9.95	89.5
Garbage	26.5	1.30	34.4			

stomach contents but sometimes the intestine and rectum are included; obviously more prey will be identified per cat when the whole gut is used.

The studies vary greatly in sample size; some present results from fewer than ten guts or scats, but others examine several hundred guts, or more than a thousand scats.

Identification of prey remains is sometimes difficult; remains in the stomach are often in large pieces and can be identified more readily than remains in the rectum or in scats, which contain only indigestible residues. The level of identification, and the amount of detail provided, vary considerably between studies; some authors identify most material to species while others list prey by type, e.g. 'small rodent' and 'passerine bird'.

Results have been expressed in various ways: most often as percentage occurrences, given as percentages of the total number of guts or scats, or of the guts with contents. Percentage occurrence underestimates the importance of large prey and overestimates the importance of small prey but has been most widely used and is therefore most useful in comparing the various studies. Ten studies give both per cent occurrence and per cent volume; comparing results by the two methods, per cent occurrences for mammals

are, on average, about equal to per cent volumes but per cent occurrences for birds, reptiles and invertebrates are increasingly greater than those for per cent volumes, probably reflecting the average size of prey in these groups. Two studies (McMurray & Sperry, 1941; Gibb, Ward & Ward, 1978) give results by per cent volume only. To standardise results from the various studies as much as possible I have converted their per cent volume figures to percentage occurrences by calculating correction factors for McMurray & Sperry (1941) from the three North American studies that presented both occurrence and volume figures (Nilsson, 1940; Hubbs, 1951; Eberhard, 1954) and for Gibb, Ward & Ward (1978) from Gibb, Ward & Ward (1969) (Table 10.1).

A few authors have presented results as percentages by weight, either by assigning a mean weight to the records for each type of prey (e.g. Fitzgerald & Karl, 1979; Karl & Best, 1982) or by applying correction factors to the weights of indigestible residues in scats (Liberg, 1984). Sometimes the numbers of individuals of each species are given as percentages of the total number of individual prey identified.

These various ways of studying the diet of cats and of expressing the results produce biases that must be kept in mind when comparing the many studies, but

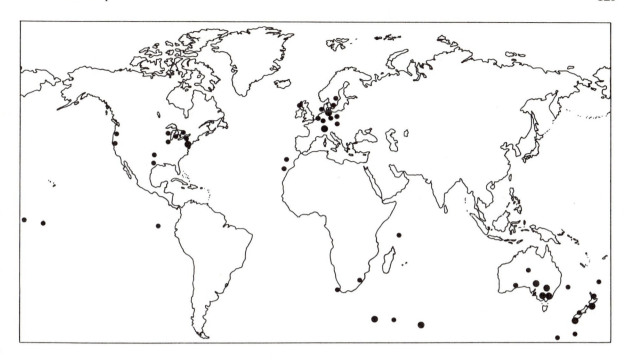

Fig. 10.1. World distribution of studies of the diet of cats, based on gut and scat analysis, and of prey brought home. Small circles indicate single studies, large circles two or more studies. (Details in Appendix 10.1).

the major features of the diet of cats are sufficiently robust to be revealed despite the differences in methods.

World distribution of studies

Quantitative studies of the diet of cats have been carried out on four continents and many islands (Figure 10.1, Appendix 10.1); continental studies are from Europe (13 studies), North America (12), Australia (9), and Africa (1). The diet of cats has also been studied on 22 islands from the equator to latitude 57°; many are remote oceanic islands. The continents have rich faunas of mammals, birds and reptiles that evolved in the presence of relatives of the domestic cat (i.e. *Felis silvestris*, *Felis lynx*, and others), or, in Australia, in the presence of similar-sized marsupial predators (*Dasyurus* spp.). In contrast, most islands where cats have been studied have few, if any, native mammals, a few species of mammals introduced recently by humans, and some have large nesting

colonies of seabirds. Their faunas have evolved without mammalian predators. Because the range of prey available on islands differs markedly from that on the continents the two groups, continents and islands, are treated separately.

The diet of cats on continents

Town and country cats compared   It is not usually possible in food habit studies to distinguish cats attached to households from feral ones though the status of the individual cat may greatly influence the range of foods it eats. Also, cats vary in their degree of dependence on people; some cats may be household pets but catch much of their food in nearby fields, and feral cats may scavenge on household scraps to varying degrees.

Liberg (1984) compared the diet of house and feral cats on farmland in southern Sweden by assigning scats collected in gardens and outbuildings of cat-owning households to house cats and scats collected at abandoned farms and other places regularly frequented by feral cats, to feral cats. The diet of house cats was similar to that of feral cats, but the former ate more household food, and tended to eat fewer lagomorphs.

A less direct means of looking at the way the diet of cats is influenced by their degree of association with people is by comparing town and city cats with country cats. In northern Germany 156 cats collected on country roads were compared with 11 house cats from a town suburb (Heidemann, 1973). Country cats took at least 14 species of vertebrates, including large numbers of voles (*Microtus* spp.), but the house cats, which were given a little food and allowed to roam in an extensive garden, held only tinned cat food and a grasshopper. In the city of Kiel, West Germany, cats were compared from the city outskirts, from the densely built-up part of the city, and from intermediate habitat (Borkenhagen 1979). Those from the city outskirts contained most prey but more birds were taken in the intermediate habitat where prey also included rabbits (*Oryctolagus cuniculus*), voles and wood mice (*Apodemus* sp.). However, in the densely built-up part of the city the cats contained almost no prey; in the 43 cats examined remains of only one rodent and one bird were found.

In the German Democratic Republic Achterberg & Metzger (1978, 1980) compared 67 feral cats from the urban district of Magdeburg with 90 cats from the city district and 113 cats from households. The feral cats contained least household food (28%) and most prey, including voles, house mice (*Mus musculus*), rats (*Rattus* spp.), hamsters (*Cricetus cricetus*), hares (*Lepus europaeus*), and birds. Those from the city district contained more household food (59%) and few prey while house cats contained most household food (66%) and virtually no prey (only three birds).

North American studies show a similar pattern. Cats from residential and non-residential areas at Ft Sills, Oklahoma were compared (McMurray & Sperry, 1941). Household food, garbage, and to a lesser extent birds and insects were more common, and rodents (chiefly cotton rats, *Sigmodon* sp.) less common, in cats from the residential area. Likewise, in Pennsylvania cats caught in fields ate more mammals (both rodents and rabbits, *Sylvilagus* sp.) and more birds than those caught in towns or thought to be pets. Household food and garbage was recorded much more frequently and in much greater quantities in town cats (Eberhard, 1954). In a poor, densely populated part of Baltimore, Maryland, cat scats contained mainly garbage plus a few Norway rats, mice and insects, whereas a few scats collected from a farm near Baltimore contained mainly Norway rat or meadow vole (Jackson, 1951).

Because the range of prey taken by cats in towns and cities is so much smaller than that on the outskirts and in the countryside, in the following analyses of the prey of cats I have excluded samples where the cats fed chiefly on household scraps and garbage.

Major groups of prey   To assess the main features of the food habits of cats, I first plotted the frequency of the main groups of prey by latitude; a few of these plots are included below to illustrate trends.

In the continental studies mammals are usually the most important prey of cats, supporting the view of Leyhausen (1979) and Fitzgerald & Karl (1979), among others, that cats are primarily predators of small mammals. Remains of mammals are usually present in 50 to 90 per cent of guts or scats. Contrary to the widely held view that cats prey heavily on birds, birds have been recorded at less than 50 per cent in all continental studies except one from Czechoslovakia (Farsky, 1944). Neither mammal nor bird predation shows a significant trend with latitude but predation on reptiles does ($r_s = -0.732$, $p < 0.01$) (Figure 10.2a). At latitudes below 35° reptiles are usually found in more than 20 per cent of guts, but above 40° are found in no more than 10 per cent. However, the samples from the different continents overlap in latitude insufficiently to show that this is a latitudinal gradient, rather than differences between the continents in the abundance of reptiles.

Other groups of prey are much less important than mammals, birds and reptiles. Frogs were recorded (rarely) in only six studies and fish (again, rarely) also in six studies from Europe, North America and Australia. Invertebrates are recorded frequently but individual items are small and usually do not contribute much to the volume of gut or scat contents. Most authors have not attempted to identify all invertebrates but usually list only the more important ones. These include a wide variety of insects but also spiders, isopods, crayfish and molluscs.

Carrion is eaten, but unless the animal is too large for a cat to capture (e.g. sheep or kangaroo), records of carrion can not be distinguished from animals the cats

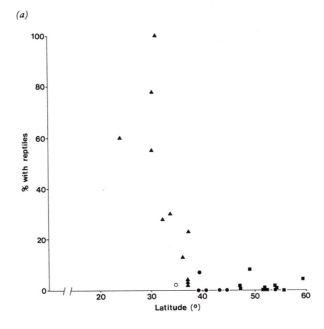

(a)

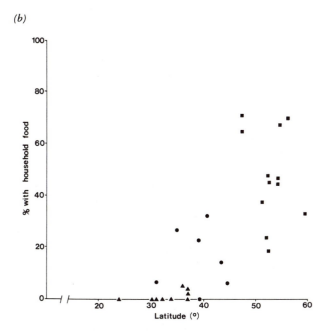

(b)

Fig. 10.2. (*a*) Reptiles and (*b*) household food in the diet of cats on continents in relation to latitude. Frequency in guts or scats of cats determined by % occurrence. (Key: triangles Australia, circles North America, squares Europe).

have killed. Even the presence of maggots with the material is not a certain indicator because cats may return later to prey they have killed and cached.

Unlike many other carnivores, cats eat virtually no fruit or other vegetable matter, apart from grass. The reasons for eating grass have not been studied but suggestions include providing trace elements and vitamins (Achterberg & Metzger, 1978), helping to disgorge indigestible material (Pettersson, 1968), and helping to void parasites (Borkenhagen, 1979).

The frequency of household food in guts or scats is strongly correlated with latitude ($r_s = 0.766, p < 0.01$) (Figure 10.2b), though this may reflect differences in the density of people, rather than differences in latitude. None of the Australian studies reported more than 5 per cent household food, though Rose (1975), in a brief account, reported picnic refuse in 29 of 31 feral cats killed in Ku-ring-gai Chase National Park, Sydney. In Europe it is difficult to find places to study the food habits of cats without access to household foods. Also, it is uncertain if cat populations could persist in northern Europe without this source of food.

Summarising the results of many studies on continents by major food types emphasises the importance of mammal prey to cats, the small, but consistent, predation on birds, and the latitudinal variations in predation on reptiles and use of household food. However, it is also important to identify the species of prey eaten if we are to try to understand the significance of predation.

Effects of sample size and latitude The number of species of mammals, birds and reptiles recorded in the various studies may be influenced by sample size and by latitude. The number of species of mammals and birds eaten increased significantly with sample size ($r_s = 0.722, p < 0.01, r_s = 0.553, p < 0.05$ respectively) and the number of reptiles decreased ($r_s = -0.497, p < 0.01$). However, this result is influenced strongly by the very small samples; when only samples greater than 50 are considered, the number of species recorded is not significantly related to sample size. Consequently, in considering the relationship between number of species and latitude the small samples (< 50) were eliminated. The number of species of mammals or birds eaten by cats does not change significantly with latitude, but there is a significant negative relationship between reptiles and latitude ($r_s = -0.644, p < 0.01$) (Figure 10.3).

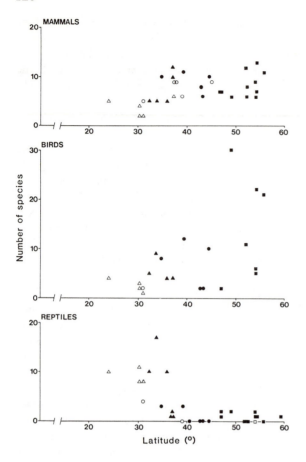

Fig. 10.3. The number of species of mammals, birds and reptiles in various studies in relation to latitude. (Key: triangles Australia, circles North America, squares Europe; hollow symbols samples 50 or less, filled symbols samples greater than 50.)

Frequency of prey species in the diet   To prepare the data for this review I first made separate lists of all vertebrates recorded as prey in the studies given in Appendix 10.1 for Europe, North America and Australia (as well as for islands). Because the species lists are very long and often contain only one record per species, they are not included here.

The number of species of mammals recorded as prey of cats on the continental land masses varies less than three-fold (5 to 13 species) in samples of more than 50 guts or scats (see Figure 10.3). In Europe and North America they usually include one or two species of lagomorph, one to three species of insectivore and

various ground-dwelling rodents, especially microtines. In Europe red squirrels (*Sciurus vulgaris*) are rarely taken but in North America various arboreal and ground-dwelling sciurid rodents are taken. In Australia mammalian prey includes introduced rabbits, native and introduced murid rodents, marsupials and bats.

In Europe lagomorphs are often an important part of the diet, mostly rabbits and a few hares in most studies, but more hares than rabbits in Czechoslovakia (Farsky, 1944) and no rabbits in Poland (Pielowski, 1976) or Switzerland (Goldschmidt-Rothschild & Lüps, 1976). As prey, lagomorphs are surpassed in frequency only by cricetid rodents (especially *Microtus* spp., but also *Clethrionomys glareolus*, *Arvicola terrestris*, *Cricetus cricetus* and *Pitymys subterraneus*); common voles (*Microtus arvalis*) are most important, though in southern Sweden where they are absent field voles (*M. agrestis*) are the most important rodent (Liberg, 1984). Because lagomorphs (even young ones) are much larger than voles (*Microtus* spp.), they often contribute more to the diet than voles do. For example, in the Netherlands, lagomorphs were found in 35 per cent of the stomachs with field prey and voles in 46 per cent, but lagomorphs contributed 58 per cent of the weight of stomach contents, and voles only 17 per cent (Niewold, 1986).

Murid rodents (*Apodemus* spp., *Micromys minutus*, *Rattus* spp. and *Mus musculus*) are less important than cricetids in the diet and may be less palatable. The numbers of the two groups brought into houses in northern Germany, and the proportion eaten have been compared by Borkenhagen (1978, 1979) (Table 10.2). Of 48 murids brought into houses by cats 18 were not subsequently eaten whereas of 89 cricetids, only 8 were not subsequently eaten. Comparing the ratio of the two groups brought in by cats with their frequencies in guts, murids formed 20 per cent of the animals of these two groups in the guts, but 35 per cent of the animals brought in. Other European studies also record murids much less frequently than cricetids.

Insectivores are evidently even less palatable. Borkenhagen (1978) recorded 23 *Sorex araneus*, 4 *S. minutus* and 21 *Talpa europaea* among 239 mammals brought in by cats (none of them subsequently eaten), but found no insectivores among 119 mammals identified in guts (Borkenhagen, 1979).

Table 10.2. *Difference in the palatability of cricetid and murid rodents as revealed by the greater numbers of cricetids eaten among rodents brought home by cats, and the higher proportion of cricetids in guts than among prey brought home (from Borkenhagen, 1978, 1979)*

	Cricetidae	Muridae
Number brought in and eaten	81	30
Number brought in and not eaten	8	18
Total	89	48
$\chi^2 = 14.68, p < 0.01$ Yates' correction		
Number brought in	89	48
Number in guts	70	17
Total	159	65
$\chi^a = 6.20, p < 0.05$		

In other European studies very few shrews or moles were identified; from gut contents 2 *S. minutus* (Heidemann, 1973) and 5 *T. europaea* (Farsky, 1944), and from 1437 scats 13 shrews, almost certainly all *S. araneus*, and 3 *T. europaea* (O. Liberg, personal communication).

Other prey rarely recorded are red squirrels (Borkenhagen, 1978), bats and stoats (*Mustela erminea*) (Liberg, 1984).

The diet of cats in North America shows a similar pattern, with rabbits (*Sylvilagus* spp.) being recorded in most studies and hares (*Lepus americanus* and *L. californicus*) less frequently (only Nilsson, 1940; Hubbs, 1951). *Microtus* spp. are important together with seven other genera of cricetid rodents. Squirrels (Sciuridae) are much more diverse in North America than in Europe and are well represented in the studies: *Tamiasciurus douglasii* (Nilsson, 1940), ground squirrels and chipmunks (e.g. Nilsson, 1940; Toner, 1956; George, 1974) and flying squirrels (*Glaucomys sabrinus*) (Toner, 1956). Other rodents recorded include gophers (*Thomomys* spp.), deer mice (*Peromyscus* spp.) and the introduced murids *Rattus norvegicus* and *Mus musculus*. One group of North American rodents, the jumping mice (Zapodidae), may be rather unpalatable; they were listed in three studies of prey brought in by cats, but were not recorded in any guts.

Insectivores, including shrews (*Sorex* spp.) and star-nosed moles (*Condylura cristata*) were recorded in all three studies of prey brought in by cats, and were found in five of the seven studies based on gut analysis. Those in the guts include *Sorex* spp., the short-tailed shrew *Blarina brevicauda*, and moles, *Scapanus* sp. They may not be very palatable but Nader & Martin (1962) found the remains of eight short-tailed shrews in the stomach of one cat and suggested that the distastefulness of shrews may be overstressed.

In Australia the variety of mammals preyed upon provides interesting contrasts and similarities with results from the Northern Hemisphere. The introduced European rabbit is important prey in most habitats except the forest (Coman & Brunner, 1972; Triggs, Brunner & Cullen, 1984). In eucalyptus forests a range of marsupials is eaten, including the small, insectivorous, *Antechinus stuartii* and *A. swainsonii* (see also Jones & Coman, 1981), the bandicoot (*Perameles nasuta*) and several larger arboreal species. Remains of the common ringtail possum (*Pseudocheirus peregrinus*) were present in 56 per cent of cat scats from NE Victoria (Triggs *et al.*, 1984) and infrequently from other forests (Coman & Brunner, 1972; Jones & Coman, 1981). Also taken are the greater glider (*Petauroides volans*), the sugar glider (*Petaurus breviceps*), possums (*Trichosurus vulpecula* and *T. caninus*), the pygmy possum (*Cercartetus nanus*) and feathertail glider (*Acrobates pygmaeus*). In arid habitats the marsupials *Sminthopsis* spp. and *Planigale* are recorded, together with native rodents (*Pseudomys hermannsburgensis*, *Leggadina forresti* and *Notomys alexis*) (Bayly, 1978; Strong & Low, 1983). Native species of *Rattus* are eaten (Triggs *et al.*, 1984) together with *R. rattus*; *Mus musculus* is recorded in most studies and is an important component of some. Two species of bats have been identified in guts and scats of cats in Australia, *Tadarida planiceps* in one study and *Nyctophilus geoffroyi* in four studies, making it the most commonly recorded bat in the diet of cats worldwide. The latter bat hunts very near to, and often on, the ground, making it vulnerable to predation (Maddock, 1983).

On all continents birds are usually much less important than mammals; birds were present on average at 21 per cent frequency of occurrence, and mammals at 68 per cent. Many species are represented by just one or two individuals. Although Farsky

(1944) found bird remains in 93 per cent of 96 guts, most of the 30 species were recorded only once or twice; but two game species, partridges (*Perdix perdix*) and pheasants (*Phasianus colchicus*), were found in 29 and 14 per cent of the guts respectively. Pheasants were also important birds in the diet of cats in southern Sweden (Liberg, 1981, 1984), the Netherlands (Niewold, 1986), and Sacramento Valley, California (Hubbs, 1951). In parts of the Netherlands, at least, the pheasant population was artificially high because birds were released and fed for sportsmen to hunt (Niewold, 1986). Other species taken frequently were starlings (*Sturnus vulgaris*) in southern Sweden, where they formed 46 per cent of bird remains (Liberg, 1981, 1984), and house sparrows (*Passer domesticus*) (Bradt, 1949; Borkenhagen, 1978). The high frequency of house sparrows in prey brought in and left uneaten, and their scarcity in gut contents suggests that they may not be very palatable (Borkenhagen, 1978, 1979). Passerine species were generally the most important group of birds eaten, forming 72 per cent of the 46 species recorded in Europe, 66 per cent of the 29 species recorded in North America and 50 per cent of 20 species in Australia. The Australian non-passerines included five species of parrots. Many of the species eaten are ground-feeding birds.

The contribution of reptiles to the diet of cats differs greatly between the three continents in frequency and in the numbers of species eaten, and is probably related to latitude, climate and species diversity. In Europe only three species of reptile are recorded, the lizards *Lacerta vivipara* and *L. agilis*, and the slow-worm, *Anguis fragilis*. In North America at least nine species of reptile (5 lizards and 4 non-venomous snakes) are recorded, all in the south and west of the continent (McMurray & Sperry, 1941; Hubbs, 1951; Parmalee, 1953). In contrast, in Australia at least 44 species (39 lizards, 4 snakes, 1 turtle) have been recorded eaten by cats. Two of the snakes are non-venomous blind snakes (Typhlopidae) and two are venomous elapid snakes, though not dangerously so (Cogger, 1983). Among the lizards eaten skinks predominate, with 21 species recorded, and lesser numbers of agamid lizards and geckos. Goannas (*Varanus* spp.) are recorded by Bayly (1976) and Catling (in press), and three species of snake-lizard (Pygopodidae) are recorded. For most species few individuals are recorded but Brooker (1977) recorded

78 *Tympanocryptis lineata*, plus 24 other reptiles, in 9 cats from the Nullarbor Plain.

Both diurnal and nocturnal lizards are taken in Australia; of those eaten by cats and listed as diurnal or nocturnal by Cogger (1983), about two-thirds are diurnal. Seven species of burrowing lizard have also been recorded (*Aprasia inaurita*, *Eremiascincus* spp., *Hemiergis decresiensis*, and *Lerista* spp.). More species of reptiles than mammals were recorded in seven of eight Australian studies where the species of both mammals and reptiles were listed (i.e. Bayly, 1976, 1978; Jones & Coman, 1981 (two of three study areas; Strong & Low, 1983; Catling, in press). In two of the studies reptiles were present in a larger proportion of the guts than were mammals (Bayly, 1976; Brooker, 1977), though they always formed a smaller proportion by volume or weight.

Diet of cats on islands

Introduced mammals   Although the islands that cats have been introduced onto differ enormously in size, climate, and native fauna, they tend to have the same few introduced mammals as prey and few, if any, native mammals. Of 22 islands where the food of cats has been studied, 15 have house mice, 10 have rabbits (*Oryctolagus cuniculus*), nine have *Rattus rattus*, six have *R. norvegicus*, and three in the South Pacific have *R. exulans*.

Where rabbits are available (on mid-latitude islands, grassland in New Zealand and on sub-antarctic islands) they usually form a large proportion of the diet; on average 55 per cent frequency of occurrence. On Hog Island, rabbits were not found in the guts of 12 cats, but a partly eaten young rabbit was found near a cat's den (Derenne & Mougin, 1976).

The frequency of rats in the diet of cats varies considerably between islands depending, at least in part, on the presence or absence of rabbits. On islands without rabbits, rats are usually present in more than 70 per cent of guts or scats, but on islands with rabbits they are the main food and rats are usually found in less than 5 per cent of samples (Table 10.3). The one locality with rat in more than 5 per cent of scats when rabbit was taken was the Orongorongo Valley, New Zealand, where rabbits were scarce and limited to a small part of the study area but rats were widely distributed. The low frequency of rats in the diet when rabbits are available may reflect the cats' preference

Table 10.3. *Frequency of rat in the diet of cats on islands with and without rabbits (references in Appendix 10.1)*

Islands with rabbits	% occurrence	Islands without rabbits	% occurrence
Grand Canary	4	Galapagos Isabela	73
N.Z. Te Wharau	3	Santa Cruz	88
Kourarau	Trace	Lord Howe	87
Orongorongo	50	Raoul	86
Mackenzie	2	Little Barrier	39
Kerguelen	0	Stewart	93
Macquarie	3	Campbell	95

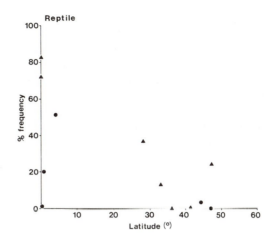

Fig. 10.4. Reptiles in the diet of cats on islands in relation to latitude. Frequency in guts or scats of cats by % occurrence. (Key: circles guts, triangles scats.)

for rabbit or low densities of rats. Perhaps rabbits sustain the cat population in sufficient numbers that the cats keep the rats at low densities.

House mice are most plentiful in the diet in studies at latitudes between 28° and 50°. Although they are present on several tropical islands where cats have been studied (Galapagos, Jarvis I. and Frigate I.), they were either not recorded in the guts or scats, or were recorded infrequently.

Birds Birds are a much more important part of the diet of cats on islands than on continents. In island studies bird remains were recorded on average at 51 per cent frequency of occurrence, and on continents at 21 per cent. Seabirds comprised a large proportion of the species of birds eaten, especially on the smaller oceanic islands; only on the New Zealand mainland and Stewart Island and on the north Atlantic islands of Grand Canary, Heisker and Helgoland did land birds predominate. Penguins were eaten on Dassen Island (Apps, 1983), Little Barrier Island (Marshall, 1961), Stewart Island (Karl & Best, 1982), Hog Island (Derenne & Mougin, 1976), Macquarie Island (Jones, 1977) and Marion Island (Van Aarde, 1980; Van Rensburg, 1985). Terns and noddies are important prey at warmer latitudes, including fairy terns (*Gygis alba*), sooty terns (*Sterna fuscata*), brown noddy (*Anous stolidus*) and grey noddy (*Procelsterna caerulea*). Petrels were the major group of seabirds recorded, including members of the following genera: *Puffinus, Bulweria, Fregatta, Oceanodroma, Pterodroma, Pachyptila, Pelecanoides, Procellaria* and *Halobaena*.

Although birds are a more important part of the diet of cats on islands than on the continents, rabbits and/or rodents are usually available and make a significant contribution. However, cat populations can persist on islands where there are no mammalian prey. On Herekopare Island, New Zealand (28 ha in size), cats were present for more than 40 years, living mainly on petrels, supplemented by some landbirds and invertebrates (Fitzgerald & Veitch, 1985). On Howland Island, central Pacific Ocean, cats were present from 1966 to 1979; terns, shearwaters and skinks were recorded eaten (Kirkpatrick & Rauzon, 1986).

Reptiles The frequency of reptiles in the diet of cats on islands shows a similar pattern to that on the continents, with high frequency at low latitudes (Figure 10.4). On Isla Isabela and Isla Santa Cruz, Galapagos, lava lizards (*Tropidurus albemarlensis*) and hatchling marine iguanas (*Amblyrhynchus cristatus*) were most important (Konecny, 1983). Laurie (1983) collected 475 cat scats on Isla Isabela for evidence of predation on marine iguanas and found remains of young, mainly hatchlings, in 20 per cent.

Frigate Island in the Seychelles has a rich fauna of reptiles and amphibians: nine species of lizard, three snakes, two caecilians and one frog (Cheke, 1984; Nussbaum, 1984a, b). Remains of two genera of skinks (*Mabuya* and *Scelotes* = *Pamelaescincus*), a gecko)*Ailuronyx*) and two snakes (*Lycoganthophis* and *Boaedon*) were found in 51.4 per cent of guts and the caecilian *Hypogeophis* in 8.6 per cent (C. R. Veitch & D. M. Todd, personal communication). The only tropical islands where reptiles were rarely recorded in the diet were Jarvis and Howland islands in the central Pacific (Kirkpatrick & Rauzon, 1986). Because of their isolation and small size these islands have impoverished reptile faunas compared with the Galapagos and Seychelles. A higher percentage of cat scats from Stewart Island contained lizard (all skinks, *Leiolopisma* sp.) than other islands and continental areas at similar latitudes (Karl & Best, 1982).

Size of prey

Prey of cats vary in size from small mammals and small birds, to adult rabbits, hares and some arboreal marsupials of similar size; pheasants, partridges and ducks are among the largest birds taken. Predation on the larger and more aggressive species of mammals falls chiefly on young animals. Rabbits taken are mainly animals less than half-grown (see e.g. Borkenhagen, 1978, 1979; Niewold, 1986). Cats often have difficulty killing full-grown rabbits and, because cats do not dig, capture young rabbits only after they emerge from their burrows (weight *c.* 200 g) (Gibb, Ward & Ward, 1978). In scats from Macquarie Island, over 80 per cent of 477 individual rabbits that could be put in size classes, weighed less than 600 g, i.e. were less than 70 days old (Jones, 1977) and in an Australian study almost three-quarters of the rabbits in cat stomachs were small young estimated at less than 50 days old (Catling, in press).

Rattus norvegicus is the largest species of *Rattus* eaten. In the laboratory Leyhausen (1979) found that few cats would fight an attacking, adult Norway rat and most of the rats caught were less than half-grown. Field observations by Childs (1986) yielded similar results: in alleys in a residential area of Baltimore, Maryland, 22 rats caught by cats all weighed less than 200 g (19 of them weighed less than 100 g) although most rats caught in live-traps weighed 300–400 g. This may explain why Elton (1953) found that cats, provided with supplementary food, kept farm buildings rat-free once rats were eradicated by other means, but cats could not eradicate established Norway rat populations. Presumably established populations contain mainly adult rats whereas colonisers are young

animals (see also below). On sub-antarctic Campbell Island Norway rats are abundant and are the main food of feral cats which are rare despite the plentiful food supply (Dilks, 1979). Perhaps many cats die when the rats are not breeding, and young rats are not available.

Selective predation on particular sex or age groups in smaller species is more difficult to determine. Christian (1975) live-trapped, tagged, and released *Microtus pennsylvanicus* and later recovered tags from scats of cats living nearby. Cats took the voles in the same proportions of males and females, and age classes, as were trapped in the population. However, Niewold (1986) found that common voles taken by cats were smaller, on average, than those trapped or flushed from their burrows.

Diet of males and females, adults and juveniles

Adult male cats are considerably larger and heavier than adult females (Borkenhagen, 1979; Niewold, 1986), and differences in their diets might be expected; but remarkably few studies have compared the diets of males and females. In the Netherlands male cats ate more lagomorphs and birds (especially pheasants), whereas females preyed mainly on microtines and other small mammals (Niewold, 1986). Similarly, in the mallee country in Australia (Jones & Coman, 1981), male cats ate more rabbit and large mammal, and less other prey than females did (Evan Jones, personal communication). In contrast, in Switzerland Goldschmidt-Rothschild & Lüps (1976) found that the numbers of mammalian and avian prey in males and females did not differ significantly. However, rabbits and pheasants were not recorded and the largest prey taken, apart from one hare, were water voles (*Arvicola terrestris*). Differences in diet of males and females might be expected to be greater in places where large prey that are difficult to capture are important (see also Chapter 9). In European studies, field prey were found in significantly more males than females in Switzerland (Lüps, 1972) but not in West Germany or the Netherlands (Borkenhagen, 1979; Niewold, 1986) (Table 10.4), and females brought home more prey than males did (Borkenhagen, 1978). These results may reflect the differing degrees of attachment that cats have to households.

Changes in diet with age are also poorly documented. Howe (1982) reported from a questionnaire

Table 10.4. *Percentages of male and female cats in Europe containing field prey. Totals (N) include animals with empty stomachs*

| Locality (Author) | Per cent with field prey | | N Males/ Females | χ^2 |
	Males	Females		
Switzerland (Lüps, 1972)	42.8	22.6	70/62	6.08, $p < 0.05$
Germany (Borkenhagen, 1979)	46.1	41.7	115/72	0.35, NS
The Netherlands (Niewold, 1986)	66.3	71.4	172/91	0.73, NS

survey that young cats (around 6–8 months old) bring home such invertebrates as spiders, craneflies, bluebottles and moths, some cats catching up to 180 invertebrates in their first year. On Herekopare Island, New Zealand, cats lived mainly on seabirds but also ate wetas (large flightless Orthoptera) (Fitzgerald & Veitch, 1985). Re-examining the data, I found wetas in 9 of 10 juveniles but only 5 of 20 adults, the difference between juveniles (i.e. those with milk teeth) and adults being highly significant (χ^2_c 1 df = 8.856, $p < 0.01$). In another small sample of 12 cats that I examined from Pureora Forest, New Zealand, in summer and autumn juveniles were feeding mainly on insects. Three juveniles weighing 0.7–1.0 kg contained remains of 14 beetles, three cicadas, one weta, one spider, and one house mouse. Three heavier juveniles (1.3–1.6 kg) all contained mice (and one a bird) as well as insects, and only the six adults contained remains of rats and rabbits. These results suggest that cats are well-grown before they kill larger prey, such as rats and rabbits. However, Catling (in press) found no significant differences in the diet of immature and adult cats collected in summer and autumn in semi-arid Australia where rabbits were important prey.

Seasonal variations in diet

Many studies provide some information on seasonal variations in diet though only the larger ones provide much detail. I have taken four studies as examples of changes in diet throughout the year, representing European, North American, Australian and island studies (Liberg, 1984; Hubbs, 1951; Jones & Coman,

1981; Evan Jones, personal communication; Fitzgerald & Karl, 1979 and unpublished data, respectively). These reveal the great variability of seasonal patterns; some prey are strongly seasonal at one locality but not at others, and at one locality some species may be strongly seasonal, and others not (Figure 10.5a–d).

In southern Sweden (Figure 10.5a) predation on rabbits was strongly seasonal, with large numbers of young rabbits eaten in spring and summer (Liberg, 1984). Similarly, in northern Germany young rabbits were taken from June to September (Borkenhagen, 1979). In California (Figure 10.5b) predation on lagomorphs, chiefly *Sylvilagus*, was recorded only between February and October (Hubbs, 1951). In Australia (Figure 10.5c) rabbits made up a large part of the diet of cats throughout the year, though reaching a peak in spring and summer (Jones & Coman, 1981; Evan Jones, personal communication) and a similar pattern was found in New Zealand (Figure 10.5d) though they were a much smaller proportion of the diet (Fitzgerald & Karl, 1979 and unpublished data).

Predation on microtine rodents in southern Sweden was not strongly seasonal (Liberg, 1984) but on California voles (*Microtus californicus*) was strongly bimodal, being important in spring and autumn (Hubbs, 1951). House mice were important prey of Californian cats from late autumn to early spring but were taken regularly throughout the year in Australia and New Zealand.

Birds were eaten most frequently in spring and early summer (Goldschmidt-Rothschild & Lüps, 1976; Borkenhagen, 1979; Liberg, 1984) but even then in Europe they were a small part of the diet whereas in California they were a large component (Hubbs, 1951). Reptiles were eaten seasonally; in California snakes were eaten from early spring to early autumn (lizards were not recorded) (Hubbs, 1951). In the mallee country of Victoria, Australia, reptiles were eaten from November to July (Evan Jones, personal communication) and at Yathong, western New South Wales, from September to May with peak amounts in December and April (P. C. Catling, personal communication).

Diet in relation to availability

Seasonal changes in diet are usually assumed to reflect changes in the numbers or vulnerability of prey, but

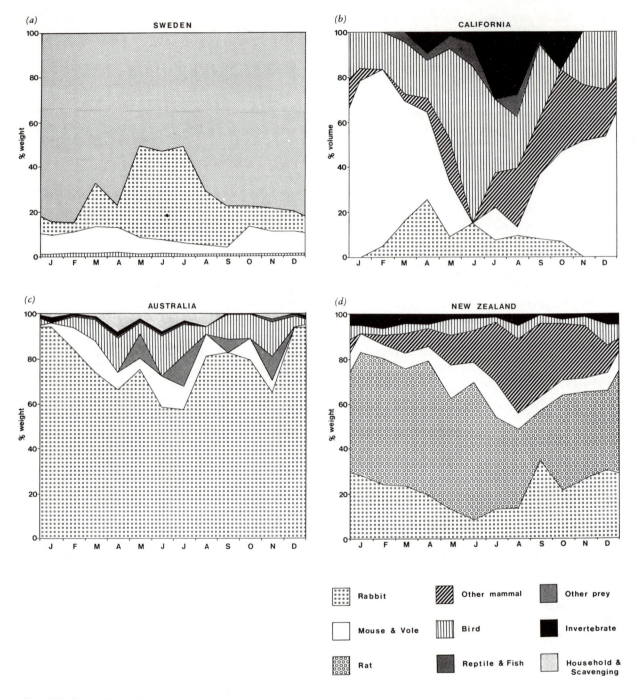

Fig. 10.5. Seasonal variation in the major categories of prey in the diet of cats in four studies (*a*) Revinge, southern Sweden (after Liberg, 1984), (*b*) Sacramento Valley, California (after Hubbs, 1951), (*c*) Mallee country, Victoria (after Jones & Coman, 1981; Evan Jones, unpublished data), (*d*) Orongorongo Valley, New Zealand (Fitzgerald & Karl, 1979, unpublished data).

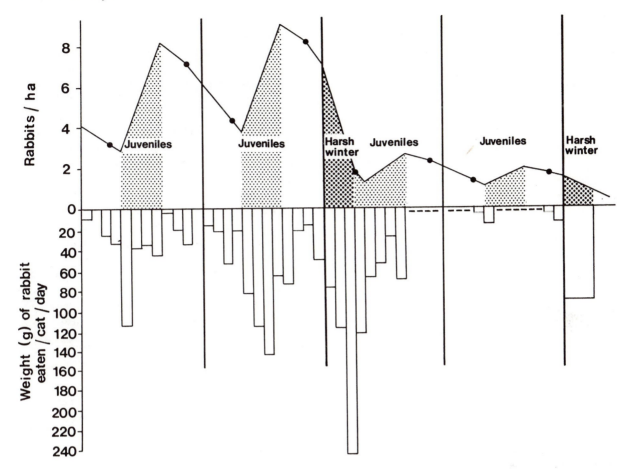

Fig. 10.6. Seasonal and annual variations in the number of rabbits at Revinge, southern Sweden, and the daily contribution, in g, of rabbit to the diet of cats, showing the increase when juvenile rabbits are available, and the heavy predation on rabbits in harsh winters. Dashes indicate periods when diet was not measured. (After Liberg, 1984.)

few studies of the diet of cats provide measurements of prey densities.

Liberg (1984) demonstrated that cats prey more heavily on rabbits when the rabbit population increases between May and September. Young rabbits entering the population then are easy prey for cats. Adult rabbits are vulnerable during severe winters; dead, dying and weakened rabbits were common in the severe winters of 1977 and 1979 and the cats fed more heavily on rabbits then than in other winters (Figure 10.6). After the winter of 1977 rabbits were

much less common and cats fed more on rodents although the rodents had not increased significantly. This example shows how changes in the numbers of a preferred prey can influence the level of predation on other prey.

In the Netherlands when voles become abundant house cats quickly move into the fields to feed on them and continue to hunt there as the vole population declines (Niewold, 1986).

Fitzgerald & Karl (1979 and unpublished data) obtained an index of the numbers of rats and mice in

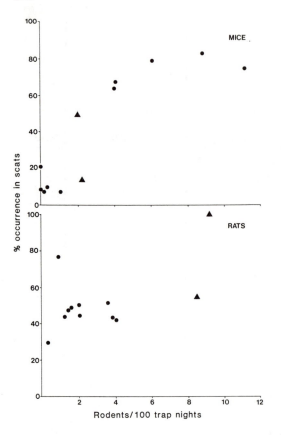

Fig. 10.7. Frequency of rats and mice in the scats of cats in the Orongorongo Valley, New Zealand, in relation to the density of rats and mice, based on snap-trapping. Circles, seasons in 1971–3 inclusive; triangles, January–June 1985 and August 1985–May 1986 (from Fitzgerald & Karl, 1979, unpublished data.)

a forest by standardised snap-trapping from 1971 to 1986. While the diet of feral cats was studied over three years (1971–3) the rat population changed very little and predation on rats also varied little. In contrast, the numbers of mice fluctuated dramatically and the proportion of the cat scats containing mice followed the changes in numbers. Since then the numbers of rats have quadrupled but the range of mouse densities has not changed. Fewer scats are now collected each month than previously and results for more months have to be pooled, but 22 scats were collected in January–June 1985 and 11 in August 1985–May 1986. A higher proportion of these scats

contained rat remains than those in 1971–3, indicating increased predation at higher densities of rats (Figure 10.7). However, contrary to Liberg's (1984) finding that cats took fewer rodents when rabbits were plentiful, we found that the proportion of cat scats containing mice did not decrease when rats were more plentiful.

The functional response of cats to changes in the density of small rodents (voles or mice) has two components; both the proportion of scats containing rodents and the number of rodents per scat can change. In the Netherlands when voles were common they were present in most cat stomachs examined and more voles were counted per stomach than when voles were scarce and infrequently eaten (Niewold, 1986). Similar results with cats preying on house mice were obtained by Fitzgerald & Karl (1979), but the number of rats per scat changed very little when the rats increased (Fitzgerald & Karl, unpublished data), presumably because one rat is a substantial meal.

Effects on prey populations

Opinions on the effects of predators on prey populations have changed over the years. Darwin (1872) clearly accepted that cats could limit the numbers of field mice when he recounted how cats, by destroying mice, limited predation by mice on nests of bumble bees, thus allowing more bees and greater pollination of clover: 'Now the number of mice is largely dependent, as everyone knows, on the number of cats'. Similarly, Elton (1927) and others contended that predators were important in controlling the numbers of their prey.

The contrary view was put forth by Paul Errington in a long series of papers, especially on bobwhite quail (*Colinus virginianus*) and muskrats (*Ondatra zibethicus*) (summarised in Errington, 1967). He considered that animals in good habitat were secure from predation and that the animals taken were a 'doomed surplus' living in poor habitat, whose removal, by one agency or another, made little difference to the populations. However, more recently, increasing numbers of studies have shown that predators play an important part in determining the population densities of their prey.

Assessing the effects of cats on prey populations is difficult because in studies on the continents the cat is usually just one of a suite of predators feeding on the prey populations and its effects cannot be isolated from those of other predators. Also, very few experiments, in which one population of cats is manipulated and another serves as a control, have been carried out to check conclusions drawn from natural history observations.

The effects of cats on prey populations are often divided into those that are beneficial, and those that are injurious to us. However, the effects on a species of prey can be injurious in one context and beneficial in another, so here each problem is treated independently.

Farmyard cats – can they control rats?

As humans learned to grow crops and store them in houses and granaries, rats and house mice would have quickly exploited the new source of food; cats probably soon moved in to prey on the abundant rodents and to scavenge (Robinson, 1984). Once humans and cats were living in close proximity the process of domestication could begin and humans probably encouraged this process in an attempt to control commensal rodents (see also Serpell, Chapter 11).

Despite this long association the effectiveness of cats in rodent control on farms has rarely been examined. In England during World War II Elton (1953) found that cats, supplied with supplementary food in the form of milk, could keep buildings free of Norway rats, once existing infestations were eliminated by other means. The effect of cats was usually restricted to areas within about 50 metres of the buildings where the cat dwelt. Their inability to eradicate existing infestations is probably explained by their predation being chiefly on young rats less than 100 g (Childs, 1986).

Even when rats are not eradicated from the buildings their seasonal population changes may be affected by the cats. In Baltimore, Maryland, Davis (1957) installed cats at farm buildings with Norway rats, and provided the cats with supplementary food; natural alternative prey were sometimes available. With cats present the rat population increased later in the spring, after the cats began preying on young pigeons, and declined earlier in the autumn than it had in previous years.

Control of rabbits in grassland

Farmers are concerned not only with the pests of stored food, but also with pests of field crops and pasture. A good example is the European rabbit which was introduced into Australia and New Zealand during the last century, and quickly reached plague numbers; although now greatly reduced in numbers, rabbits continue to be a concern for farmers.

In a 10-year study of a population of rabbits in an 8.5 hectare enclosure (reduced to 4.3 ha after 6 years), Gibb, Ward & Ward (1978) provided an excellent demonstration of the effects of predators (cats, ferrets *Mustela furo* and harriers *Circus approximans*). The rabbit population passed through two population cycles; in the first predators had free access, and in the second cats and ferrets were mostly excluded (Figure 10.8). After the first two years the rabbit population briefly reached about 120 rabbits per hectare and then declined over the next three years. The numbers of cats (and ferrets) seen hunting in the enclosure increased more slowly than the rabbits, and they were seen most commonly when the rabbit population was decreasing rapidly. In contrast, the more mobile harriers more or less tracked the rabbits and as rabbits became scarce, moved elsewhere. Through the long decline in numbers of rabbits (1960–3) there was ample evidence that the rabbits were breeding (many pregnant females were live-trapped) but in the breeding season 1961–2 only two young rabbits were seen above ground and few, if any, were seen in the following two seasons. However, during this period cats continued to prey on the few young rabbits emerging above ground and ferrets killed them in their burrows; as rabbits became scarcer the predators, especially ferrets, took increasing amounts of other prey. By mid-spring 1963 fewer than 3 rabbits per hectare remained (11 males and 2 females in total!). The cats and ferrets were trapped and removed and the enclosure fence was electrified to prevent predators from entering. Two weeks later young rabbits appeared above ground and survived (the first to do so in more than two years) and for the next three years survival rates of older rabbits were far higher than previously. The population increased dramatically for two years after most predators were excluded, reaching a peak of 172 rabbits/ha in the summer 1965–6. During the summer and the following winter many young rabbits died of starvation – the only time in 10 years that this happened. The rabbit population increased steeply again the following spring and early summer, whereas earlier, when predators were present, the rabbit population continued to decline to very low levels (Gibb, Ward & Ward, 1978).

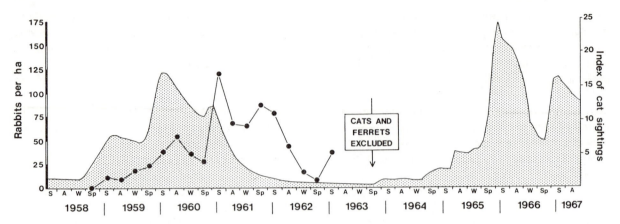

Fig. 10.8. Fluctuations in the numbers of rabbits in the Kourarau Enclosure, Wairarapa, New Zealand, in sightings of cats (—●—), and in the numbers of rabbits after cats and ferrets were excluded. Area of the enclosure 8.5 ha 1958 to mid-1962, reduced to 4.3 ha mid/1962 to 1967. (After Gibb, Ward & Ward, 1978).

Over much of New Zealand the high rabbit populations in the 1940s and early 1950s were reduced to low levels by poisoning and by night-shooting from four-wheel drive vehicles fitted with spotlights. Night-shooting was continued because it was considered to be an effective, if costly, method of destroying rabbits. In an experiment to test its effectiveness Gibb, Ward & Ward (1969) had night-shooting withdrawn from an area of about 1200 hectares of hill pasture and scrub for three years. At the beginning of the experiment rabbit populations were sparse, and distributed patchily in small groups. After three years there were slightly fewer rabbits on both the experimental and the adjacent control area. The rabbit population on the experimental area had relatively fewer young and more old animals than did the population on the control area, probably because cats and other natural predators favoured young rabbits and man shot mostly adult rabbits. Gibb, Ward & Ward (1969) concluded that the sparse rabbit population, operating at densities far below the food limit, 'was controlled primarily by predation, especially by feral cats'.

In a much larger Australian experiment the effect of carnivores on rabbit populations was examined at Yathong in western New South Wales (A. E. Newsome, I. Parer & P. C. Catling, unpublished). On a study area of approximately 300 square kilometres the numbers of rabbits were assessed by warren surveys and spotlight counts and the numbers of cats and foxes by spotlight counts. Rabbits built up to high densities in spring 1979, then crashed and remained at low densities for more than two years. During this fluctuation the numbers of cats and red foxes (*Vulpes vulpes*) increased and subsequently declined more slowly than the rabbits did; predation pressure was greatest in the six months after rabbits reached their lowest numbers.

Carnivores were then shot on an area of 70 square kilometres, later extended to 160 square kilometres, and 288 foxes and 112 cats were killed in 20 months. The spotlight counts and greater number of young animals killed in the second half of the experiment indicate that shooting was effective in reducing the carnivore populations. The rabbit populations on the areas where carnivores were shot increased significantly faster and reached higher densities than those on areas where carnivores were left. However, the effect of predators was confined to the period of population growth, the declines in the populations being imposed by the effects of severe summer droughts.

At Yathong the effects of predation were studied on a rabbit population that was occasionally devastated by summer drought; those results can be contrasted with ones from a rabbit population at Revinge, southern Sweden which was sometimes subjected to severe winters with snow on the ground for much longer than usual (Liberg, 1981, 1984; Erlinge *et al.*, 1984a). At Revinge rabbits were the main food of cats, and some other predators, but field voles were an important supplementary food, especially in winter, when young rabbits were not available. In years when rabbits were abundant, they formed half of the food of generalist predators, but were less important after the numbers of rabbits declined during a harsh winter; predators then ate more rodents. The authors estimated that 99 and 84 cats were present in spring 1975 and 1976 when the rabbit population was increasing and high, and 87 and 101 cats were present in the two subsequent years when rabbits had declined to about a quarter of their earlier numbers. The numbers of the five other species of generalist predators also changed very little despite the dramatic decline in the numbers of rabbits, and the predation pressure on the rabbits after they were reduced by the severe winter must have been intense.

Because Erlinge *et al.* (1984a) estimated that all predators together consumed only about 20 per cent of the annual production of rabbits (cats accounted for less than 4%) they considered that the rabbit population was not regulated by predators, but 'fluctuated stochastically (adverse winter weather and myxomatosis)'. However, the pattern shown in their Figure 1 is remarkably like those described by Gibb, Ward & Ward (1978), and A. E. Newsome, I. Parer & P. C. Catling (unpublished). In all three studies the rabbit populations increased over two or three years, declined very rapidly in the adverse conditions of drought or snow (Australia and Sweden), or less rapidly without adverse weather causing direct mortality (New Zealand), and then remained low for a further two years. This suggests that in southern Sweden, as in New Zealand and Australia, rabbit populations are, for much of the time, regulated by predators.

Rodents – voles in grassland, rats in forest

A species may be affected differently by predators, depending on whether it is their major food, or a secondary food. This is well illustrated by studies of predation on voles. In the studies in southern Sweden described by Erlinge *et al.* (1984a), the six species of generalist predators, including cats, preyed heavily on

rabbits; field voles formed a small proportion of their diet but the annual predation on voles and other rodents was of the same magnitude as the calculated annual production of rodents. Under these circumstances the vole population remained fairly stable between years and did not fluctuate cyclically as it does in northern Scandinavia, beyond the distributional range of rabbits (Erlinge *et al.*, 1983, 1984a).

In contrast, in California voles were the main prey of generalist and/or specialist predators, alternative prey were taken mainly later in the decline and trough in vole numbers and the vole population showed cyclic fluctuations (reviewed by Pearson, 1985). In a detailed study of a cyclic population of the California vole, Pearson (1964, 1966, 1971) measured the predation by feral cats, gray foxes (*Urocyon cinereoargenteus*), raccoons (*Procyon lotor*), striped skunks (*Mephitis mephitis*) and spotted skunks (*Spilogale putorius*) during three cycles. Predation pressure was greatest when the vole population was near the end of its decline and predation on alternative prey (gophers *Thomomys bottae*, brush rabbits *Sylvilagus bachmani*, and wood rats *Neotoma fuscipes*) allowed predators to remain longer on the area, preying on the remaining voles and reducing them to extremely low densities. Pearson (1966, 1971) concluded that predators were responsible for the timing and amplitude of the 3–4 year vole cycle. Here alternative prey were secondary in importance to voles, whereas in southern Sweden voles were secondary to rabbits and the interactions stabilised the vole populations.

In Poland intensive studies on the interactions between the common vole and its predators have been undertaken in agricultural land with its associated small woods and shelterbelts (Ryszkowski, Goszczynski & Truszkowski, 1973; Goszczynski, 1977). Common voles were the major prey of most predators, including cats, and the number of cats in the fields was strongly correlated with the density of common voles. When voles became plentiful cats increasingly left farm buildings to hunt in the fields and as voles became scarce returned to the buildings. The vole population fluctuated dramatically over four years; when they were abundant predators took a small proportion of the population, but as voles became scarce predators took a larger proportion and also took more forest rodents (*Clethrionomys glareolus* and *Apodemus* spp.). This pattern resembles that described by Pearson (1966, 1971) but here

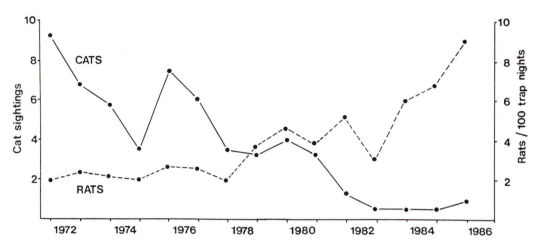

Fig. 10.9. Changes in the frequency of sightings of feral cats, and in the trapping index of rats (*Rattus rattus*) in the Orongorongo Valley, New Zealand, 1971 to 1986. Annual points are the means of the four seasonal figures. (B. M. Fitzgerald & B. J. Karl, unpublished data.)

alternative prey (forest rodents) are in different, but adjacent habitat.

In a 15-year study of predation by cats on forest rodents in the Orongorongo Valley, New Zealand (Fitzgerald & Karl, 1979 and unpublished data) the numbers of rats (*Rattus rattus*) and house mice were measured by snap-trapping for three nights each season, the numbers of cats by an index of sightings, and the diet of cats by scat analysis. Annually over the same period the sparse population of rabbits that lives along the edges of the river was censused by J. A. Gibb (unpublished data) by pellet surveys and by counts of rabbits on some areas; he also surveyed the vegetation in the rabbit habitat.

For the first three years of the study when the rat population was low and stable, rat remains were found in 40 to 50 per cent of scats in most seasons, rabbits were second in order of importance in the diet, and mice, whose numbers fluctuated irregularly, were eaten in relation to their availability (see Figure 10.7) (Fitzgerald & Karl, 1979). Since then the number of cats seen has progressively declined and they were very scarce during the last four years (Figure 10.9). (Some of our tagged cats were caught in gin traps set by possum trappers and we attribute the decline in cat sightings to trap mortality.)

The number of rats has increased four-fold over this same period (Figure 10.9) and the mouse population fluctuations have changed; earlier mice fluctuated markedly, reaching high numbers after heavy seeding of beech trees (*Nothofagus* species), and declined rapidly to low numbers again soon after. Recently the mouse populations have increased and declined slowly, apparently independently of beech seeding, a pattern not seen when cats were abundant. The rabbit population has also changed. The amount of habitat for rabbits has varied during the study, sometimes being reduced when floods destroy feeding areas. Now, with few cats, there are more rabbits relative to the amount of suitable habitat and vegetation than there were in the early phase of the study (J. A. Gibb, personal communication). These changes in the populations of three species of prey, differing in size, habits, importance as prey, and in the case of rabbits, in habitat, show patterns that might be expected if predation is important in their population dynamics.

Small game species – do cats compete with hunters?

Although much has been written about the effects of predators on small game species, few quantitative studies of the effects of predators have been conducted and even fewer of them have involved cats. Finding that a certain proportion of the guts of predators contain game species does not, on its own, make a good case for arguing that the predators are limiting the numbers of game. One also needs to know the density of the game species, its productivity, and mortality from predators and from other sources.

One study that provides such details has been carried out on brown hares and ring-necked pheasants in southern Sweden (Erlinge *et al.*, 1984b). Foxes and cats were the chief predators, taking about 90 per cent of the hares, and 80 per cent of the pheasants consumed by predators, though these prey formed only about 3 and 1 per cent respectively of the predators' diet. Predators ate at least 40 per cent of the annual production of hares and almost 60 per cent of pheasants; hunters shot far fewer hares, and less than half as many pheasants, as were taken by predators. The authors concluded that removing predators would probably increase the hunting bag for these species but were uncertain if it would increase the breeding density of hares and pheasants.

Hares, mostly young, formed a similar proportion of the diet of cats in Poland (Pielowski, 1976); foxes were the main predators, taking about 10 per cent of the young hares but few adults. Removing predators had little effect in hunting fields where hares were plentiful (Pielowski & Raczyński, 1976).

Effects on bird populations on continents

Predation on songbirds by domestic cats is noticed because it takes place during the day, whereas much predation on mammals takes place at night. People generally enjoy having birds in their gardens, and by providing food in winter may increase the numbers of birds. When cats kill some of these birds, people assume that cats are reducing the bird populations. However, although this predation is so visible, and unpopular, remarkably little attempt has been made to assess its impact on populations of songbirds.

A little information is available from the records of the fate of banded birds (Mead, 1982). In Britain 31 per cent of the recoveries of dunnocks (*Prunella modularis*) and robins (*Erithacus rubecula*) were of birds caught by cats, and for another four species more than a quarter of the recoveries were of birds caught by cats. For most species, age or sex of the bird had little effect on the risk of being taken. All six species feed on the ground or low vegetation and regularly live in gardens. The author considered that there was no

evidence that cats harmed the overall population levels of these birds; perhaps the populations of some species might be greater in the absence of cats, but no-one seems to have attempted to demonstrate this experimentally. It might also be argued, as Fitzgerald & Karl (1979) have done for feral cats in New Zealand, that cats may suppress the populations of other, more damaging predators such as rats, and thus allow denser populations of birds than would exist without them.

Another example of the complexity of indirect interactions between cats and birds is given by George (1974). He showed that domestic cats are important predators of voles and other small mammals in southern Illinois and suggested that because cats are also provided with food by their owners they can continue to hunt sparse populations of small mammals, and reduce their numbers much further than wild carnivores would be able to do. In southern Illinois this may leave insufficient prey to support wintering raptors, including red-shouldered hawks (*Buteo lineatus*), red-tailed hawks (*B. jamaicensis*), marsh hawks (*Circus cyaneus*), and American kestrels (*Falco sparverius*) in the numbers previously encountered.

As Mead (1982) emphasised, the birds in suburban and rural parts of Britain have coexisted with cats for hundreds of generations, and they may now be under less pressure from cats than they were in the past from the assorted natural predators. Any bird populations on the continents that could not withstand these levels of predation from cats and other predators would have disappeared long ago but populations of birds on oceanic islands have evolved in circumstances in which predation from mammalian predators was negligible and they, and other island vertebrates, are therefore particularly vulnerable to predation when cats have been introduced.

Effects on wildlife on islands

Endemic species of mammals were present on few of the islands where cats have been introduced but where they were present they have declined in numbers or become extinct. Hutias, rodents of the genus *Geocapromys* (family Capromyidae), are known this century from only three Caribbean islands. They disappeared from Little Swan Island, Honduras, after cats were released in the 1950s and are rare on Jamaica where the mongoose (*Herpestes auropunctatus*) may be a significant predator, but are still abundant on East Plana Cay, Bahama Islands, where they are undisturbed (Clough, 1976).

In the Galapagos Islands the endemic rodents (*Oryzomys* spp.) are now found only on those islands without cats (Konecny, 1983), although those islands also probably lack introduced *Rattus rattus*, which may compete with *Oryzomys*.

Birds (both landbirds and seabirds) have been affected most by the introduction of cats to islands but the impact is rarely well documented. In many cases the bird populations were not well described before cats were established and the possible role of other factors in changes in the bird populations are treated inadequately. Some island species have become extinct after cats became established on the islands, and island populations of other, more widespread species have been eliminated. An often quoted example of extinction is the Stephens Island wren (*Traversia lyalli*) from Stephens Island off the New Zealand coast, that was discovered, and exterminated, by the lighthouse keeper's cat in 1894. Only about 15 specimens are known, all brought in by the cat (Oliver, 1955). A more recent example of extinctions comes from Socorro Island, Mexico, where an endemic dove (*Zenaida graysoni*) became extinct and an endemic mockingbird (*Mimodes graysoni*) was reduced to the verge of extinction after feral cats were introduced by a small military garrison on the island in the late 1950s (Jehl & Parks, 1983).

Many other species have become endangered after cats were introduced to their island, and in time may become extinct. The kakapo (*Strigops habroptilus*), a large, flightless, endemic parrot, is almost extinct on the South Island of New Zealand and the small population on Stewart Island is endangered; feral cats are the major known source of mortality and remains of kakapo were found in 5 per cent of cat scats collected in the areas where kakapo are present (Karl & Best, 1982).

Many of the species of island landbirds that have been exterminated by cats are ground-feeding species. On Herekopare Island, New Zealand, five of the six species of landbirds that disappeared after cats became established, dwelt or fed on the ground, whereas of the six species of landbirds persisting, only two feed much on the ground (Fitzgerald & Veitch, 1985). Another New Zealand example of a species that feeds to a considerable extent on the ground being affected by cats is the saddleback (*Philesturnus*

carunculatus), which disappeared from three islands (Little Barrier, Cuvier and Stephens) soon after populations of cats were established in the last century. Saddlebacks have been successfully re-established on Cuvier Island since cats were removed in 1960–4 (Veitch, 1985).

The effects of cats on seabird populations have been even more dramatic. Many islands that had teeming colonies of breeding seabirds have become desolate places since cats were introduced. Ascension Island in the Atlantic Ocean had vast populations of nesting seabirds but by 1823 feral cats were abundant and now only the wideawake or sooty tern breeds in significant numbers on the island. Remnant populations of other seabirds breed only on isolated rocks and stacks around Ascension Island, particularly on Boatswain Island where ten species of seabird are found breeding, including the endemic frigate bird (*Fregata aquila*). Wideawake terns still breed on Ascension despite the cats, probably because they breed in large, dense colonies and leave the island entirely for three months after each breeding season, thus preventing the cat population from increasing beyond the numbers that can be supported during this lean period (Stonehouse, 1962).

On Raoul Island cats were introduced before 1870 and populations of the Kermadec petrel (*Pterodroma neglecta*) and black-winged petrel (*P. nigripennis*) among others have been exterminated. Sooty terns still breed there but their numbers appear to be declining, perhaps because, when the terns are away, cats have a more plentiful alternative food supply (*Rattus norvegicus* and *R. exulans*) than is available on Ascension Island (Taylor, 1979).

Sometimes these changes happen slowly (Fitzgerald, in press). Cats were introduced to Little Barrier Island, New Zealand, between 1867 and 1880; the grey-faced petrel (*Pterodroma macroptera*) was being preyed on heavily in the 1940s and ceased breeding there after 1963. Cook's petrel (*P. cooki*) and the black petrel (*Procellaria parkinsoni*) still suffered heavy predation in the early 1970s and their populations were declining, a century after cats were introduced.

The effects of cats on seabirds have been documented in some detail on Herekopare Island, New Zealand, where cats eliminated dense breeding populations of diving petrel (*Pelecanoides urinatrix*) and broad-billed prions (*Pachyptila vittata*) in about 45 years (Fitzgerald & Veitch, 1985). On other, sub-antarctic islands, diving petrels seem one of the species that disappears most quickly in the face of predation by cats. They were common on Marion Island in 1951–2 when cats were introduced, but no nests could be found by 1965–6 and they were very rare in 1976 although still abundant on nearby, cat-free Prince Edward Island (Van Aarde, 1980).

Another way of examining the changes that have taken place on islands after cats were introduced is by comparing present populations of seabirds on the islands with those of adjacent, cat-free islands. Major differences in the bird populations of cat-free and cat-inhabited islands are seen at Ascension (Stonehouse, 1962), in the Kermadecs (Merton, 1970), Macquarie Island (Brothers, 1984), Marion Island (Van Aarde, 1980) and Hog Island in the Crozet Archipelago (Derenne & Mougin, 1976). Species that are most vulnerable are small species that nest on the surface or in shallow burrows, and larger burrow-nesting species whose burrows cats can enter (Derenne & Mougin, 1976).

A further method of assessing the effect of cats on islands at the same latitude is by comparing the number of species of seabirds eaten by cats with the length of time cats have been present. We can compare three sub-antarctic islands, Marion, Hog, and Macquarie, between latitudes 46° and 54° S, where cats have been present since 1948, by 1887, and by 1820 respectively. Predation on seabirds was determined by gut analysis and by collecting and identifying remains of large numbers of seabirds killed and partly eaten by cats (Derenne & Mougin, 1976; Jones, 1977; Van Aarde, 1980; Van Rensburg, 1985). On these three islands the longer cats have been present, the fewer species of seabird they are eating (Figure 10.10).

Although we have seen that reptiles can form a significant part of the diet of cats on islands at low latitudes, few studies have related declines in reptile populations to predation by cats. In the Caribbean, an island population of the Turks and Caicos Islands iguana (*Cyclura carinata*), estimated in July 1974 at more than 15 000 individuals, was exterminated between 1976 and 1978 after a large hotel was built and feral cats and dogs increased in numbers. By 1978 predation on smaller lizards (*Anolis scriptus* and *Leiocephalus psammodromus*) was also noted and their populations had declined (Iverson, 1978). This

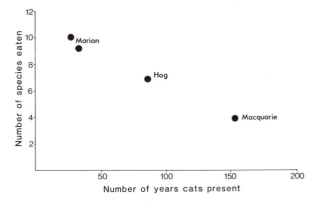

Fig. 10.10. Number of species of seabird eaten by feral cats on three subantarctic islands, based on gut contents and the uneaten remains of prey, in relation to the length of time cats have been present on the island. (Data from Derenne & Mougin, 1976; Jones, 1977; Van Aarde, 1980; Van Rensburg, 1985.)

case was better documented than most because the iguanas were exterminated at a time when their natural history and social behaviour were being studied. On other larger islands the process is often slower or happened so long ago that indirect evidence has to be considered.

On the Galapagos Islands the endemic marine iguana is in danger of extinction on some islands. Introduced cats, dogs, rats and pigs all feed on marine iguanas and their eggs; on islands with these predators the populations of marine iguanas are sparse and contain few, if any, juveniles. Remains of young, mainly hatchling, iguanas were found in 20 per cent of 475 cat scats on Isla Isabela and locally were more frequent (Laurie, 1983). Remains of hatchling iguanas were also found regularly in cat scats by Konecny (1983).

In the Fijian Islands dense populations of iguanas (*Brachylophus* spp.) and the large species of *Emoia* skinks are now found only on islands without cats; feral cats are present on virtually all islands inhabited by humans (Gibbons, 1984).

Concluding remarks

Predators can be categorised into several types, on the basis of their degree of specialisation (specialist or generalist) and mobility (resident or nomad) (Andersson & Erlinge, 1977). A review of the quantitative studies of the diet of house and feral cats shows that they are versatile generalist predators, exploiting a wide range of prey, and are able to switch readily from one prey to another. Andersson & Erlinge describe feral cats as partially migrating generalists because they switch from small rodents to domestic subsistence at certain times but they are probably better considered as resident generalists. Household food can buffer cats from population declines when field prey becomes scarce and they can continue to exert heavy predation pressure on favoured prey until the prey reach extremely low densities.

Cats on the continents are chiefly predators of small mammals, especially of young lagomorphs and of microtine rodents; birds form only a small part of their diet, and reptiles are even less important except at low latitudes, where they can be more important prey than is usually acknowledged. In contrast, where cats have been introduced to islands they live on a few species of introduced mammal (*Oryctolagus cuniculus*, *Rattus* spp. and *Mus musculus*) and birds, especially breeding seabirds. In the long term they usually eliminate the seabirds; the extinction of some endemic species of landbird has also been attributed to introduced cats. Every effort should be made to remove feral cats from islands that do not have permanent human settlements, and to ensure that cats are not released onto other islands.

The effects of cats (and other predators) are often ignored in studies of the population dynamics of small mammals but several studies on rabbits and rodents show that predators (including cats) strongly influence the population dynamics of their prey. The few experimental studies in which cats have been excluded or removed have been particularly informative. Cats are often able to reduce rabbit populations to low levels and maintain this trough in numbers for two or more years. Predation by cats on voles can be stabilising or destabilising. Where voles are their major food they, with other predators, may be responsible for generating the characteristic 3–4 year cycle in abundance, but where voles are secondary prey they may suppress the cyclic fluctuations and hold the population at low levels.

In his characteristically positive approach to research on predation, Pearson (1985) lists the variables that need to be measured if we are to understand the consequences to prey populations of predation, some of the methodologies that need to be developed or improved, and reminds us of the value of exploiting the many 'natural experiments' that are available, including islands with and without predators. There are, he suggests, some fascinating predator–prey interactions waiting to be revealed – and some of them I am sure will involve cats. Cats are ideal subjects for studies of predation. They are widespread, often at high densities, are sometimes tame and cooperative, and can be studied in varied circumstances and habitats.

Acknowledgements

I am indebted to many people who have helped with this review. Among them, Brian Karl has worked with me for many years and contributed much to our knowledge of cats in New Zealand. Peter Catling, Brian Karl, Alan Newsome, Ian Parer, Ray Pierce, David Todd and Dick Veitch provided unpublished data, and Michael Brooker, Evan Jones and Olof Liberg willingly delved back through their records to supplement published work. Phil Moors and Rachel Harvie provided translations, and Deirdre Garland and Patricia Sheehan library assistance. Jocelyn Berney typed the manuscript and Jocelyn Tilley prepared the figures. John Gibb and Dennis Turner gave constructive criticism of the manuscript.

Appendix 10.1

Studies of the food of cats, giving locality, latitude, whether the study is based on guts (stomach, intestine and rectum), scats or prey, sample size (for guts both the total sample and the number with contents) and whether results are presented as % occurrence, % volume, % weight or by the number of individual prey identified

Author(s)	Date	Locality		Guts, scats or prey	N = (N with contents)	Method of analysis
Europe						
Achterberg & Metzger	1978	Magdeburg, E. Germany	52°08'N	Stom., int.	67; 113; 90	occ., ind.
Achterberg & Metzger	1980	Haldensleben, E. Germany	52°18'N	Stom., int.	62	occ., ind.
Borkenhagen	1978	Kiel, W. Germany	54°20'N	Prey	309	ind.
Borkenhagen	1979	Kiel, W. Germany	54°20'N	Stom., int., rect.	187 (117)	occ., ind.
Farsky	1944	Czechoslovakia	c.49° N	Guts	96	occ.
Goldschmidt-Rothschild & Lüps	1976	Bern region, Switzerland	c.47° N	Stom.	257 (189)	occ., ind.
Heidemann	1973	N. part of W. Germany	c.54° N	Stom., int., rect.	156 (145) 11	occ., ind.
Heidemann & Vauk	1970	N. part of W. Germany	c.54° N	Stom., int., rect.	53 (47)	occ., ind.
Liberg	1984	Southern Sweden	55°42'N	Scats	1437	occ., wt.
Lüps	1972	Canton Berne, Switzerland	c.47° N	Stom.	135 (83)	occ., ind.
Niewold	1986	The Netherlands	c.52° N	Guts	337 (284)	occ., wt
Pettersson	1968	Stockholm, Sweden	59°20'N	Stom., int., rect.	70 (69)	occ., ind.
Pielowski	1976	Czempin, Poland	52°08'N	Stom.	500 (383)	occ.
Spittler	1978	N. Rhine Westphalia, W. Germany	c.51° N	Stom.	300 (224)	occ.
North America						
Bradt	1949	Michigan	c.42°45'N	Prey	1690	ind.
Davis	1957	near Baltimore, Maryland	c.39°20'N	Scats	129	occ.
Eberhard	1954	Pennsylvania	c.40°30'N	Stom., scats	202 (154) 32	occ., vol.
Errington	1936	S. Wisconsin	43°15'N	Stom.	50	ind.
George	1974	S. Illinois	37°30'N	Prey		ind.
Hubbs	1951	Sacramento Va., California	c.39°20'N	Stom.	219 (184)	occ., vol., ind.
Jackson	1951	Baltimore, Maryland	c.39°15'N	Stom.	500	occ.
Llewellyn & Uhler	1952	Patuxent, Maryland	39°05'N	Scats	15; 25	occ., vol.
McMurray & Sperry	1941	Oklahoma	c.34°40'N	Stom.	107 (84)	vol.
Nilsson	1940	Willamette Va., Oregon	c.44°30'N	Stom., scats	147 (86) 63	occ., vol.
Parmalee	1953	East-Central Texas	c.31° N	Stom.	33 (31)	occ., ind.
Toner	1956	Haliburton Co., Ontario	c.45° N	Prey	?	ind.
Australia						
Bayly	1976	South Australia	c.31'00'S	Stom.	14 (?)	occ., vol.
Bayly	1978	South Australia	c.30°20'S	Stom.	21 (20)	occ., vol.

Author	Year	Location	Latitude	Material	N	Notes
Brooker	1977*	Nullarbor Plain, WA	30°20'S	Stom.	9	occ., ind.
Catling	in press	Yathong Nature Reserve, NSW	33°45'S	Stom.	113 (104)	occ., wt
Coman & Brunner	1972	Victoria	c.37° S	Stom.	128 (80)	occ., vol.
Jones & Coman	1981	S.E. Australia	32°–37°S	Stom., int.	(131) (65) (117)	occ., wt.
Mahood	1980	W. NSW	c.33° S	Guts	<79	occ.
Strong & Low	1983	S. Northern Territory	c.24° S	Stom.	22 (20)	occ.
Triggs, Brunner & Cullen	1984	S.E. Victoria	37°25'S	Scats	48	occ.
Africa						
Rowe-Rowe	1978	Natal, S. Africa	c.29° S	Stom.	9 (8)	occ.
Islands						
Apps	1983	Dassen I., S. Africa	33°25'S	Scats	77; 131	occ.
Cook & Yalden	1980	Deserta Grande, Madeira	32°32'N	Scats	8 + frags	occ., wt
Corbett	1979	Heister, Monach Is, Scotland	57°32'N	Scats, prey	561; 451	occ.
Derenne	1976	Kerguelen	49°15'S	Stom.	89	occ.
Derenne & Mougin	1976	Hog I., Crozet	46°06'S	Stom., prey	12	occ.
Dilks	1978	Campbell I.	52°32'S	Scats	20	occ.
Fitzgerald & Karl	1979	Orongorongo Valley, N.Z.	41°21'S	Scats	677	occ., wt
Fitzgerald, Karl & Veitch	unpubl.	Raoul I., Kermadecs	29°15'S	Guts	(57)	occ.
Fitzgerald & Veitch	1985	Herekopare I., N.Z.	46°52'S	Stom., scats	32(30), bulk	occ., ind.
Gibb, Ward & Ward	1969	Te Wharau, Wairarapa, N.Z.	41°11'S	Scats	68	occ., vol.
Gibb, Ward & Ward	1978	Kourarau, Wairarapa, N.Z.	41°07'S	Scats	279	vol.
Heidemann	1973	Helgoland, North Sea	54°09'N	Stom., int., rect.	11 (10)	occ.
Heidemann & Vauk	1970					
Jones	1977	Macquarie I.	54°30'S	Stom., int., scats	41; 756	occ.
Karl & Best	1982	Stewart I., N.Z.	47°10'S	Scats	229	occ., wt
Kirkpatrick & Rauzon	1986	Howland I., C. Pacific	0°48'N	Stom.	8 (5)	occ., vol.
		Jarvis I., C. Pacific	0°23'S	Stom.	141 (73)	occ., vol.
Konecny	1983	Galapagos I.	0°15'–0°34'S	Scats	640	occ.
Marshall	1961*	Little Barrier I., N.Z.	36°12'S	Scats	94	occ.
Miller & Mullette	1985	Lord Howe I.	31°33'S	Stom., scats	(4) 12?	occ.
Pascal	1980	Kerguelen	49°15'S	Stom.	866	occ.
Pierce, R. J.	unpubl.	Mackenzie Basin, N.Z.	c.44° S	Guts	146 (133)	occ., wt, ind.
Santana, Martin & Nogales	1986	Grand Canary I.	28°00'N	Scats	588	occ.
Van Aarde	1980	Marion I.	46°50'S	Stom., prey	125 (116) 1224	occ.
Van Rensburg	1985	Marion I.	46°50'S	Stom., prey	(143) 429	occ.
Veitch, C. R. & D. M. Todd	unpubl.	Frigate I., Seychelles	4°35'S	Stom.	35	occ.

*plus additional information (Brooker, pers. comm.; Marshall, unpublished data of the late J. S. Watson in Ecology Division files).
Data for all New Zealand studies are given in Fitzgerald (in press).

V

Cats and people

11

The domestication and history of the cat

James A. Serpell

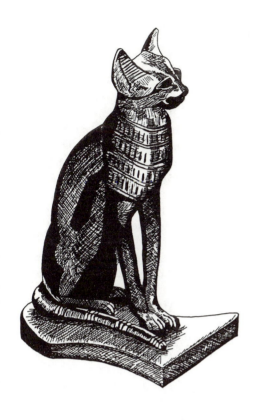

Origin

The systematic classification of small cats is still somewhat controversial. Kerby (1984) has recently grouped the European wild cat, the African wild cat and the domestic cat together as a single species, *Felis silvestris*. The domestic cat (*Felis silvestris catus*) is probably descended from the African subspecies (*Felis s. libyca*), although some authorities (see Zeuner, 1963; Clutton-Brock, 1981) have argued in the past in favour of a certain amount of hybridisation between the domestic cats and European wild cats (*Felis s. silvestris*), jungle cats (*Felis chaus*) and even Pallas's cat (*Felis manul*). Uncertainty about the precise origins of the domestic cat arise for several reasons. In terms of the morphology of its skeleton, the domestic cat differs relatively little from its wild relatives. In several modern breeds the skull tends to be broader and the facial region shorter than in many wild cats, but these characteristics are highly variable and generally unreliable as a means of distinguishing between the remains of wild and domestic forms. In general,

the archaeological contexts in which cat remains are found are often more informative than osteological evidence (Zeuner, 1963). Domestic cats have only recently been bred intentionally for specific characteristics and, compared with dogs, they appear to be genetically resistant to extreme modification. Domestic forms also hybridise, on occasions, with their nearest wild relatives. These various factors combined may help to account for their relative lack of morphological divergence from ancestral forms (Todd, 1977; Clutton-Brock, 1981).

Behavioural evidence also supports the subspecies *libyca* as the most likely ancestor of the domestic cat. The northern wild cats have a reputation for fierceness and timidity, even when hand-reared as kittens. Experimental attempts to rear them and tame them from an early age have been largely unsuccessful; the adults remain exceptionally shy and intractable. First generation hybrids between European wild cats and domestic cats also tend to resemble the wild parent in behaviour (Pitt, 1944). Although *silvestris* is unlikely to be entirely untameable, its domestication would have been a discouragingly long and time-consuming business. The African subspecies, however, appears to possess a far more docile temperament, and they often live and forage in the vicinity of human villages and settlements. During a visit to Africa during the nineteenth century, the botanist–explorer, George Schweinfurth, observed the local people catching and rearing young wild cats and keeping them, as adults, around their huts and enclosures (Guggisberg, 1975). Schweinfurth himself 'procured several of these cats, which, after they had been kept tied up for several days, seemed to lose a considerable measure of their ferocity and to adapt themselves to an indoor existence so as to approach in many ways to the habits of the common cat.' Similar observations on the comparative docility of *libyca* have been made more recently by Smithers (1968).

Finally, there are etymological reasons for believing that the cat is of north African or Near Eastern origin. The English word 'cat', the French 'chat', the German 'Katze', the Spanish 'gato', the fourth century Latin 'cattus', and the modern Arabic 'quttah' are all probably derived from the Nubian word 'kadiz', meaning a cat. Similarly, the English diminutives 'puss' and 'pussy' and the Romanian word for cat 'pisicca' are thought to come from Pasht, another name for Bastet, the Egyptian cat goddess (Beadle, 1977). Even the tabby cat is named after a special kind of watered silk fabric, once manufactured in a quarter of Baghdad known as Attabiy (Chambers 20th Century Dictionary).

Domestication

Fragments of bone and teeth, identified as belonging to *Felis s. libyca*, have been excavated from Proto-neolithic and Pre-Pottery Neolithic levels at Jericho, dating from between 6000 and 7000 BC (Clutton-Brock, 1969). There is no osteological evidence that these animals were domesticated, and it is probable that they represent the remains of wild cats killed for food or pelts (Clutton-Brock, 1969, 1981). Cat remains have also been recovered from the Indus Valley site of Harappa (*c.* 2000 BC) but, again, there are no conclusive signs of domestication.

On the basis of current evidence, it is likely that the cat was first domesticated in Egypt, although the probable date of this event is, at best, an approximation. The earliest pictorial representations of cats from Egypt date from the third millennium BC, but it

is often difficult to ascertain whether these animals were wild or domestic. One notable exception was found in the fifth dynasty tomb of Ti (*c.* 2600 BC), where a cat is depicted wearing a collar – a fairly positive indication of captive if not domestic status. More convincing evidence has come to light from a later tomb (*c.* 1900 BC), where the bones of seventeen cats were recovered together with little pots for offerings of milk (Mery, 1967; Beadle, 1977). From about 1600 BC onwards paintings and effigies of cats become increasingly abundant in Egypt, and it is likely that these animals were fully domesticated. Cats were illustrated sitting under their owners' chairs, eating fish, gnawing bones, playing with other animals, and even helping people to hunt birds among the papyrus swamps of the Nile Delta (Zeuner, 1963; Mery, 1967; Beadle, 1977).

The actual process that led to the domestication of the cat in Egypt has been the subject of considerable speculation. Kipling's Just-So Story, *The Cat that Walked by Himself* (see Macbeth & Booth, 1979 and Chapter 5), has stimulated some authors to argue that cats more or less domesticated themselves. The scenario runs roughly as follows. Like that of most of the ancient civilisations, the Egyptian economy was based largely on the cultivation and storage of grain. The abundance of stored grain in urban areas is likely to have attracted rodent pests and, if the Old Testament can be relied upon, these incursions of rats and mice occasionally reached plague proportions. Encouraged by the large and concentrated biomass of prey species, local wild cats will have taken to foraging in and around Egyptian homes, villages and temples. Meanwhile, the Egyptians, recognising the value of cats as pest-controllers, will have tolerated and promoted this mutualistic association until it became increasingly intimate and permanent (see Zeuner, 1963; Messent & Serpell, 1981).

While it clearly appeals to those who appreciate the cat's proverbial self-sufficiency and independence of spirit, this story portrays the people of Egypt in an uncharacteristically passive role. One of the more outstanding facets of Egyptian social and religious life was their overriding obsession with animals. From the earliest dynasties onwards, animal taming and pet-keeping seems to have been one of the principal Egyptian leisure activities, and it is unlikely that a people who tamed and kept monkeys, baboons, hyaenas, mongooses, crocodiles, lions and various wild ungulates (Smith, 1969) would have allowed wild cats to escape their attentions. As earthly representatives of gods and goddesses, and as the objects of religious cults, many of these species were well fed and cared for in captivity. Those, such as cats, that responded well to this sort of treatment, may eventually have bred and given rise to domestic strains, more docile and sociable than their wild progenitors. No doubt their hunting and rodent-catching abilities added to the value of early domestic cats, but it is likely that the Egyptians would have kept them as cult objects and as household pets regardless of any practical or economic advantage.

History

To the uninitiated, the religious beliefs of the ancient Egyptians appear little short of chaotic, with innumerable gods and goddesses; half human, half animal; merging, hybridising and diverging over time to produce a dazzling kaleidoscope of bizarre and exotic deities. It is likely that many of these gods and their animal representatives originated in predynastic times as tribal emblems or *totems* which were then consolidated, under the Egyptian State, into a single pantheon along the lines of those found in ancient Greece and Rome. As might be expected from their tribal (and regional) origins, the shifting status of these different gods often reflected the changing political fortunes of particular areas and groups within Egypt (see Mackenzie, 1913).

Cats played an important, if somewhat confusing, part in the Egyptian pantheon. The male cat was sacred to the sun god, Ra, and it was in the guise of a tomcat that the sun god battled each night with the typhonic serpent of darkness, Apep (Howey, 1930). The Egyptians were doubtless familiar with the sight of cats killing snakes, so perhaps they assumed that Ra would adopt the form of this animal when required to do likewise. Cats and lionesses were also associated with the warlike goddess, Sekhmet. According to Howey (1930), the use of the cat as a symbol of Ra was a late embellishment. The original conflict, she argues, involved the primordial Mother Goddess, variously invoked as Isis, Atet or Mut, and the Serpent of Evil. This idea makes sense in so far as the cat acquired far greater prominence in the Egyptian religion as a representative of the cat goddess, Bastet, and as a feminine symbol of fertility, fecundity and motherhood. Indeed, in early texts Bastet is referred to as the

daughter of Isis and Osiris, and some authors regard her as simply one of the later manifestations of the original Mother Goddess (Howey, 1930; Dale-Green, 1963). Like Isis, Bastet was associated with the moon, the source of the earth's fertility, and with lunar and menstrual cycles. Cats, with their nocturnal or crepuscular habits (but see Chapter 9), and their reputation for fertility and attentive maternal behaviour, were well-suited to be her earthly representatives.

One popular explanation for the association between cats and the heavenly bodies involves the widespread belief that a cat's eye changes in shape and luminescence according to both the height of the sun in the sky, and the waxing and waning of the moon. Plutarch and several other early authors refer to this characteristic of cats and, centuries later, the English naturalist, Edward Topsell, described the phenomenon in some detail in his *Historie of Foure-Footed Beastes* (1607):

The Egyptians have observed in the eyes of a Cat, the encrease of the Moonlight, for with the Moone, they shine more fully with the ful, and more dimly in the change and wain, and the male Cat doth also vary his eyes with the sunne; for when the sunne ariseth, the apple of his eye is long; towards noone it is round, and at the evening it cannot be seene at all, but the whole eye sheweth alike.

Nineteenth-century Chinese peasants apparently shared this belief, and actually used cats' eyes as a means of telling the time of day. The missionary, Pere Evariste Huc described the practice in his book *The Chinese Empire*, and observed that he had 'some hesitation in speaking of this Chinese discovery, as it may, doubtless, injure the interests of the clock-making trade.' The conspicuous eyeshine produced by cats' eyes at night intrigued many early writers. The majority seem to have believed that cats were able to generate this light themselves by storing light collected during the day (Aberconway, 1949). Many found the phenomenon disconcerting. Topsell, for example, states that the glittering eyes of cats, when encountered suddenly at night, 'can hardly be endured, for their flaming aspect.'

Although Bastet was worshipped in a small way from early times in Egypt, her cult did not achieve real prominence until the twenty-second dynasty (*c.* 950 BC). This change in status was associated with a political takeover by the Libyan Pharaoh, Sheshonk; a vigorous military ruler who established peace in Egypt after a long period of internal strife. He also, incidentally, formed an alliance with the Hebrews by marrying his daughter off to king Solomon. Sheshonk made his capital at Bubastis, east of the Nile Delta, and turned the local goddess, Bastet, into the official deity of the entire kingdom (Mackenzie, 1913). The cult later spread to Thebes, and continued to exert a powerful influence until Roman times.

Information about the cult of Bastet and Egyptian attitudes to cats are derived almost entirely from the writings of Herodotus, who visited Bubastis around 450 BC, and from those of the Roman writer Diodorus Siculus. According to Herodotus, the city contained a vast temple dedicated to the goddess, surrounded by two concentric enclosures and canals 30 metres wide. The vestibule of the temple was 20 metres high and beautifully ornamented with handsome figures. At the very centre stood an immense statue of the goddess. The temple also contained thousands of cats which were fed and cared for by the priesthood. The annual festival of Bastet, during April and May, was probably the largest in Egypt. As many as 700 000 people attended having first performed a pilgrimage by water along the Nile. The atmosphere was apparently festive, involving a lot of singing, dancing and good-natured bawdiness, and culminating in animal sacrifice and a sort of orgiastic drinking session (Howey, 1930; Dale-Green, 1963; Mery, 1967). There is little reason to doubt the authenticity of Herodotus's account as he was a remarkably keen observer. Among other things, he was apparently the first to record the phenomenon of male infanticide in cats. 'Females' he wrote, 'when they have kittened, no longer seek the company of males; these last, to obtain once more their companionship, practise a curious artifice. They seize the kittens, carry them off, and kill them, but do not eat them afterwards. Upon this the females, being deprived of their young, and longing to supply their place, seek the males once more' (see Krutch, 1961).

The status of cats during this period of Egyptian history seems to have been roughly equivalent to that of cows in present day India. Many people owned pet cats, and the death of one sent the entire family into mourning, shaving their eyebrows as a mark of respect. Those who could afford to had their pets embalmed and buried in special cat cemeteries, vast underground repositories containing the mummified remains of hundreds of thousands of these animals. In 1888, one of these sacred burial grounds was accidentally uncovered by a farmer, and the remains inside proved to be so numerous that an enterprising businessman decided to ship them to England for conversion into fertiliser. One consignment of nineteen tons of mummified bones arrived in Manchester which was estimated to have contained the remains of 80 000 cats (Beadle, 1977). The new soil additive, however, was mysteriously unpopular with English farmers, and the business venture proved to be a failure.

Live cats were a protected species in Egypt, and causing the death of one, even by accident, was a capital offence. Consequently, anyone encountering a dead cat fled immediately from the scene, lest others should think that they had a hand in its demise. Diodorus, writing in about 50 BC, recorded a diplomatic incident involving a cat during a rather sensitive period in Romano–Egyptian relations. A Roman soldier made the mistake of killing one and 'neither the officials sent by the king to beg the man off, nor the fear of Rome which all the people felt' were sufficient to save him from being lynched by angry mobs. The Egyptians also restricted the spread of cats to other countries by making their export illegal. They even sent special agents out to neighbouring parts of the Mediterranean to buy and repatriate cats that had been illicitly smuggled abroad (Howey, 1930; Aberconway, 1949; Dale-Green, 1963; Mery, 1967; Beadle, 1977). Despite all these precautions, cats did eventually spread to other areas although, initially, progress was slow.

An ivory statuette of a cat, dating from about 1700 BC, was found by archaeologists at Lachish in Palestine. Egypt and Palestine enjoyed strong commercial links at this time, and it is likely that Egyptian entrepreneurs lived there and brought their cats with them. A fresco and a single terracotta head of a cat (*c.* 1500–1100 BC) are also known from late Minoan Crete, another area with which Egypt probably had strong maritime connections. The cat does not appear to have reached mainland Greece until somewhat later. The earliest representation of the animal from Greece is on a marble block (*c.* 500 BC), now in the Athens Museum. It depicts two seated men, together with various onlookers, watching an encounter between a dog and a cat. There is an atmosphere of tense expectation to this bas-relief, as if the observers were anticipating, and perhaps looking forward to, a fight. Cats were not apparently common at this time and were kept largely as curiosities, rather than for any practical purpose. When troubled with rodents, both the Greeks and the Romans used domestic polecats or ferrets in preference to cats. During the fifth century BC the Greeks introduced cats to southern Italy but, again, the animal does not seem to have been particularly popular, except as a rather unusual and exotic pet. An attractive Neapolitan mosaic, dating from the first century BC, shows a cat catching a bird but, apart from this, there are few literary or artistic depictions of the species. The Romans failed to recognise the cat's vermin-destroying capabilities until around the fourth century AD when Palladius recommended the use of cats, rather than the more traditional ferret, for curbing the activities of moles in artichoke beds (Zeuner, 1963; Beadle, 1977). Cats were also slow to reach Asia. The earliest reference to cats in India dates from about 200 BC, and they probably reached the Far East and China somewhat later. Judging from contemporary illustrations, all of these early cats possessed the wild-type, striped or spotted tabby coat colour, and many feral cats around the Mediterranean still retain this ancestral *libyca* appearance.

The Romans were almost certainly responsible for introducing cats to northern Europe and other outposts of their Empire. Domestic cats were already present in Britain by the middle of the fourth century AD, and their remains have been found in various Roman villas and settlements in southern England. At Silchester, an important Roman site, archaeologists found a set of clay tiles bearing the impression of cat footprints. By the tenth century, the species appears to have been widespread, if not common, throughout most of Europe and Asia (Zeuner, 1963). Todd (1977) has pointed out that the cat owes much of its colonising abilities to the fact that it adjusts well to shipboard life. Judging from its present distribution, for example, the sex-linked-orange colour mutant (i.e. ginger, ginger and white, calico and tortoiseshell) appears to have originated in Asia Minor, and to have then been transported, possibly in Viking longships, to Britanny, northern Britain and parts of Scandinavia. Similarly, the tenth century, English, blotched tabby mutant seems to have spread down a corridor through France along the valleys of the rivers Seine and Rhône. For centuries these rivers have formed part of an important inland barge-route between the Channel Ports and the Mediterranean.

Changes in attitude

The gradual extinction of the pagan gods and goddesses, and the rise and spread of Christianity, produced a dramatic change in attitude to cats throughout Europe. From being essentially benevolent symbols of femininity and maternity associated with the Mother Goddesses Bastet, Minerva, Diana and the Norse goddess Freya, they became, instead, the virtual antithesis: malevolent demons, agents of the Devil, and the traitorous companions of witches and necromancers. In part, this change may have been politically motivated. In order to consolidate its power, the medieval Church found it necessary to employ extreme ruthlessness in suppressing unorthodox beliefs and in extirpating all trace of earlier pre-Christian religions. Because of its links with the widespread cult of the Mother Goddess, the cat was simply caught up in a wave of wholesale persecution and terror which swept through Europe and took centuries to dissipate.

During the thirteenth century, nearly all the major heretical sects – the Templars, the Waldensians, the Luciferans, the Manichaeans, the Paturini and the Albigensians – were accused of worshipping the Devil in the form of a black cat. Anti-heretical propaganda, inspired and disseminated by the agents of the Inquisition, described how their rituals involved the sacrifice of innocent children, cannibalism, grotesque sexual orgies, and obscene acts of ceremonial obeisance toward cats which were often kissed on the anus (*sub cauda*). Many heretics, needless to say, admitted to engaging in such practices when under torture.

As a degenerate survival of the ancient fertility cult, witchcraft was also closely associated with cats. Witches, most of whom were women, were believed to ride to their Sabbats on the backs of giant cats. They were also thought to be able to transform themselves into cats in order to disguise their diabolical activities and engage in nocturnal sexual orgies with demons (Howey, 1930; Dale-Green, 1963; Mery, 1967; Beadle, 1977). Topsell, writing in 1607, reaffirmed popular beliefs in the malevolent character of cats. He maintained, in what is perhaps an early reference to allergic asthma, that 'the breath and favour of Cats consume the radical humour and destroy the lungs, and therefore they which keep their Cats with them in their beds have the air corrupted, and fall into several Hecticks and Consumptions.' In parts of England and Scotland, until as late as the nineteenth century, cats were still viewed as the archetypal witch's familiar – demonic companions who carried out their mistress's evil designs in return for protection and nourishment (Serpell, 1986). Unfortunately for cats, these fantastic stories were all too effective in moving public opinion.

Throughout the Middle Ages and the early modern period, cats, particularly black ones, became the victims of enthusiastic persecution. On feast days all over Europe, as a symbolic means of driving out the Devil, they were captured and tortured, tossed onto bonfires, set alight and chased through the streets, impaled on spits and roasted alive, burned at the stake, plunged into boiling water, whipped to death, and hurled from the tops of tall buildings, all in an atmosphere of extreme festive merriment. And anyone encountering a stray cat, especially at night, felt obliged to kill or maim it in the belief that it was probably a witch in disguise (Howey, 1930; Dale-Green, 1967; Darnton, 1984). By associating cats with the Devil and bad luck, the Church provided the underprivileged and superstitious masses of Europe with a sort of universal scapegoat; something to blame and punish for all the numerous hardships and misfortunes of existence.

There also seems to have been an element of misogyny embedded in this hatred of cats. In contrast to the ancient religion of the Mother Goddess, Christianity was, and still is, an essentially patriarchal cult, dominated by an all-powerful male priesthood, and associated with distinctly ambivalent attitudes toward women. This love–hate relationship with women is exemplified by the image of the Blessed Virgin, on the one hand, and Eve, the begetter of original sin, on the other. The early Christian Church seemed to idealise women but, at the same time, portrayed them as lascivious temptresses who use their sexual charms to beguile, bewitch and subvert men. As symbols, cats fitted this negative perception of women rather well. They solicit physical intimacy and enjoy being stroked and caressed. But they are also notoriously coy and unpredictable; demanding affection at one moment, scratching or running away the next. Sexually, the female cat is highly promiscuous, unashamedly inviting the attentions of several males. But she is also a back-biter, and will often turn and attack her partner immediately after copulation. For centuries, proverbial wisdom has identified cats with women and the more threatening aspects of female sexuality (Darnton, 1984). The unmitigated cruelty cats have received as a result of this metaphor doubtless speaks volumes about the sexual insecurities of European males.

Europe was not, however, the only region to view cats negatively. Malevolent, spectral cats were a common element of oriental folklore, and in Japan popular legends existed of monstrous vampire cats which assumed the forms of women in order to suck the blood and vitality from unsuspecting men. The Japanese also applied the word 'cat' to Geishas on the grounds that both possessed the ability to bewitch men with their charms. According to superstition, the tail was the source of the cat's supernatural powers, and it was common practice in Japan to cut off kittens' tails to prevent them turning into demons later in life (Dale-Green, 1963). This belief may also help to explain the origin of the genetically-unique, bob-tailed cats of Japan.

The cat's somewhat ambivalent relationship with human society provides another possible clue to its victimisation. Together with the dog, the cat is one of the few domestic species which does not need to be caged, fenced in, or tethered in order to maintain its links with humanity. Cats, however, tend to exhibit a degree of independence which is uncharacteristic of dogs, and which inclines them to wander at will, and indulge in noisy sexual forays, particularly during the hours of darkness. In other words, cats lead a sort of double life – half domestic, half wild; part culture, part nature – and it was perhaps this failure to conform to human standards of proper conduct that led to their subsequent harassment. According to the psychoanalyst Carl Jung (1959), animals are often 'the expressions of the unconscious components of self.' Whether they are perceived in positive or negative terms as a result of this self-identification, however, depends presumably on the individual moral perspective of the person or culture involved. At the time of the medieval Inquisition, the Christian Church did everything in its power to suppress anyone or anything that tended to blur the physical, social or moral distinctions between human beings and the rest of brute creation (Thomas, 1983; Serpell, 1986). Perhaps by exploiting the comforts of domestic existence while, at the same time, enjoying the pleasures of a wild night on the tiles, the cat provided a metaphor for the unbridled, animal side of human nature, and thus encouraged its own remorseless persecution. Attitudes to dogs during this period differed according to class. Like the cat, ordinary street dogs, mongrels and curs became symbols of man's baser qualities – gluttony, crudity, lust, etc. The pets and hunting companions of the nobility, on the other hand, represented loyalty, fidelity, obedience and other desirable human attributes (Thomas, 1983). The latter image of the dog is nowadays prevalent in Western countries. But the image of the cat, it seems, is still tarnished by its earlier unruly reputation.

Although behavioural characteristics of animals often provide the basis for intolerant or disparaging attitudes, it should be emphasised that such effects are highly culture-specific. In the majority of Islamic countries, for instance, attitudes to dogs and cats are more or less reversed. The dog is regarded as unclean, and touching one results in defilement. Cats, on the contrary, are tolerated and, to some extent, admired.

Modern attitudes

From its sacred origins in ancient Egypt, the domestic cat has now spread to virtually every corner of the inhabited world. Indeed, modern statistics suggest that this species is now rapidly overtaking the dog as the most popular companion animal in Western countries (Messent & Horsfield, 1985). This trend, however, is very recent. In nineteenth-century zoological literature, cats were the most frequently and energetically vilified of all domestic animals. Whereas the dog was admired for its loyalty and obedience, the cat was despised and distrusted for its lack of deference and its failure to acknowledge human domination. Cats were also negatively portrayed as 'the chosen allies of womankind' (Ritvo, 1985). Attitudes to cats remain ambivalent to this day. In a massive survey of contemporary American attitudes to animals, for example, Kellert & Berry (1980) found that 17.4 per cent of those questioned expressed some dislike of cats, as against only 2.6 per cent who disliked dogs. The popularity of anti-cat literature seems to reflect these views. The small book of cartoons entitled *A Hundred and One Uses of a Dead Cat* (Bond, 1981) became a world best-seller, and sold over 600 000 copies in the first few months after publication. Various similar titles, such as the *I Hate Cats Book*,

The Second Official I Hate Cats Book and *The Cat Hater's Handbook*, were also highly successful (Van de Castle, 1983). (It is somehow difficult to imagine *A Hundred and One Uses of a Dead Dog* or a *Dog Hater's Handbook* achieving the same levels of popularity, and the fact that such books have not appeared in print suggests that publishers do not regard them as viable commercial propositions.) Many people still regard the sudden appearance of a cat as a sign of bad luck, and others fear or dislike these animals, perceiving them as furtive and untrustworthy. The cat's traditional association with women and female sexuality is still implied by the slang use of the term 'pussy' and, although research in this area is sparse, it is also tentatively confirmed by the results of some attitudinal surveys. A study of 3862 children aged between 8 and 16, for example, found that 18 per cent of girls questioned described the cat as the animal they would most like to be, while only 7 per cent of boys gave the same response. Dogs, on the contrary, were chosen with almost equal frequency – 34 and 32 per cent – by both sexes (Freed, 1965). One author has also recently claimed that homosexual males are more inclined to keep cats than so-called *real* men (see e.g. Fogle, 1983). Presumably this entire legacy of negative attitudes and perceptions will continue to decline, as people gradually learn to accept the benefits of living with this clean, affectionate and essentially companionable species.

Concluding remarks

Since it is based on extremely limited archaeological evidence and a fragmentary historical record, much of what can be said about the domestication and history of the cat is largely speculative. Judging from the evidence that exists, however, cats were probably domesticated in Egypt some 4–5000 years ago from the north African wild cat, *Felis silvestris libyca*. Cats have been valued since antiquity for their rodent-catching abilities and they have also acquired religious or symbolic importance in many societies. Attitudes towards them as symbols, however, have ranged from reverence to abhorrence. We have seen that in ancient Egypt, cats were worshipped and jealously protected as representatives of Bastet or Pasht, a goddess of fertility and motherhood. In medieval and early modern Europe, on the contrary, cats became a metaphor for many negative human attributes, and were persecuted and despised for their alleged links with necromancy and witchcraft. In symbolic terms, cats still appear to excite a certain ambivalence of feeling in many Western countries although, within the last 50–100 years, they have attained unprecedented popularity as companion animals.

12

The human–cat relationship

Eileen B. Karsh and Dennis C. Turner

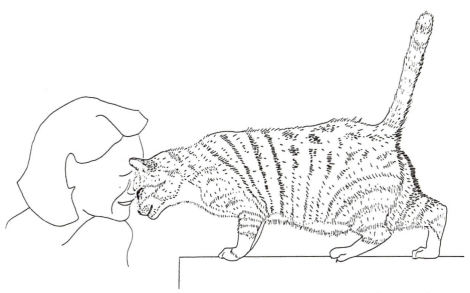

Introduction

Cats and people seem to have a natural affinity for each other. Yet historically, the relationship between people and cats (which goes back as far as we have records) has been an ambivalent one (Leyhausen, 1985b). During some periods such as the contemporary one, the attitude toward cats has been positive, characterised by long-term attachment, while at other historical times it has been negative with much hatred shown toward cats. The Egyptians seem to have been genuinely attached to their cats. Not only were cats worshipped and protected, but families kept cats as companion animals. When an Egyptian family's cat died, it was mourned (grief at loss – a sign of attachment) and mummified (an expensive procedure – another sign of attachment, Zeuner, 1963). At the same time there is evidence that Egyptian priests raised colonies of cats, which were sacrificed, mummified, and sold.

Later, when cats spread over Europe, they were loved and appreciated as companion animals for some time. Celtic monks were fond of cats and made beautiful cat illustrations; Chaucer wrote of pampered cats in England (Wright & Walters, 1980). Then a widespread persecution of cats began in the thirteenth century, encouraged by the Church, and it lasted for about 450 years. Thus by medieval times, the pendulum had swung back to a predominantly negative attitude. Cats were feared as associates of witches and embodiments of the devil. Cats were burned ritually on bonfires, boiled, or roasted alive. People hunted and killed cats. A person who kept a cat was in danger of being burned as a witch. (See Serpell, Chapter 11, for a more detailed history.) At the present time cats are popular again. The number of households with cats in the USA has been increasing rapidly and has recently surpassed the number of households with dogs. Books featuring Garfield, an overbearing cartoon cat, have been runaway best-sellers for more than five years. Yet the attitude is not completely positive, as can be seen by the successful publication of a cartoon book detailing many uses for a dead cat. How has this relationship between people and cats developed? This chapter reviews the scientific evidence concerning the cat-to-person relationship and also what is known about the person-to-cat relationship.

Socialisation

Socialisation refers to the process by which an animal develops appropriate social behaviour toward conspecifics. Typically, an infant animal (or person) first relates to its parents (usually the mother), then to litter mates or siblings, next to peers, and finally to other members of its species. To study the normal socialisation process, scientists have frequently interfered by taking an infant animal away from its mother and/or litter mates (deprivation or isolation experiments), or by exposing the infant to an unnatural substitute or caretaker. This substitute has sometimes been an object, sometimes a member of another species, and sometimes a person. For example, Konrad Lorenz (1935), in an early demonstration of imprinting, divided a clutch of goose eggs in half and, after hatching, left half the goslings with the mother and exposed the other half to himself. Upon testing, the goslings that had been exposed to Lorenz followed him.

Scott and his associates have done extensive work on the development and socialisation of dogs. Virtually all of the testing of social behaviour involved social responses toward human handlers. In an early paper describing developmental stages which were observed in 73 puppies over a four-year period, Scott & Marston (1950, p. 25) stated that 'the behaviour patterns exhibited by dogs toward human beings are essentially the same as those exhibited toward dogs.' In a more recent paper, Scott (1980, p. 134) acknowledged that 'most of the experiments with social attachment in dogs have concerned their attachment to humans.' He further stated that the attachment process is normal for dogs and not peculiar to the dog–human relationship.

In these studies, the use of a person as a socialising agent seems to have been a convenient accident; the experimenter was there and easily available. It is only very recently, within the past six years, that we have begun to focus on the relationship between animals and people as an important problem in its own right for both pure and applied science. Therefore, although we will review many relevant studies, we will concentrate our attention in this chapter on those experiments which have been specifically designed to investigate the relationship between cats and people.

Socialising cats to other species

The earliest work in socialising cats to other species was done by the Chinese biologist Zing Yang Kuo in the late 1920s and 1930s. Kuo wanted to demonstrate that so-called 'instinctive' behaviour patterns were a product of environmental as well as genetic components. In his first, and most well known paper, Kuo (1930) showed that when kittens were reared with rats, they grew up to be cats that did not kill their cagemates and usually did not kill other similar rats. Kuo wrote another paper which was not published until 1960, although the work had been done much earlier. In this later study, Kuo raised kittens with other species (puppies, rabbits, rats, and birds) for 10 months in large enclosures. He had different combinations of animals, for example five kittens and one puppy or one kitten and five puppies, in different groups. He found that animals were more likely to become attached to conspecifics, if they were available. Without conspecifics, a single kitten would become attached to the puppies. He measured attachment in the following way: he would take all the animals out of the pen except for one kitten, who would become restless, cry and look as if it was in great distress. If the kitten lived with five puppies, as soon as he put in a puppy, the kitten calmed down. However, when the kitten lived with four other kittens and one puppy, the kitten remained restless and distressed in the presence of the puppy until another kitten was put in the cage.

Separation distress has been a traditional measure of attachment. The first author has measured separation distress in her earlier studies (Karsh, 1983a) for comparability to other experiments (see Rheingold & Eckerman [1971]) and found that a person reduced crying in both handled and non-handled kittens almost as much as the presence of the mother, but not as much as the presence of a litter mate.

A colleague of the first author, Luci Paul (unpublished studies), repeated part of the earlier Kuo experiment. Paul raised groups containing a kitten and a rat, two kittens, or a kitten alone. In both the kitten-with-kitten and kitten-with-rat groups, Paul got clear evidence of attachment. When a kitten's cage-mate was removed, the kitten emitted distress cries and became agitated. This was followed by cessation of movement, lack of play, and failure to eat. Paul found no difference in kitten-to-rat *vs* kitten-to-kitten attachment. However, she did not have a condition where kittens were exposed to both another kitten and a rat, which was the type of condition where Kuo found greater attachment to the conspecific.

Another study raising kittens with puppies was done by Fox (1969). Fox found that kittens that were raised with a Chihuahua pup starting at four weeks of age, played with other pups without showing fear when they were 12 weeks old. On the other hand, kittens that had had no experience with pups until 12 weeks, avoided pups and behaved defensively when approached by them.

Cat-to-person attachment
Socialising cats to people

In a series of early handling studies in the late 1950s, investigators of early experience focused on the increased stimulation provided by handling infant animals. Although this handling experience was momentarily stressful to the young animal, it seemed to have beneficial effects. The handled animals showed accelerated development in maturation of the central nervous system and in physical development. Several studies investigated this type of handling effect on cats. For example, Meier (1961) found that handling Siamese kittens for 20 minutes daily for the first 30 days of life increased their rate of development. Handled kittens opened their eyes one day earlier, emerged from the nesting box 2.6 days earlier, and developed Siamese coloration earlier. The effects of early handling have subsequently been reinterpreted. It appears that handling rat pups causes them to emit distress cries which, in turn, stimulate the mother to increase her maternal behaviour (Thoman & Levine, 1970). Meier's maturational acceleration may also have been mediated through the mother.

A later study (Wilson, Warren, & Abbott, 1965), ostensibly on the effects of infantile stimulation, really produced evidence of cat-to-person attachment. Twenty cats that were handled (for 5 minutes daily from birth to 45 days) approached a person (sitting on a chair in the middle of a 3.6 square metre enclosure) sooner (35 sec for handled *vs* 105 sec for non-handled) and contacted the person more frequently than the non-handled cats did. The first author (Karsh, 1983a)

replicated these results closely. She found that eight cats that were handled for five minutes daily approached a person faster (32 sec) than seven non-handled cats (128 sec).

Shortly after Wilson *et al.* (1965), Collard (1967) also did a study where kittens were handled but now the handling was regarded as a social experience. Collard was interested in the effects of handling on fear of strangers and on play behaviour. Kittens, from 5½ to 9½ weeks of age, were handled by one person, by five different people, or by no person. During the first week of the experiment, the kittens were carried for one minute and held in the lap and stroked for three minutes. For the next three weeks, the kittens were carried or held for only one minute and then were called by the experimenter or were enticed to play with a string. Collard found that the five-person kittens showed the least fear of strangers (as measured by number of escape attempts when held by a stranger). However, the one-person kittens played more and showed more social behaviour, particularly toward the person who had handled them. They purred, played with the familiar person's hands or clothing, and made over twice as many playful or affectionate contacts (climbing on, rubbing against, mouthing, etc.) as the other kittens. These are striking findings when the small amount of handling is considered.

The early handling studies, such as Meier's (1961), looked at the effects of handling from birth to weaning on precocious development. However, in this paper, we are mainly concerned with the effect of handling during the socialisation period on attachment of cats to people, as initiated by Wilson *et al.* (1965) and Collard (1967).

Sensitive period of socialisation

The changing concept of the sensitive period The term 'critical period', taken from embryology, was introduced to animal behaviour by Konrad Lorenz (1937) in relation to imprinting. Imprinting refers to the development of a strong social attachment by precocial infant animals to their mother (or a substitute, initially Lorenz himself) and frequently involves a following response. Precocial young (typically birds such as goslings, ducklings, chicks, but also some mammals like lambs and goats) are born in a well developed state (they are able to walk the same day they are born) and they typically follow the first moving object they see, normally their mother, and develop a strong attachment to her. The imprinting process in precocial young was thought to be confined to a short critical period very early in life, which had a definite onset and an equally well defined offset. The social attachment or preference was presumed to be permanent and irreversible. Bateson (1987a) has characterised this early version of imprinting as based on a permanent image left by experience on the 'soft wax' of the developing brain. Slower-developing altricial young (such as kittens, puppies, and human infants) also form social attachments but during a longer period of time, beginning a little later in life due to their slower maturation.

In a well known laboratory experiment, Hess (1959) exposed isolated mallard ducklings to a male decoy and found a sharply defined period for imprinting from 12 to 18 hours after hatching. Fear responses to strange objects, which appeared at age 20 hours, seemed to be the limiting factor. This type of result was usually explained by an internally-determined sensitive period which Bateson (1987a) likened to a window opening on the external world for a pre-determined time and then closing.

Subsequent research in the 1960s and 1970s (reviewed by Bateson, 1979 and Immelmann & Suomi, 1981) has led to a number of changes. The term 'critical period' has been replaced by 'sensitive period', with the latter term implying a less definitive onset and offset. Evidence for an extended gradual decline in sensitivity was generated by a series of experiments by Immelmann (summarised in Immelmann & Suomi, 1981) who misimprinted male zebra finches on Bengalese finch foster mothers and was then able to alter their sexual preferences for the foster species by extensive cohabitation with zebra females. The older the male was when exposed to his own species, the longer the contact required to change his preference.

Both Bateson (1979, 1987b) and Immelmann & Suomi (1981) agree that the onset of the sensitive period is primarily determined by the sensory and motor development of the animal but can be altered by environmental changes. For example, birds exposed to patterned light can learn earlier than dark-reared birds. Bateson (1981a, 1987a) has proposed a two-stage model based on competitive exclusion to explain the offset of the sensitive period. The first stage, called the recognition system, has a large capacity to deal

with learning about familiar objects. The second-stage executive system controls behaviour and has a limited capacity. Bateson (1981a) attributes the narrowing of responsiveness to familiar objects, which occurs in imprinting, to the connection from a particular store in the recognition system gradually dominating access to the executive system which controls social behaviour. This domination by the first object is not necessarily irreversible if a second object can also gain access to the executive system. The second object can come to be preferred at a later time if the majority of connections between the first object and the executive system become inactive. The rate at which a stimulus gains control of the executive system seems to be related to a richness–impoverishment dimension. A rich stimulus, such as the bird's natural mother, dominates the executive function rapidly, while an impoverished stimulus, such as the pattern of the walls of an isolation cage, gains access much more slowly. As the limited-access connections to the executive system are completed, the sensitive period draws to a close. The differential rate of gaining access for more and less biologically suitable stimuli can explain the lengthening of the sensitive period which is found when animals are isolated or their stimulation is restricted. We will apply this model, in a later section, to the first author's data for the sensitive period of socialisation in the cat.

Another important distinction between the 'critical' and 'sensitive' period is in restrictiveness. The critical period concept confined the development of attachment within its boundaries, while the sensitive period definition deals with relative difficulty and relative probability of forming social attachments. Within the sensitive period, attachments are formed easily and fairly rapidly. At other times, attachments may be formed, or preferences may be changed, but it is a much more tedious process involving extensive exposure.

Bateson (1983) discusses different instances where adult social and emotional behaviour patterns are dramatically altered late in the life of both humans and animals. Of particular interest is the stress-induced attachment, which is much like imprinting, but occurs in adults. Bateson's example of a Soay sheep, undergoing a difficult birth, that had to be anaesthetised in order to remove the lamb, and who forever after followed people, is not that unusual. The first author has encountered this type of stress-induced attachment in cats. Her most striking example was a male breeding cat, obtained from another laboratory as an adult, who became ill with a high fever, and after being medicated and recovering, began to follow her around and continues to do this whenever possible. The stress-induced attachment appears to be mediated by nor-adrenalin which facilitates neural plasticity (Bateson, 1983) and essentially recreates the conditions under-lying imprinting.

Social isolation studies   A number of studies by other researchers have demonstrated the profound effects of raising animals in total isolation, with no contact with any member of their own species or with any other living thing. Most of this work has been done on dogs and monkeys. Harlow & Harlow (1962) found that total isolation during the first 6–12 months of life produced asocial monkeys that exhibited bizarre behaviour and none of the social, sexual, or defensive behaviour that is typical of the species. Scott (1970) also found that puppies that were isolated during their socialisation period (3–12 weeks) did not develop attachments to other dogs or to people.

Much less has been done in isolating cats, perhaps because cats have been generally believed to be less social to begin with (Leyhausen, 1979). Kuo, in his last study (1960), isolated cats for a long period of time (from birth to 10 months). The cats were then tested twice weekly for their reactions to a strange animal (cat, dog, rabbit, rat, guinea pig, canary, parrot, sparrow). Kuo described the reactions of the isolated cats to other animals as predominantly hostile and attacking. Seitz (1959), in an early weaning study, did not seem to realise that in addition to weaning, he also subjected his kittens to isolation. He took kittens that were two weeks old, separated them from their mothers, and put each kitten in an individual cage for the rest of its life. Other kittens were weaned and separated at 6 and 12 weeks. When all the cats were tested at nine months, the early-weaned and isolated cats displayed excessive undirected activity, disorgan-ised behaviour, fear of novel situations, and inability to tolerate delay in feeding. In a conflict situation they were not deterred by discomfort. Their hyperactivity, disorganisation, and tolerance of discomfort were similar to the behaviour of totally isolated dogs (Thompson & Melzack, 1956). Seitz's early-weaned cats showed aggression and non-cooperation in a food-competition test, while cats from the other two

groups cooperated. This is hardly surprising since the early-weaned cats were isolated throughout the entire socialisation period to be described in a following section.

Sensitive period of socialisation in dogs   Scott and his associates originally observed the development of 73 puppies (Scott & Marston, 1950) and classified their early development into three periods: the neonatal period, the transition period, and the period of pri-mary socialisation when attachments are formed to conspecifics, to other animals or people, and to places.

Freedman, King & Elliot (1961) tested Scott's critical period hypothesis by handling different groups of puppies, beginning at 2, 3, 5, 7 and 9 weeks. The puppies in the control group were not handled for 14 weeks. During testing, the 5 and 7 week dogs were the most responsive to human contacts while the control dogs never formed close attachments to people and were extremely fearful of human contacts. Scott (1970) claimed that he had somewhat arbitrarily placed the end of the critical period at 12 weeks (between the 9 and 14 week groups) and that a major limiting factor was the development of a fear response to strangers. This increase in fear response had also been thought to limit socialisation in other species (Hess, 1959). Scott, Stewart & DeGhett (1974) con-cluded that they could define the period of primary socialisation as extending from 3 to 12 weeks for the dog.

Sensitive period of socialisation in cats   Fox (1970) was the only investigator who had described the socialisation period in cats. He characterised it as beginning at 17 days of age (compared with 23 days for the dog), when increased sensory abilities and improved locomotor abilities enable the kitten to interact with the environment and with litter mates. In a later, popular book, Fox said, 'As in the dog, there seems to be a critical period early in life (ranging from four to eight weeks) when kittens are most easily socialized with people. The attachment can be enhanced by giving the kitten a lot of handling' (Fox, 1974, p. 139). No published experiments were cited in support of this statement. Later, Beaver (1980, p. 83), in a book on feline behaviour, stated that the socialis-ation period in cats . . . 'probably ranges from three to nine weeks of age.' She referred to Scott's (1962) work with puppies and also to the Fox (1974) book, so there appear to be no published data on the timing of the socialisation period for cats prior to that described below.

In what follows, we present an investigation into the sensitive period of socialisation for the cat by the first author. A pilot study and three subsequent experiments, involving over 100 kittens, were carried out during the period from 1981 until 1986.

The first experiment used three groups of kittens which were handled at times that were chosen to represent the presumed beginning of the socialisation period (three weeks), the middle (seven weeks), and after the end (no handling for 14 weeks). The middle value of seven weeks for onset of handling represents a time when many people adopt kittens and begin handling them. It is about the age represented in most pet care books as the best time to begin handling, although this may indeed be too early an age to adopt cats as pets (see Chapter 13).

All the cats used by the first author were British shorthair cats. They were born and reared in the Feline Behavior Laboratory at Temple University. Newborn kittens were caged with their mothers in large maternity cages until 8 weeks of age. The other cats and kittens lived in groups in a free environment in colony rooms. All the cats in these studies lived with other cats from birth to maturity. All cats, handled or not handled, had exposure to people working in the laboratory for routine feeding and cleaning procedures every day. Some observation and testing took place in the cat's home room (holding) while other tests were conducted in an enclosure (1.8 m × 1.8 m) in a testing room.

Shortly after birth, kittens in each litter were randomly assigned to three treatment groups. One group had early handling from 3 to 14 weeks, the second group had late handling from 7 to 14 weeks, and the third group had no handling during the 3 to 14 week period. The handling procedure consisted of an experimenter holding a kitten on his/her lap and stroking or petting it for 15 minutes daily. Each kitten was handled by four experimenters on different days.

Two response measures that have been found to be highly related to a cat's friendliness or attachment to people were used (Karsh, 1983a). The first measure involved one assistant holding a cat while a second assistant recorded how long the cat stayed with the

person. The person did not actively restrain the cat. Holding started after fourteen weeks and continued every 2–4 weeks until each cat was one year or older.

The second measure involved approach to a person in the testing enclosure. First the cat was adapted to the test situation; then the cat was removed and a person was seated at the far corner of the room on the floor, with a chalk line drawn at a distance of 15 centimetres around the person. The cat was introduced and the time taken to reach the person (latency) was recorded. Trained observers also recorded time spent with the person within the chalk line during a three minute test period and other friendly responses such as head and flank rubs, purrs and chirps. Approach testing also started after 14 weeks and was done every 2–4 weeks until the cats were one year or older.

For the holding measure, the early-handled cats stayed over twice as long (41 sec) as the non-handled cats (15 sec). This difference was significant ($p < 0.001$). The early-handled cats also stayed longer than the late-handled cats (24 sec, $p < 0.025$).

In the approach-to-person test, the latency measure (time taken to reach the person) was shorter for the early-handled cats (11 sec) than for the non-handled cats (39 sec), and this difference was significant ($p < 0.025$). The mean latency for the late-handled cats (42 sec) was close to that of the non-handled cats (39 sec). In observing and interacting with these cats during testing and in their home rooms, it was obvious to everyone working in the lab that the late-handled cats behaved more like the non-handled controls.

Since the sensitive period for cats appeared to taper off much sooner than had been surmised, it seemed reasonable that it might begin earlier also. Moelk (1979) had reported striking effects of handling and talking to kittens when she started interacting with them shortly after birth. Considering this, in the second experiment, kittens were handled earlier, at the end of the first week, and these very-early-handled kittens were compared with kittens handled starting at three weeks of age, as before; in both cases handling continued to 14 weeks of age.

In the second experiment the handling procedure was the same as in the previous one except that these kittens were all handled for a longer period of time (40 min daily). This was because longer handling seemed to increase attachment, as found in another experiment which will be described in a subsequent section.

The mean scores for the very-early-handled cats and the early-handled cats in this experiment were not significantly different for any measure. But they were in the direction one might expect if the sensitive period were to begin before three weeks. For holding, the mean for the very-early-handled cats was 77 seconds and for the early-handled cats it was 70 seconds. For latency to approach a person, the very-early-handled cats averaged 9 seconds while the early-handled cats averaged 13 seconds. In time spent with the person in the approach test, the very-early-handled cats spent 94 seconds while the early-handled cats spent 91 seconds.

The results of this study and the previous one suggested that there is a sensitive period of socialisation for cats which seems to begin sooner, reach its peak sooner, and taper off sooner, than the comparable socialisation period for dogs. The small (although non-significant) differences found between the two groups handled starting at 1 week or at 3 weeks suggest that the sensitive period may start between these values, perhaps at 2 weeks. The greater and reliable differences between groups where the handling began at 3 and 7 weeks indicated that the most receptive time (peak period) for socialising cats to people is earlier than 7 weeks. This contrasts with the finding of peak social receptivity at 7 weeks in dogs (Freedman et al., 1961). Finally, the closeness of the group handled from 7 to 14 weeks and the non-handled control group would argue that the socialisation period for cats has tapered off greatly by 7 weeks.

The third and most supportive experiment involved 75 kittens. In the two prior experiments, kittens were handled for different numbers of weeks. The group started at 3 weeks was handled from 3 to 14 weeks, the group started at 7 weeks was handled from 7 to 14 weeks. In this study each kitten was handled for exactly 4 weeks, and different groups were handled from 1–5, 2–6, 3–7, and 4–8 weeks.

If the sensitive period were from about 2 to 7 weeks as implied by the two previous experiments, then cats handled from 2–6 and 3–7 weeks would show higher attachment scores than the other 2 groups, and this appears to be true. The average scores for each group, using data from all 75 subjects, with 17–21 cats per group, are shown in Table 12.1. The mean holding scores of the cats handled from 2–6 weeks (109 sec) and 3–7 weeks (108 sec) are longer than those of the

Table 12.1. *Holding scores in seconds as a function of handling period*[a]

| | Handling period (weeks) | | | |
	1–5	2–6	3–7	4–8
For all cats				
Group size	18	21	19	17
Holding scores	86.88	108.96	108.06	87.35
For non-timid cats				
Group size	13	17	16	13
Holding scores	109.98	126.05	120.45	103.57
For timid cats				
Group size	5	4	3	4
Holding scores	26.82	36.32	42.02	34.64

[a]Values for Experiment 3: see text.

cats handled from 1–5 weeks (87 sec) and 4–8 weeks (87 sec).

A one-way analysis of variance did not show a significant main effect of the different handling periods, even with the large number of subjects per group (17–21), because of great individual differences among the cats. Karsh, who had been investigating temperament/personality variables for other reasons (as discussed in the following section), hypothesised that about a dozen timid cats were causing excessive variation in the data. The analysis of variance was redone as a factorial, keeping handling periods as the first factor and adding timidity (timid vs non-timid) as a second factor, using an adjustment for unequal numbers of subjects in groups (Winer, 1962). Sixteen timid cats, 3–5 in each handling group, were chosen by using ratings from three assistants who had known all the cats well. Only cats that were rated as very timid by all three raters were designated as timid.

Timidity proved to be a significant factor ($p < 0.001$) which did not interact with handling periods ($F < 1$). This can be seen by examining mean holding scores for timid and non-timid cats in each handling condition, shown in Table 12.1. The overall mean for non-timid cats was 116 seconds, over three times as large as the mean for timid, 34 seconds. The planned comparison between cats handled from 2–6 and 3–7 weeks vs those handled from 1–5 and 4–8 weeks was significant ($p < 0.05$) for non-timid cats. Thus the results of this experiment indicate that the sensitive period of socialisation for cats to people is from 2 to 7 weeks of age. The data from this experiment are quite compatible with an explanation using Bateson's (1981a, 1987a) competitive exclusion model. Kittens that are reared with their mother and littermates are exposed to strong, rich, biologically suitable stimuli. Those stimuli are expected to promote rapid growth of neural connections and thus gain access to the executive system controlling social behaviour. Since the executive system has limited access and rich stimuli can capture this access rapidly, other potential attachment objects, such as a person or persons must be present near the onset of the socialisation period in order to gain access to the executive system (i.e. to have social behaviour directed toward them). As objects become familiar to the kittens and capture access to the executive system (control social behaviour) the sensitive period draws to a close. This means it will be more difficult, but not impossible, for new objects to control social behaviour at a later time.

How should socialisation be carried out in life situations? Should kittens be adopted when they are very young (2–4 weeks of age)? We say emphatically 'no'. Kittens should *not* be adopted before they are weaned naturally at about 8 weeks. The stress of early separation from the mother and littermates can cause later behavioural problems such as hyperactivity (Seitz, 1959) or excessive sucking and wool-chewing. Karsh has found that as long as kittens are handled by people during the socialisation period, it is relatively easy for them to relate closely to other people when they are placed in homes one, two, or even three years later. Cats that have not been handled at all during the sensitive period of socialisation can be rehabilitated but it is a laborious task requiring much time and patience.

Factors affecting cat-to-person attachment

This section covers several factors which can affect the degree of attachment which develops between a cat and a person (or persons). Studies have been conducted in different cat colonies where the amount of time a kitten was handled varied between less than one minute per week (Rodel & Turner, unpublished) to 40 minutes daily (Karsh, 1983b). Additional variables such as the number of handlers, experience after the sensitive period, the presence of the kitten's mother, and feeding also influence the development of a cat–person relationship.

Amount of handling The first author became interested in the influence of amount of daily handling upon attachment in the context of another study. She had placed kittens born in her laboratory in private homes at younger than usual ages (4 weeks) to see whether early adoption increased the kitten's attachment to their person. When these kittens were brought into the laboratory to be tested monthly, it was apparent that their behaviour in relation to a familiar person was both qualitatively and quantitatively different from the behaviour of laboratory kittens. For example, in the approach-to-person test, a laboratory-reared kitten would approach the person, give the person a few head rubs, then leave the person's vicinity and come back several times. The home-reared kittens would go directly to the person, climb on the person's lap, purr, and go to sleep. These home-reared kittens had been handled for 1–2 hours daily, while the laboratory kittens were only handled for 15 minutes per day. Karsh (1983b) then performed an experiment to see whether longer handling would increase attachment responses in laboratory cats. She found that cats which had been handled for 40 minutes stayed significantly longer (73 sec) in the holding test than cats handled for only 15 minutes (43 sec) did. They also approached a person significantly faster (10 sec *vs* 30 sec) but did not stay with the person much longer (88 sec *vs* 81 sec). The home-reared cats performed better than the 40-minute-handled, laboratory-reared cats on both tests: their mean holding score was 111 seconds, and time spent with the person was longer (127 sec); both these differences were reliable but the difference in approach time (7 sec for home-reared *vs* 10 sec for 40 minute lab-reared) was not significant ($p < 0.10$). It is quite clear that increasing the daily handling time (from 15 to 40 min) increased attachment responses for the laboratory cats. However, differences still remained between the home-reared cats and the longer-handled laboratory cats. Whether these differences were due to still longer handling or to other factors is uncertain. The adopters of the home-reared cats reported that one or more family members interacted with the cats between one and two hours daily. This is similar to Turner's (1985b) findings that cat owners in Zürich said they were occupied with their cats (including feeding and cleaning as well as petting) for an average of 86 minutes per day. Besides possible longer daily handling, and almost certainly more handling at later ages (Karsh's cats were never systematically handled beyond the period specified in the experiment), home-reared cats have opportunities to interact with people that do not exist for laboratory cats. For example, laboratory cats usually do not have a chance to follow people around (they are not allowed in the hallways), to come when called, to 'help' with meal preparation, or to engage in extended interactions with people.

Number of handlers Considering Kuo's (1960) findings cited earlier, that a kitten reared with only puppies became very attached to the puppies while a kitten reared with other kittens and a puppy became much more attached to the other kittens, the first author decided to produce maximum cat-to-person attachment by placing kittens at an early age (4 weeks) and having them handled exclusively by one person. The first case went well. Two kittens that were semi-rejected by their mother and were completely weaned during their fourth week, were adopted by a student who kept them at home and was the only person to handle them until they were 14 weeks old. In two subsequent cases, Karsh found that she could not control the number of people handling the kittens once they were adopted, so she moved the study back to the laboratory. It then became an experiment where the number of handlers was varied: eight kittens were handled by one person while eight littermates of these kittens were each handled by four people. Collard (1967), also cited earlier, had shown that kittens handled by one person made more social responses than kittens handled by five persons. Collard's kittens were handled only very briefly during the first 4 weeks. Collard began handling more toward the end of the socialisation period. Kittens were handled from 5½ to 9½ weeks and they were tested once weekly during this same period. Even though Collard found that her one-person kittens averaged over twice as many 'playful or affectionate contacts' (climbing on, rubbing against, etc.) as her five-person kittens, it was not clear that these differences would persist when the kittens matured. Karsh's kittens were handled from 3 to 14 weeks (including most of the socialisation period). Most kittens were handled for 40 minutes daily. When Karsh considered all ten one-person cats (8 from the lab, 2 home-reared by the student) she found that the one-person cats could be held significantly longer (81 sec) by their person than by another person (48 sec, $p < 0.001$). If only the eight

laboratory-reared cats were used for comparison, the results are similar; they stayed for 84 seconds when held by 'their person' and only 49 seconds when held by someone else, again a reliable difference ($p < 0.01$). Five of the 10 one-person cats showed very strong differences between their handler and another person, three showed moderate differences, and two had little or no difference. This was even true for the two home-reared litter mates; one was strongly attached to her person and the second showed less difference between her person and a stranger. In the group of eight laboratory cats, four showed great attachment to their person and the others showed weaker attachment or no measurable attachment. The two cats who did not react differentially to the handler and other people were both very active cats and Karsh (1983b) has found that active cats do not test well. When holding scores for the eight one-person lab cats, held by their handler (84 sec) were compared with the holding scores of their littermates (77 sec) who were handled by and tested by four different people, they were similar. The one-person cats seemed to react negatively to non-handlers (49 sec) rather than more positively to handlers. The non-handlers were not strangers, they were lab assistants who were familiar to the cats.

Mother presence during early contact with humans Most studies on the effects of early handling (petting) of kittens on their later attachment to humans have ignored the fact that the mother cat is normally present during early kitten–human contact periods and may influence the course of events leading to the establishment of her kittens' relationships with humans. Turner (1985b) proposed looking at the effects of both mother presence and early handling together; Rodel (1986) has done this in her recently completed thesis at the University of Zürich-Irchel. She found that when the kittens' mother was present (but restrained) in the encounter room along with the test person, the kittens entered the room on their own at an earlier age than those kittens tested without their mothers; but they went directly to and stayed near their mothers and not the test person. However somewhat later, these kittens were still the first ones to start exploring the encounter room with the test person. It is Rodel's interpretation that at the beginning the mother cat and human can be viewed as competitors for the kitten's attention and that the more familiar mother wins at this stage. If the mother has been socialised to humans, her calm presence may reduce the kitten's anxiety (build up its confidence), allowing exploration of the environment, and through this, may actually facilitate establishment of a relationship between the kitten and human. If, on the other hand, the mother is shy (a condition Rodel did not have), she might induce her kittens to be even more frightened by humans than if they were exposed to people without their mother. Additionally, the trauma of being exposed to the test person in the absence of the mother might also have been expected to promote attachment to the human; but apparently this was not the case.

The mother may also indirectly influence her kittens' attachment to humans in another way, if she has free access to areas outside of the house. Turner (1988) suggests that if she hides her nest with kittens for a sufficiently long period the first human contact may come after the sensitive period for socialisation; and an interesting but, to date, unanswered question is whether mother cats who tend to do this are themselves less attached to their owners. But we caution the reader from assuming that only 'indoor' mothers produce candidates for well-attached kittens; for example, the second author has found many such human-attached cats on farms.

Effects of later experiences with humans Although early experience with humans during the sensitive period probably produces more lasting effects on attachment than experiences gained after that period, the latter should not be completely ignored. In a field study Meier & Turner (1985) were able to classify 35 cats that Meier had encountered outside their houses into either 'shy' or 'trusting' behavioural types, based on their reactions to her. Later, the cats' owners qualitatively classified 32 of these 35 into the same type as the authors did. During the interviews, eight owners were able to answer the question, 'Has your cat had a negative experience with a stranger?' precisely and describe that experience. Six of their cats had been classified as 'shy', based on their reaction to the test person; two, as trusting. And for one of the latter two, the owner related that ever since her cat had been struck by a family member, the cat was only trusting toward strangers. The second author is currently developing a model to explain the interplay between early and later experience on attachment to humans, which will be tested in the field.

Feeding and the human–cat relationship For many cat owners, especially owners of cats free to roam outside the house, feeding time may represent one of the regular contact periods between the human and the cat. Additionally, owners often suggest that the family member who feeds the cat has a 'better' relationship with the cat than other family members. The second author recently directed a study on this by Geering (1986), who set up the following experiment. The cats in a research colony were fed by an animal caretaker in a large outdoor enclosure. During a control phase of 11 days, two persons unknown to the cats entered the enclosure immediately after they had finished feeding and stood 'motionless' (without interacting with the cats) equidistant from the food trays on opposite sides of the enclosure. From day to day their positions were assigned randomly to eliminate any side-preferences the cats might have for the enclosure. During this control phase, one of the two test persons was statistically preferred by the cats, i.e. approached more often ($p < 0.005$). Then, during the following experimental phase, the non-preferred test person fed the cats without speaking to or touching them. He left the enclosure right away; then both test persons entered it again and took up their randomly assigned positions. During the first half of this experimental phase, the new 'feeder' was statistically preferred; during the latter half neither test person was preferred. Geering interprets these results as follows. The act of feeding a cat can enhance the establishment of a relationship, but it is not sufficient to maintain it. Other interactions (petting, playing, vocalising, etc.) are required to cement a newly founded relationship.

On the other hand, regular feeding at the home base certainly influences the potential for a long-lasting human–cat relationship by ensuring that a free-roaming cat more or less regularly returns to that home base. Liberg & Sandell (Chapter 7) have concluded that the spacing of females in an area is determined by the distribution of food (provided at households) and that male spatial organisation, especially during the mating season, is determined by female distribution. However, when males are also fed at home, their ranging behaviour is certainly influenced by the supplemental feeding (see Turner & Mertens, 1986).

Cat temperament/personality and attachment to people

About 60 years ago, Pavlov (1927) observed different temperaments in his dogs and he classified them into two categories: excitable and inhibited. Pavlov also concluded that the excitatory temperament could interfere with conditioning. If there were not enough stimulus changes, excitable dogs would get bored during conditioning and fall asleep.

More recently Hart & Hart (1984) have attempted to assess the suitability of different breeds of dogs as companion animals by developing behavioural profiles for each breed. The data used were forced-choice rankings made by 96 veterinarians and obedience judges. Their most prominent trait, in terms of reliability, was excitability which was combined with several other traits in a cluster dimension called reactivity. This excitability–reactivity dimension seems highly similar to Pavlov's (1927) excitatory temperament, although no reference is made to Pavlov by these authors. In the same paper, Hart & Hart presented a brief description of breed-specific behaviour of cats based on the opinions of four cat-show judges. For example, Siamese cats were described as outgoing, demanding of attention, and vocal, while Persians were described as lethargic, reserved, inactive and not desiring close contact due to their heavy coats.

Abyssinians were called shy, fearful, and too nervous for children. Although Hart & Hart pointed out that the judges emphasised that there are major individual differences between cats of the same breed, they nevertheless concluded that 'the value of selecting a pure-bred rather than a mixed breed is that one has more success in predicting what a cat will be like as an adult' (1984). The association of different personality types and behaviour patterns with different breeds of cats is an interesting question, but the answer would require standardised observations of many cats of each breed by trained observers.

Feaver, Mendl & Bateson (1986) assessed the distinct individual style or personality of 14 female cats living in a laboratory colony by observers' ratings and also by direct behavioural measurements. The two observers, who did not initially know the cats, familiarised themselves with the cats' behaviour through both formal and informal observations in the cats' living quarters over a three-month period. At the end of this period, both observers rated each cat on 18 dimensions. Ten of these dimensions (e.g. active, aggressive, curious, equable) were adopted from a list developed by Stevenson-Hinde *et al.* (1980b) for rhesus monkeys and the other eight (e.g. agile, fearful of people, hostile to cats, vocal) were chosen by the authors. The correlations between the observers'

ratings were significantly positive for 15 of the 18 rated items, but only those seven items where the inter-observer correlations were 0.70 or greater were used for further analysis. When inter-item correlations were calculated, the seven items fell into three groups: (a) alert = (active + curious) / 2, (b) sociable = (sociable with people − fearful of people − hostile to people − tense) / 4, (c) equable. These three groupings seemed to be independent personality dimensions. Cats that scored similarly on the three dimensions had obvious, shared characteristics. For example, three cats that had positive scores on alert and sociable but negative on equable were active, aggressive, 'bossy' cats, three other cats with negative scores on all three dimensions were timid, nervous cats, and a third group that had positive scores on all three dimensions were sociable, confident, 'easy-going' cats.

When five of the personality scores obtained by ratings were compared to observational categories that were judged by the authors to be equivalent (e.g. sociable with people = approach + sniff + head and body rub observer), the correlations ranged from 0.60 to 0.85 and were all significant beyond the 0.02 level. Thus the rating of personality dimensions, which is usually regarded as subjective, seems to be reasonably reliable (inter-observer correlations) and valid (correlations between ratings and direct observations) when done by well-trained observer/raters.

The first author has also done some work on personality assessment. Since kittens in her laboratory have been handled and/or tested at two weeks of age (or younger) for the past five years, she and her students have noticed pronounced individual differences in very young kittens, particularly in the amount of activity and vocalisation that they show. The activity dimension seemed very much like Pavlov's (1927) excitatory temperament. Karsh then became interested in predicting adult cat behaviour from kitten behaviour and in developing a temperament/personality profile for cats particularly in regard to dimensions that make later placement difficult, such as high activity and severe timidity. One of her students, Heidi Wolfson, measured two aspects of behaviour of 25 very young kittens and related these to later adult behaviour of the same cats at 5–7 months of age. The behaviour measured was number of escape attempts and number of cries made while the kitten was being handled (on the handler's lap) for 40 minutes daily during the four-week handling period.

Wolfson found significantly negative correlations between number of escape attempts and two measures of later attachment: the time an adult cat allowed itself to be held by a person during the holding test and the duration of time spent with a person in an approach-to-person test. The number of escape attempts, i.e. the number of times a kitten attempted to leave the lap of the person handling it, was directly related to activity level. A very active kitten tried to leave more often than a less active kitten. Karsh (1983b) has previously observed that highly active cats had low test scores on attachment measures. In Wolfson's study also, the cats that had tried to leave her lap more when they were kittens had lower holding scores and less time spent with a person as adults. The early vocalisation scores were not related to number of escape attempts nor were they related to later attachment measures, but they were predictive of later vocalisation. Thus activity and vocalisation seem to be independent aspects of cat behaviour which are discernible early in life and remain stable during development.

Because of a cat placement study (to be described in the following section), Karsh then became interested in identifying cats that were shy, timid, or fearful. To test cats for timidity, she added a starting component to the apparatus used for approach testing, reasoning that timid cats would be more reluctant to emerge into the test situation. Some time before this testing, she began having her most experienced assistants who had been working with the cats for more than a year, rate the cats on several dimensions, including timidity.

When starting times (time to emerge from the starting compartment) were examined for cats rated timid and confident (by three experienced observers) there were large differences. Table 12.2 shows starting times for timid and confident cats in approaching a person (labelled person) and in a control condition when the test compartment was empty (labelled alone). The timid cats took 86 seconds starting to a person while the confident cats started in 3 seconds, which was significantly faster ($p < 0.001$). The timid cats were equally slow whether a person was there (86 sec) or they were alone (75 sec), but the confident cats started faster when there was a person present (3 sec *vs* 18 sec), and this difference was also significant ($p < 0.025$).

The timid cats also showed more reaction than the confident cats did when both were tested by a strange person. Table 12.3 shows that in the holding test, the

Table 12.2. *Starting time in seconds for approach to person and for empty test area (alone)*

Timid cats			Confident cats		
Subject	Person	Alone	Subject	Person	Alone
Hector	26.25	21.19	Josephine	1.06	18.88
Ebony	134.77	131.48	Graham	4.27	48.84
Tracy	12.27	4.54	Kafka	6.33	9.90
Dorian	2.21	4.96	Zanzibar	3.11	2.74
Willow	168.80	180.00	Voltaire	1.29	1.55
Boris	150.22	127.97	Othello	2.39	4.26
Thorndike	2.33	1.11	Bausond	4.01	1.47
Wilding	46.05	47.59	Radcliff	1.58	12.06
Millay	166.32	168.69	Marmalade	4.61	9.81
Finley	67.64	61.20	Clyde	3.36	64.50
Natasha	92.36	90.65	Napoleon	3.18	31.73
Ivan	154.00	63.68	Tuxedo	3.04	17.58

scores of the timid cats declined substantially, typically by more than 50 per cent, while the scores of the confident cats decreased less and sometimes increased. The mean percentage decrease was significantly greater for the timid cats (72.72%) than for the confident cats (1.21%, $p < 0.001$).

The second author and his students have also conducted experiments in which personality dimensions have been identified. Meier & Turner (1985) were able to distinguish between two basic behavioural types in a housing-area population of free-roaming cats, operationally labelled the 'shy' and 'trusting' types. Although they *initially* used the criterion of being, or not being able to approach and pet the cats during first encounters to distinguish the two types, they found evidence that cats representative of each type showed other consistent behavioural differences and were not merely being assigned to the one or the other type because they allowed, or did not allow petting. Both the 'shy' and 'trusting' cats were encountered at various distances away from their homes; 'trusting' cats were trusting regardless of where they were encountered, while the 'shy' cats ran away from the test person at greater distances, the further away from home they were encountered.

Mertens & Turner (in press) conducted a more detailed ethological study of first encounters between 231 test persons and 19 adult colony cats in a standardised encounter room and were able to qualitat-

Table 12.3. *Reaction (in seconds) of timid and confident cats to holding by stranger*

Timid cats			Confident cats		
Subject	Mean score	Stranger score	Subject	Mean score	Stranger score
Hector	22.94	4.35	Josephine	99.67	180.00
Ebony	37.98	29.29	Graham	166.17	152.76
Tracy	33.78	3.84	Kafka	169.94	180.00
Dorian	15.34	4.25	Zanzibar	144.98	132.04
Willow	15.35	3.00	Voltaire	180.00	124.16
Boris	33.62	2.59	Bausond	93.63	69.24
Thorndike	66.85	11.46	Radcliff	155.79	80.21
Wilding	40.20	15.57	DD	172.97	180.00
			Othello	123.27	180.00

ively distinguish between two friendly (trusting, above) types – initiative/friendly and reserved/friendly – depending on whether the cat or the human initiated the interaction, and a rebuffing/unfriendly type. Still, individual differences between the cats (things affecting their 'personality', see Mendl & Harcourt, Chapter 4) proved to be the most significant factor affecting the cats' behaviour towards the humans, more so than the sex of the cat, or the behaviour, age or sex of the human test partner (Figure 12.1).

Thus researchers in three widely separated laboratories, using different methods, have identified two common personality types: (a) Feaver, Mendl & Bateson's 'sociable, confident, easy-going', Karsh's 'confident', and Meier & Turner's 'trusting'; (b) Feaver *et al.*'s 'timid, nervous', Karsh's 'timid', and Turner's 'shy' and 'unfriendly'. A third personality style, like Pavlov's (1927) a excitatory temperament, is exemplified by Feaver *et al.*'s 'active, aggressive' and Karsh's 'active'.

Given such individual differences in the behaviour and temperament of cats, we can begin searching for sources of that variation. Turner *et al.* (1986) have located one rather surprising source using the methods developed by Feaver *et al.* (1986). Independent observers rated adult female cats and their offspring at two research colonies on the trait 'friendliness to people', defined as willingness to initiate proximity and/or contact. The persons showed high inter-observer reliability and, as in the Feaver *et al.* study,

such global assessments of friendliness correlated well with measured behaviour towards humans. Turner *et al.* found that at both colonies the friendly ranked offspring were disproportionately distributed between one of two fathers, although the offspring had never come into contact with their fathers at either colony. Only in the colony where the various mothers had lower coefficients of relatedness (greater genetic variability) could they find a significant mother-effect on this trait, which of course, could be modificatory and/or genetic. The authors stated that they did not find evidence for direct inheritance of the behaviour involved, since it is just as likely that shared genes from the father could generate common personality characteristics in the offspring through an effect on e.g. the growth rate and thereby, on their socialisation to humans. Nevertheless their results demonstrate that offspring from a particular male are reliably different from those of another particular male; variability on the trait 'friendliness to humans' is at least partly explained by paternity.

Person-to-cat attachment

There is even less scientific evidence regarding the person-to-cat attachment than there is on the cat-to-person relationship. The paucity of data is undoubtedly due to the fact that the concern with beneficial, possibly even therapeutic effects of bonds between people and animals is of very recent origin. In 1961, when Boris Levinson, a clinical psychologist, proposed to the American Psychological Association that an animal (a dog) could be used to help disturbed children relate to a therapist, he was ridiculed (Levinson, 1961). Twenty years later, shortly before his death, the retired Levinson was finally honoured for his pioneering efforts in animal-facilitated therapy (Levinson, 1983). In the present decade, people in general (and the scientific community more reluctantly) have finally become interested in examining relations between people and animals. The popular interest has focused on programmes that unite two groups of our society's castaways: the elderly, usually in nursing homes, with animals from shelters. Unfortunately, these programmes of relatively infrequent visitation (once or twice a month) seem to have little or no lasting results; a fairly recent review of the literature found no hard evidence of beneficial effects of human–animal interactions (Beck & Katcher, 1984). We think that the problem here is that there have been

(a)

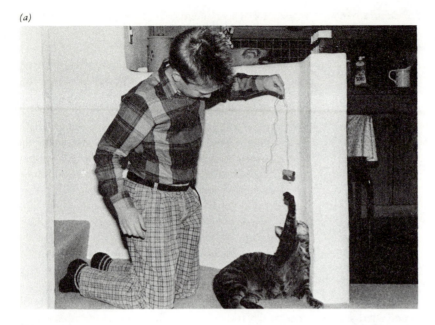

(b)

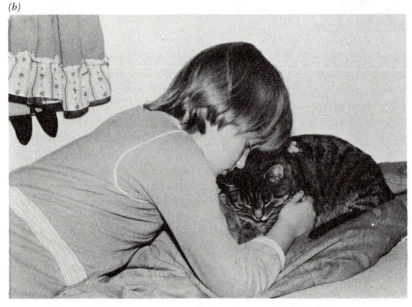

Fig. 12.1. Mertens and Turner (in press) have found that some friendly cats are of a more playful nature (*a*), while others prefer being cuddled and petted (physical contact) rather than engaging in play (*b*). (Photos: D. Turner.)

no well-designed longitudinal experiments. The relationships which generate the benefits cannot develop during brief exposures.

Companion cats: a longitudinal study

The first author will discuss a number of important factors in the person-to-cat relationship which she has encountered during an ongoing cat-placement programme (Companion Cats), which includes some preliminary studies. Karsh has been placing cats with families for over 10 years, but it was not until 1983 that she along with Robert Moffatt and Carmen Burket began a study that would follow the cats and their adopters for at least a year and possibly longer.

For this longitudinal study, Burket interviewed 20 persons who lived alone in the Philadelphia area. The majority of these people were over 60 (average age 59.3). Seventeen of the 20 people adopted cats and eleven kept their cats for over a year. These cat owners were followed up at six-month intervals with an interview/test procedure. Burket also retested five of the six people who no longer had cats and two of the three people who did not adopt cats a year after their original interview. Thus, they compared 11 long-term cat owners and seven short-term or non-owners after a one-year period.

At the end of the first year, there were striking differences between the long-term cat owners and the non-owners on all measures. (Short-term owners and non-owners were grouped together as non-owners.) To measure feelings of well-being, they used the Life Satisfaction Index (Neugarten, Havinghurst & Tobin, 1961). The cat owners showed increased scores (they felt better) while the non-owners' scores decreased (they felt worse) and the difference was statistically significant. Karsh and Burket asked all their prospective owners to rate themselves on scales of loneliness, anxiety, and depression before adopting a cat and several times afterwards. At year's end, the long-term owners felt less lonely, less anxious, and less depressed. Although the owners and non-owners did not differ initially in loneliness, anxiety, and depression, they did differ significantly by the end of one year. Karsh and Burket also found evidence of physiological benefits. Four of the elderly cat owners had high blood pressure before the adoption and two were also diabetic. All four showed reduced blood pressure that has been maintained for over two years. One women showed a dramatic drop from 175/70 to 120/70 and was able to discontinue her medication. The two diabetics showed a drop in blood sugar levels. Five of the non-owners were also hypertensive, and one of these was diabetic. Two of these people showed increased blood pressure, the diabetic had the same pressure but had a substantial increase in blood sugar level, one person remained the same, while the fifth showed reduced blood pressure. Although these results are provocative, it must be pointed out that this was a preliminary study dealing with only nine hypertensive and three diabetic people. A follow-up study should be done on a much larger sample.

The psychological and physiological benefits depend not on the presence of a cat in the household but on the social bond that develops between the person and the cat. Karsh and Burket propose that the amount of positive change is directly related to the strength of attachment. All of their long-term cat owners seem to have 'special' relationships with their cats. For example, during a follow-up interview, one of their long-term adopters was talking to the interviewer about her three children: Barney (her cat), Tina (her daughter), and John (her son).Obviously, the people who returned their cats did not develop a strong bond. To test this difference, Karsh and Burket gave a pet attachment index (Friedmann, Katcher & Meislich, 1983) to the cat owners and former owners. Not surprisingly, all the owners scored much higher (averaging over 80%) than any of the former owners (averaging less than 50%) and this difference was statistically reliable.

The most meaningful change, however, is not the decreased loneliness nor the decreased blood pressure but rather an increase in the quality of life for the cat owners. A house with a cat is not an empty house. A companion cat provides fun and companionship and helps people take their mind off their ailments, worries, and problems. The cats are all exceptionally smart, according to their owners. One had even trained himself to be a hearing-ear cat. He would come to his person and walk to the telephone or the door when she (the person) did not hear it ring.

Factors influencing choice of a cat

The first author placed over 80 cats during the three-year period between 1983 and 1986. During the first few months it became evident that the appearance of the cat, particularly the cat's colour, was an extremely important factor in choice. Sometimes people are aware of choosing a cat because of its appearance, as when they mention that the cat looks like or reminds them of a cat they once had. Others seem to be relatively or totally unaware of using the cat's appearance as their basis for choosing a cat. One women told the first author that only the personality of the cat was important to her. When she was shown the first few cats, she remarked that she couldn't relate to a cat that was all white or all black. When questioned about this, she responded that she related better to cats that were grey or striped. So, although she first chose cats on the basis of their colour, she continued to believe that only personality factors were important to her.

Size is frequently a secondary or sometimes a

limiting factor. People in their late 70s or older, tend to be somewhat frail and usually do not want a large or heavy cat they could not lift. City apartment dwellers seem to prefer small cats and sometimes request cats that can only be described as dwarfs.

To further investigate the importance of the cat's appearance, a student of the first author, Shirley Olson, conducted a study on the attractiveness of cats. She asked each of 20 undergraduate student volunteers first to rank eight different coat colours and patterns in order of preference. Then, she asked them to rank colour, weight, and size of the cat in order of their importance to the appearance of the cat. Then the subject was shown, one at a time, eight pairs of short-haired cats and one pair of long-haired cats. Each pair of short-haired cats had similar colouring but differed in size and weight. The two long-haired cats differed in both size and colour. After seeing each cat, the subject rated the attractiveness of the cat's colour, the size and weight of the cat, the cat's overall attractiveness, and stated whether he/she liked the cat and why. When the colour rankings were averaged, grey turned out to be the most preferred colour, with black second, and striped and black and white tied for third. Orange was least preferred, with calico as second lowest in preference. Most subjects (75%) chose colour as the most important factor in appearance, with size chosen as second (by 70%) and weight as third (by 80%). In ratings of the attractiveness of the colour of the cat, and the general appearance of the cat, and in statements of whether the subject liked the cat or not, the order of the cats was similar. Colour was obviously an important factor. The correlation between the colour ranking (before seeing the cats) and the rated attractiveness of the colour of each cat was 0.74. The correlation between the ratings of attractiveness of colour and general appearance of the cats was 0.90. The correlation between the rating for general appearance and the number of subjects that liked the cat was 0.87, so that appearance accounted for over three-fourths (76%) of the variance in liking the cat. Another, lesser factor, was the cat's weight. Size did not seem to be a factor at all. The cats had been chosen so as to have a large and a small cat in each colour category (except calico) and also large and smaller long-haired cats.

Thus the results of Olson's study are generally in agreement with the first author's placement experience. Appearance and particularly colour, are usually very important factors in selection. Often people seem to have a prototype or idealised image of what a cat should look like. This image is usually based on a cat they have known and liked: a cat from the recent past, the family's cat when they were young, or a friend's cat. Typically this image only presents a problem when a person's cat has recently died and they are trying to replace it prematurely before they have finished grieving.

Karsh has found size to be more important (in her placement experience) than Olson's study indicated. This may reflect an age difference in the subjects.

Matching the cat to the person

In placing cats, the first author and her associate in the Companion Cat programme, Carmen Burket, an experienced clinician, have used a technique called adoption counselling. They developed this procedure for prospective adopters who were not familiar with a variety of cats. The structured interview consists of describing, in some detail, a number of important dimensions of appearance, personality, and temperament, the variation that occurs along these dimensions, and getting the prospective adopter to express a preference on each dimension. For example, activity is a very salient dimension that most people do not consider when adopting a cat. A person who wants a lap cat should adopt a cat on the lethargic side of the activity dimension, a relatively inactive cat. On the other hand, active cats are more interesting, they play games, sometimes of their own devising, but they are more likely to get into trouble.

In addition to assessing preferences, it would be interesting as a next step, to get personality profiles of both the person and the cat and relate them to each other. For example, Karsh has found that people who lack self-confidence find it difficult, even impossible to relate to a shy or timid cat. In this situation the cat's inclination to hide triggers feelings of rejection in the insecure person and the problem can easily escalate to the point where the person gives up the cat. Nurturant people, however, provide good homes for timid or even fearful cats. Karsh has placed 10–12 real problem cats (non-handled or timid and fearful) usually with students, and in two or three instances with young couples, and these cats, with time and patience have usually turned out to be good companions. Karsh envisions, as an ideal person-to-cat match, placing aggressively friendly cats (those who come up and repeatedly initiate cat–person interactions) as therapy for mild to moderately depressed persons.

Some problems in the development of person–cat relationships

On the basis of their experience in adopting cats to people, Karsh and Burket have found three areas of usually insoluble problems in person-to-cat attachment. The first, and most common, is when a person tries to replace a beloved cat, who has recently died, without sufficient grieving. In this situation, the new cat never seems to measure up to the dead cat and is eventually rejected. The only solution here is for the person to complete the grieving process and then adopt a different cat, not a replacement.

A second type of problem occurs when one person tries to persuade another (relatively unwilling) person to adopt a cat. Usually it is an adult, married child (or children) who tries to get an aged, widowed parent, living alone, to get a cat as a companion. This rarely works. The mother (or occasionally the father) is pushed and prodded to apply for a cat, select a cat (she usually cannot make up her mind so the daughter/son selects one), and take the cat home. A week or two later, the cat is rejected because it 'spilled its food when it ate' or 'it didn't like me' but really the person is not trying to establish a relationship with the cat.

The third problem situation is when a person's personality or emotional problems interfere with the development of a person–cat relationship. One example was described in the previous section on matching the cat to the person. People who lack self-confidence have great difficulty in relating to a cat that shows any sign of timidity. The insecure person would find it much easier to relate to a confident cat who initiates interactions with the person.

Different types of person–cat relationships

There is some scientific evidence, as well as much anecdotal and case-history evidence which indicates the existence of several different types of person–cat relationships:

Strong person–cat attachment (cat lovers)   The first author, in a study described in a previous section, found that people who had adopted and kept cats for a year or longer, scored significantly higher on an attachment index (Friedmann *et al.*, 1983) than people who had adopted cats and given them up.

These adopters all showed a great deal of love and concern for their cats and generally regarded their cat as a family member. Voith (1985) described the results of a questionnaire, returned by 872 cat owners who had brought their cats to the Veterinary Hospital of the University of Pennsylvania in 1981 and 1982. Almost all (99%) considered their cat a family member, 89 per cent reported that their cat slept on their bed, 97 per cent talked to their cat at least once daily and 91 per cent believed their cat was aware of their moods. As another indication of attachment, Voith emphasised that cat owners kept their cats despite behaviour problems (mainly elimination and destructive behaviour) reported by almost half (47%) of them. As a follow-up to the questionnaire, Voith collected specific information from 38 cases where cats were brought to their clinic that deals with behaviour problems. When the clients were asked why they had kept their cat this long, 55 per cent answered with a statement such as 'I love him', and frequently owners would say that the cat was a member of the family or 'you wouldn't get rid of a child because it had a behaviour problem would you?' (Voith, 1985, p. 291). Voith proposed that people become attached to their animals (cats and dogs) because people may be predisposed to become attached to other people, particularly children, and cats (or dogs) can exhibit many of the same characteristics that influence person-to-child attachment. For example, like children, your cat (or dog) is dependent upon you for survival and care and, in this respect, is a perpetual child. Your cat appears to miss you when you are away and be happy to see you when you return. And your cat relates to you as an individual in a non-judgmental way, independent of your professional, social, or financial success or failure.

Weak person–cat attachment (low involvement cat adopters)   In her first cat placement study, described in a previous section, Karsh found that six of the original 17 placements (35%) failed, i.e. the adopters would not keep their cats. Obviously, these six people did not develop strong bonds with their cats; their scores were all less than 50 per cent on the Pet Attachment Index (Friedmann *et al.*, 1983). Karsh had made arrangements for the adopters to contact her in case of problems, so these cats were re-placed, but, in the normal course of events, cats such as these are usually given to shelters, where most of them are euthanised.

Arkow (1985) estimated that in the United States there are over 55 million dogs and over 52 million cats and that about 13 million unwanted animals (probably 5–6 million cats) are put to death during the year by municipal and private shelters. Arkow & Dow (1983) reported, from a survey of people giving up their dogs to shelters, that the typical reasons for disposing of the dog were changes in the owner's lifestyle, the animal's behaviour problems, or because its care required too much time or responsibility. Another finding was that a free dog was kept for an average of 17 months, while a dog that cost over $100 was kept more than twice as long for an average of 36 months.

We believe that the situation is the same or possibly worse for cats. Most cats (like the dogs profiled by Arkow) are probably acquired free, as kittens from a friend, neighbour, or from a 'free to a good home' advertisement in a local paper. The kitten is probably selected on the basis of appearance, mainly coat colour and pattern, with little thought about other characteristics, except friendliness. Probably all kittens born in someone's house (as opposed to many farm cats or most feral cats) will be acceptably friendly as kittens. However, if they have not been handled during the socialisation period (and some people do not handle them), they will typically grow up to be much more aloof. Also, unless one observes many kittens, it is difficult to tell an overly active kitten from an ordinarily active one, since all kittens are active. Therefore, if a kitten is selected impulsively, it may very well mature into a cat that differs from the adopter's expectation, and may be rejected. We believe that acquainting people with the different cat personality types and persuading them to make a deliberative rather than an impulsive choice, can decrease the large number of expendable cats.

Negative attitudes toward cats   Some people appear to dislike cats because cats are too independent and cannot be trained or controlled as easily as dogs can. Leyhausen (1985b) has proposed that cats have domesticated themselves. Cats have bred freely and have developed differences in appearance (coat colour, size and body type) and in personality characteristics. Moreover, cats are able to establish a variety of complex social systems (see Leyhausen, 1979, 1985b and other chapters of this volume) and can therefore live with people (as companion animals) or

can live close to people (e.g. farm cats) or can live totally on their own (feral cats). Leyhausen believes that cats have been controversial through the ages because they display these behavioural and personality traits which many people feel no sub-primate animal has a right to display.

Other people seem to be afraid of cats, particularly black cats. The fears of the Middle Ages, that devils and witches appear as cats, seem to persist today as an irrational fear of cats. The first author has on a number of occasions encountered groups of workmen who are afraid to enter cat colony rooms, where 10 or 15 cats live uncaged, unless the cats are removed or someone accompanies the workmen to fend off possible attacking cats.

As far as we know, the extent of these and possibly other negative attitudes toward cats has never been assessed in the general population. Once the prevalence of such negative attitudes has been determined, there are many attitude-change techniques that could be used. However, the best programme for the future would be to prevent such negative attitudes by early positive educational experiences with cats and other animals.

Concluding remarks

In this chapter, we have presented many different factors which can affect the relationship of cats toward people and people to their cats. This information has been derived from various sources: from laboratory and field experiments and controlled observations by the authors and other researchers and from surveys, questionnaires, case histories, and clinical experience. Information from all these sources contributes toward fostering a stronger bond between people and cats. For example, it is now clear that the sensitive period of socialisation for kittens is earlier than previously thought, from about 2 to 7 weeks. Kittens that have been handled during that time will be friendly to people, while kittens that have not been handled then will be extremely difficult to socialise at a later date. When people adopt kittens, it is important for them to find out whether or not the kittens have been handled.

Cats differ enormously in characteristics of personality and temperament. This has been suggested by Leyhausen (1985b) and recently documented by laboratory and field studies (see Chapter 4), as well as by interviews and case histories of cat owners. It seems that many people are not aware of these differences in personality and style among cats (even among litter mates) and tend to select cats mainly on the basis of their appearance. This can lead to disappointment. Our answer to these problems is to inform people about the research findings regarding cat socialisation and cat personality which underlie the formation of a strong cat-to-person and person-to-cat attachment relationship.

Acknowledgements

The research of Karsh's group has been supported by grants from the Geraldine R. Dodge Foundation and Kal Kan Food Inc., and by product donations from the following companies: Beecham, Dad's, Hartz Mountain, Superior and Waverly. Research by Turner and his associates has been funded by the Swiss National Science Foundation (Grants 3.338.82 and 3.247.85) and Effems Beratung für Kleintierhaltung, Zürich.

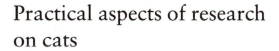

13

Practical aspects of research on cats

Claudia Mertens and Rosemarie Schär

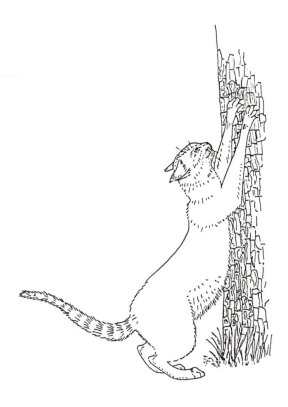

Introduction

The population of pets is growing all over the world (FEDIAF, 1982; Klamming, 1983), and human preference for cats over dogs seems to be increasing in a number of countries. In 1983, about 20 per cent of all households in sixteen countries kept cats (Messent & Horsfield, 1985), although some interesting differences exist between countries. Incredible sums of money are spent for pets, and the petfood and related industries have become important businesses (Beck, 1983). At the same time human living conditions in general are changing, with progressive urbanisation and its ramifications as a main characteristic (Freye, 1985). This is perhaps one reason why pets, especially cats, play an increasingly important role in man's life. Pets are kept under various conditions (Messent & Horsfield, 1985), which sometimes differ greatly from natural or semi-natural environments.

Domestic animals adapt to a variety of conditions; nevertheless their adaptability has limits. Cats, which were domesticated several thousand years after the dog (Messent & Serpell, 1981) and have only been systematically bred for about a century, may not adapt equally well to all conditions under which they are kept. As those conditions diverge even further from the natural environment and/or even more emphasis is placed on the selective breeding of extreme forms, we can expect an increase in the number of problems within individual human–cat relationships.

Veterinarians, who are most often confronted with these problems, are best qualified to handle the health aspect. But they often lack scientifically funded knowledge of (a) normal cat behaviour, (b) the minimum living conditions 'acceptabale' to the cat, (c) the causes of behavioural disturbances, (d) what humans expect from their cats and the ability of cats to satisfy those expectations. This is, however, usually not the veterinarian's fault! The scientific basis of our ethological, ecological, sociological and even psychological knowledge of domestic cats and the human–cat relationship is limited, and many of the existing studies summarised in this volume have not been accessible to veterinarians or the interested layman.

179

On the other hand, popular cat books generally are not written by scientists and most often are not up-to-date (to say the least).

The increasing popularity of cats over dogs, which is partly due to changes in age, family structure and living conditions of pet owners (Messent & Horsfield, 1985), should induce more studies on cats and their owners. More scientific data on normal cat behaviour and ecology are needed, as well as studies on the owner–cat relationship, if we are to 'manage' the growing cat population on a private, communal or national scale. Additionally, the latest findings on these topics should be synthesised and made accessible to the practitioner.

Based on both the information contained in this volume and our own experience and observations while advising cat owners with 'cat problems', we have attempted to summarise the most important aspects for a harmonious companionship between man and cat in everyday life.

Three main factors influencing the cat and the human–cat relationship

Since people and their pets live close together and the pet is dependent on its owner, their mutual relationship should be as harmonious as possible. This requires that the needs and expectations of both partners are satisfied. We believe that there are three main factors, which affect the relationship between people and their cats:

the general housing conditions;
the cat owners and their attributes;
characteristics of the cat itself.

Housing conditions

With respect to general housing conditions there are again three factors, which require examination and are probably very important for a harmonious cohabitation of man and cat:

The quantity and quality of space we offer our cat
The two extreme forms of cat keeping that come to mind are farm cats, which are not spatially restricted by man (but occasionally have no access to the house), and cats living in a one-room flat for their entire life. The home range of an unrestricted cat is not unlimited, but certainly much larger than the 25 square metres of an average apartment. With respect to the quality of

the respective environments we can say that farm cats have a rich milieu, whereas strictly indoor cats often, though not always, live in poorer environments. Between these two extremes we find many intermediate forms of cat keeping (cats in small flats, but with access to the surroundings; indoor cats in a large house; outdoor walks on a leash, etc.).

The intraspecific social system, in which the cat lives
Here again, a wide variety of social systems exist, in which cats can be found. At one end of the scale are the free-ranging cats which live in large groups (same primary home, same food resource) with all possible age- and sex-classes represented. If they want, these cats also have opportunities for social contact with members of neighbouring groups. At the other end, we have the solitary cats, kept in such a way as to prohibit any contact with conspecifics. In between are the cats in closed social groups (more than one cat living exclusively indoors in a household), where the sex and age of the social partners are selected by the owner.

The interspecific social system, in which the cat lives
Family size and age structure of the owner-family probably have an influence on both human behaviour towards the cat, and vice versa. The cat may live in a large family with grandparents, parents and children, or in a one-person household. Further, the amount of time each family member alone and all together devote to the cat will vary greatly.

In other words, each of the three main factors under housing conditions that influence the cat's life, contains a number of variants, which result in an even larger number of combinations. And cats can be found living under each combination of conditions. When studying cat behaviour and human–cat relationships, we need to take into account these differences.

The cat owners and their attributes

There are different characteristics of pet owners, which are suspected or known to have an effect on their behaviour and on their attitude towards the pet (Brown, 1984; Kellert, 1984). Personality profiles have been developed for pet owners in general (Friedmann *et al.*, 1984; Ory & Goldberg, 1984) and for the owners of some pet species specifically (Kidd, Kelley & Kidd, 1984), but not for cat owners.

Even if significant personality differences between cat owners and non-owners (Friedmann *et al.*, 1984), or between cat owners and the owners of other pet species are not found, we would expect that demographic variables such as age, gender, race, geographic location, household composition, type of residence and socioeconomic status will influence the relationship. A farmer wants his cat to catch mice. A lonely senior citizen in the city prefers a cat that will listen to him or her and allows petting and nurturing. A cat means different things to adults and children (Kellert, 1984), and different experiences (quantitative and/or qualitative) will cause different attitudes, expectations and behaviour (Quigley, Vogel & Anderson, 1983).

Characteristics of the cat

It is well known to cat owners, that cats differ greatly among themselves in various ways. Feaver, Mendl & Bateson (1986) present two methodological approaches to determine such individual differences in behavioural styles. These differences may be attributed to different causes and a number of studies investigates the origin of variation in the behaviour of kittens and adult cats (see Chapters 2, 4 and 12).

We suggest that seven factors are particularly worth considering, when searching for causes of behavioural differences between animals: age, sex, breed, personality, early experience, learning and castration.

Since personality is a very complex factor, which partly depends upon the other factors mentioned, it deserves more attention: certainly, heredity influences personality, but early experience and learning may also be decisive. Unfortunately, the scientist as well as the practitioner are rarely in a position to consider, to determine or even to control all variables influencing the personality. Nevertheless, an increasing number of studies indicates that the concept of personality best explains observed differences between individual cats. Personality and individuality are terms which describe the individual as a whole and not just single behavioural patterns. For example the 'shy' and 'confident' cat represent such personality types, and these two terms include a series of behavioural characteristics (see Karsh & Turner, Chapter 12). However, individual differences on a single behaviour will still be correlated with specific personality types. Up to now most studies have dealt with relatively small sample sizes; it is likely that with larger samples, personality could be replaced by one or more of the other six factors listed above.

When we speak of *early* experience we mean events

or those situations occurring during a sensitive period at the beginning of the kitten's ontogeny, which have a long-lasting effect on the animal's subsequent behaviour. 'Early experience' is a special form of learning and is therefore looked at separately. We remind the reader of imprinting mechanisms, probably operative in human–pet relationships too.

When we refer to learning, we mean all the processes occurring after the sensitive period, by which the cat changes its own behaviour, which are not due to maturation or aging. A cat learns best in terms of speed and efficiency when it is young, but learning can occur throughout its life.

Differences between cats on quite a number of specific behavioural elements have already been related to the influence of one or more of the factors listed above. It would be important and helpful to know how those behavioural patterns that are of crucial importance for the establishment or maintenance of a good owner–cat relationship are influenced. But first, the most important cat attributes from the owners' standpoint have to be determined, as has already been done for the dog (Serpell, 1983). Such 'key-attributes' of the cat, as well as the factors potentially influencing a specific cat behaviour, are not only important for good owner-to-cat matching and a harmonious relationship, but also have to be considered when behavioural problems arise. But before we look at some of the more frequent problems with cats, we need to review what we can deduce from various studies on the spatial and social (both intra- and interspecific) requirements of our cats, and how the most frequent medical manipulation – castration – affects their lives.

Spatial requirements: quantity and quality

More and more cats are being kept in 'home ranges' (areas regularly used by an animal) artificially restricted by man, i.e. in small flats and apartments without outdoor access. Many people living in urban areas, without much personal space themselves, keep a cat because they are convinced that cats are better suited to such a life-style than dogs. Working singles and couples without children would also often like to have a pet. Since a cat does not have to be walked, and is often thought to be solitary, it appears to be the ideal pet for those people. Further, dogs are often forbidden in large apartment houses, whereas cats are more often tolerated if not let out.

What are the consequences for the cat? Unfortunately, scientific studies have not yet been conducted to determine what the minimum amount of space required by a cat is, and how that requirement changes with increased quality of the space offered. However, the fact that behavioural problems arise especially with indoor cats suggests that a lower space limit and/or minimal quality level exist, beyond which physical and behavioural disturbances are inevitable.

We do have estimates of the amount of space used by semi-free-ranging cats. Studies of farm cats or feral cats, which live under the most natural conditions, can give us a clue to normal home range size for the species, and of the variability of the parameter. Here, we fortunately are provided with field data from different habitat types and cat densities (see Liberg & Sandell, Chapter 7, for a detailed treatment of range size).

Clearly, we observe larger home ranges in males than in females. This holds for all habitat types and cat densities. The factor by which male ranges exceed female ranges varies between just over one (Turner & Mertens, 1986) and ten (Tabor, 1983). Male ranges may vary between 0.4 and 990 hectares, those of females between 0.02 and 170 hectares (see Chapter 7).

The core area of the range of farm cats, which is of great importance to the animals in terms of time spent there, is usually about 0.1 to 0.45 ha large. It includes the feeding place and resting places, and especially females spend most of their time there (81%; see Panaman, 1981). Individuals which belong to the same primary home, have 100 per cent overlapping core areas.

What is important to the practitioner is, that range size is quite variable (depending on several factors), and that male ranges are larger than female ranges at the same cat density. For application to indoor conditions, this means that cats are adaptable with respect to range size, and that females may be generally better predisposed to indoor conditions, since they require less space than males. Also, we suspect that a switch from outdoor to indoor conditions may be less difficult for a female than for a male, although it is not advisable to impose such a basic change in the life of an adult cat of either sex.

Still, the question of minimum spatial requirement persists and additional experimental investigations are needed. If we compare the smallest ranges found in semi-feral suburban female cats (200 sq m; Tabor, 1983) with a medium sized two-room apartment (60 sq m) we are disturbed by this discrepancy.

Since it will take a while until we have scientifically determined lower space limits, for the time being we would recommend an apartment with *two rooms* as the absolute minimum for strictly indoor cats. This recommendation also takes into account the question of space quality. A two-room apartment will probably allow installation of enough objects (furniture, etc.) to satisfy the cat's needs and at the same time, take care of the following problem: a cat that can see and control every point of its surroundings from one position, without moving or searching, is certainly not stimulated enough. Dividing the space into two separate rooms allows the cat to separate spatially its various activities and promotes movement. And the cat's natural curiosity is satisfied by having to 'control' each room occasionally.

Since more and more cats live under restricted conditions, we should focus our attention on space quality, when quantity is at a minimum. High space quality may be generally achieved by enriching the cat's environment. One way is to provide several good resting places and observation posts. From our studies on farm cats, a good resting place should be warm, dry, protected from one or better two sides, and preferably elevated. Farm cats lie on straw, hay, shavings, sacks or clothes, which they find in the various buildings of the farm. Their sleeping places are often (but not always) concealed, whereas observation posts allow a good view of what is going on around them. Outside the buildings, the cats choose a sunny place, but avoid being too far from cover (Schär, 1986).

Another good way to improve room quality, and at the same time enlarge living space for the cat, is to install wall-shelves at different heights in the room. Indoor cats which have the opportunity to do so, also choose window sills to rest and observe the inaccessible environment. And because of the already restricted room to move of indoor cats, one should seriously consider allowing the cat to use all possible space (including the kitchen, bathroom, etc.) without creating taboo zones.

Farm cats also hunt and explore, and they interact with conspecifics to different degrees. All of these activities are severely limited in a small apartment. Nevertheless, there are different ways of compensat-

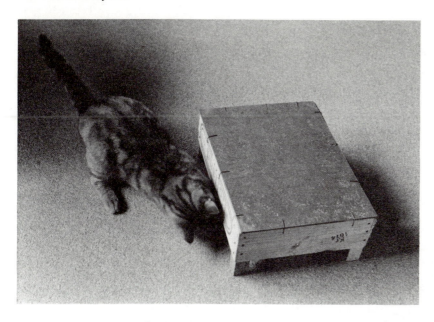

Fig. 13.1. It is certainly not expensive or difficult to enrich the quality of space for indoor cats; exploration can be promoted by simply offering the cat a box to examine. (Photo: D. Turner.)

ing for these deficiencies. There are play objects and games, with which the owner can stimulate simulated hunting behaviour in the cat. For some cats it is essential that the owner participates in this play, since they are stimulated mostly by movements or moving objects; others activate their prey surrogates themselves by throwing them into the air. Exploration can be promoted by placing new objects in the room, e.g. a cardboard box, packing material or new play objects (Figure 13.1). A dripping water-tap also fascinates many cats. Social partners (human and conspecifics) can also stimulate the cat, but this will be discussed separately later on.

The main problem confronting many indoor cats (and their owners) is how to prevent 'boredom'. Lack of things to do and see is a major cause of psychic stress for the animal, which manifests itself in various behavioural disturbances (e.g. food refusal, eating poisonous plants instead of 'cat grass', damaging furniture) and can jeopardise the owner–cat relationship.

We have discovered from the cat's utilisation of space in field studies that while farm and feral cats don't necessarily have fixed places for defecation and urination, they won't soil their feeding or sleeping places, and they seldom defecate *and* urinate at the same place. So, it is inappropriate to place all of the

cat's infrastructure in the same corner of one room. We suggest having two litter boxes per cat (preferably in two different rooms), and placing the food dish, waterbowl, resting shelves and litter boxes as far apart as possible.

We conclude that it is not necessarily abusive to keep cats in restricted environments *per se* (e.g. indoor apartment cats), since they are very adaptable with respect to home range size and not that active even when free. Nevertheless we are aware that a minimum amount of space is necessary to enable increasing the quality of the space. When behavioural disturbances exist, the amount and quality of space available to the cat should be examined right away.

The significance of social partners for a cat

The belief that domestic cats are solitary animals is widespread among cat owners and propagated by many popular cat books, as well as some scientific volumes (Fox, 1975; Hart & Hart, 1985). This belief arises from the fact that, apart from the lion and possibly the cheetah, all wild felid species are solitary or said to be solitary (Guggisberg, 1975; Schaller, 1972).

As a rule, domestic cats and especially indoor cats are kept singly, and this is thought to be good for the cat. Sixty-nine per cent of Swiss cat owners in 1984 kept a single cat (EFFEMS, 1984). But when we consider recent field studies (see Chapters 6 and 7), we are forced to revise our concept. P. Leyhausen (personal communication) has stated that the disposition to solitude is never wholly absent in cat species. For domestic cats we must admit that many can live well by themselves, without suffering (even dying) from the lack of social partners, as is known for other group-living species (Rasa, 1975). But if we look at cat groups which belong to the same primary home, we can likewise say that a disposition to sociality is also present in the domestic cat. Cats vary greatly with respect to their individual sociality, and the term 'generic behaviour' used by Leyhausen (see Chapter 5) seems appropriate for what we observe.

Thus, the differences in social organisation found by various researchers are not incompatible, but rather reflect the cat's adaptations to different conditions. The question of how such different organisations form in a given environment or during individual lives, is of interest from the scientific as well as the practical point of view.

Cats which belong to the same primary home share the feeding place, resting places (although there may be individual preferences) and generally the whole core area. They may aggregate at specific places without apparently interacting, but also sleep in physical contact, lick each other, suckle other females' kittens, play or even coordinate hunting tours. The quantity and quality of social interactions differ, depending on ecological factors such as food availability or population density, and/or on personal characteristics such as age, sex, social status of the cat, and the degree of relatedness between potential partners.

Most social interactions occur within the core area, e.g. around the farm buildings; outside the core area, on hunting or exploration tours, the same animals behave as solitary beings, avoid social contacts, and show more intolerant reactions if an encounter occurs (Schär, 1986). So the origin and expression of different organisation types may be sought in the primary homes.

Schär's (1986) data indicate two factors which probably influence the tendency of a cat to be social or not: the number of potential interaction partners present during the kitten's ontogeny (i.e. cat density in the area or in the primary home), and the willingness of those partners to answer a kitten's approach in a socio-positive manner (i.e. group sociality in the natal group). Kittens are known to be curious, and their readiness to interact with other cats (including unknown individuals) is high. A kitten growing up in a group of adults which have frequent positive interactions will most likely be positively reinforced when it interacts. When the group is large and especially when it includes other kittens, there will be many opportunities to interact and the kitten will develop into a social individual. On the other hand, a kitten growing up without playmates, or constantly being rejected by the adults it encounters will sooner or later stop trying to interact positively or even to establish contacts at all. In other words, a kitten will develop the same social tendency as the group in which it grows up.

According to Rosenblatt, Turkewitz & Schneirla (1961) a sensitive period for *cat-to-cat* socialisation occurs between their third and sixth week of life. Since a kitten's social partners at this age are normally its own mother and siblings and those interactions are mostly positive, the effect of social learning in subsequent ontogeny periods must be high and also long-lasting. The behavioural patterns which are most often followed by further social interactions are play, comfort and resting behaviour; those inhibiting further social contacts are hunting, exploring and aggression (Schär, 1986).

We must caution the reader that aggression is a normal part of social life, even within social groups. Whereas aggression was rare in Macdonald & Apps' (1978) social group, Schär (1986) found a much higher frequency of aggression within her social groups. Even animals that often slept in physical contact were capable of showing aggression towards each other. That cats from different groups exchange mostly aggressive behaviour, if they meet at all, is less surprising; still, many owners of single cats with outdoor access are shocked when their cat is involved in a fight with the neighbour's cat.

The question of dominance or social rank in cats is discussed by various authors and in different contexts (e.g. Leyhausen, 1979; Liberg, 1981). But our knowledge about dominance relationships between cats of the same or opposite sex is poor and should be improved by more detailed experimental studies. Many owners maintaining a group of several indoor cats report social problems among group members, which they relate to dominance. It is possible that social stress becomes greater, or at least more visible, in a restricted environment where opponents can't withdraw from each other. It is difficult to say to what extent dominance is involved in such situations.

'Riding up' (one cat mounting another) in a context other than sex, which is quite common among dogs, has also been observed in cats (e.g. Schär, 1986). Although the behaviour is reported by only a few authors, it does not seem to be an aberrant behaviour due to the lack of receptive females, homosexuality or to a special learning effect, since it has been reported in unrestricted farm cats too. The social function of riding up has never been investigated in the cat. In wolves and dogs it represents a clear sign of dominance (Mech, 1970; Scott & Fuller, 1965), and Schär (1986) has hypothesised that it has the same function in cats. It is certainly not just a sign of hypersexuality or male 'heat' as Leyhausen (1979) proposed.

What are the practical consequences of our knowledge on social organisation among cats? Just as we found for space utilisation and home range size, there is great variation in the sociality of individuals, groups and possibly even populations. Many factors can influence social behaviour, some with long-lasting effects, e.g. early experience, some with temporary effects, e.g. mating season.

Although no proof exists yet that cats which are social in intraspecific contexts are also social towards humans, we should still prefer social cats as companions. One reason is the increasing cat density in housing areas. Free-ranging cats of the social type are better able to cope with frequent encounters, even when many of these are aggressive. Secondly, for indoor cats, especially those whose owners are frequently absent, two (or more) cats can stimulate each other and reduce boredom in many ways. But this only works when both partners are of the social type! [Non-social (or solitary) individuals will hardly interact at all.] In other words the therapeutic value of a conspecific as a means of enriching a cat's housing conditions depends very much on the partner's social characteristics. That aggression sometimes occurs between social cats in the same household shouldn't upset us, since we now know that this is normal for unrestricted cats too. Of course, each indoor cat should still be able to avoid its partner(s) and to withdraw or hide. This, in turn, means that it is of no use to the cats to keep dozens of animals in an apartment.

To increase the chance of 'producing' social cats (intraspecifically speaking), owners of a litter should keep at least two kittens rather than the usual one offspring, so that they can interact intensively and form social bonds; and potential owners should consider taking two young cats at the same time, preferably siblings, if they are going to be away much of the day. But we should not forget that solitary cats will continue to exist for various reasons. A free-ranging cat of this type is best suited for low cat density areas. The solitary cat is also capable of living alone indoors, but in this case the owner must be more considerate of the cat's needs and provide sufficient non-social stimulation. The value of social contacts with humans *to the cat* has not yet been investigated. But it is clear that humans stimulate and activate the animal and many cats actively seek contact with humans.

The cat in its relationship with humans

The cohabitation of humans and cats very much depends upon the quality of the owner–cat relationship. Relationships between members of different species have only recently begun to attract scientific attention, but their importance is already gradually being accepted (see e.g. Fogle, 1983; Serpell, 1986). From the list of seven factors probably influencing the cat's behaviour (see p. 181), two are particularly important for the human–cat relationship: early experience or the cat's socialisation towards humans, and personality.

Cats not only socialise to cats, but also to other species including humans. One sensitive period for the socialisation of kittens lies between two and about seven weeks of age (see Karsh & Turner, Chapter 12). But a potential causal connection between cat-to-cat and cat-to-human socialisation has not yet been examined. Is a positive intraspecific socialisation essential for a positive cat-to-human socialisation? Does an intensive human–cat relationship have a negative influence on cat-to-cat relationships? Can a human social partner be a good or even superior surrogate for an intraspecific partner?

Although these are still unanswered questions, it is clear that both intra- and interspecific socialisation start very early, around two weeks after birth.

People in general prefer cats which are 'friendly' with them. From an ethologist's viewpoint, friendliness might mean, or be correlated with any one of the following: a quick and confident approach by the cat to the person; few attempts to escape; tolerates being held; frequent initiation of social interactions; few distress-calls in the presence of a person; and/or preference of a human over a conspecific partner in a choice situation. Of course, not all of these features really measure the cat's attachment to a human; but they are often perceived as an expression of attachment by the person involved.

We now know that the earlier and more a kitten is handled, and the more persons handling a kitten during the sensitive period, the more friendly and attached to people it will be later on (see Karsh & Turner, Chapter 12). Further, speaking to a kitten favours its socialisation to humans (Moelk, 1979). But this socialisation phase ends before one should take a kitten away from its mother; social learning continues even after weaning and we therefore recommend not removing a kitten until at least eight weeks (better, ten or twelve weeks) old. Therefore, it is the responsibility of the 'breeder' to ensure a good cat-to-human socialisation.

Both the professional and the involuntary cat 'breeder' can influence the kitten's intra- and inter-specific socialisation, and should take advantage of this for the sake of the cat and its future owner. It is important to note that socialisation to humans does not have to take place with the future owner. A kitten forms a general attitude towards people in its sensitive period, which is more or less stable over time and affects its behaviour to both familiar and unfamiliar persons (Meier & Turner, 1985; Turner *et al.*, 1986). Potential owners should pay more attention to the kitten's previous life history (how it has been handled), since an important part of its socialisation has already occurred when they acquire the young animal. In spite of such long-lasting effects of early experience, a cat is able to learn during its entire life, and it is therefore possible to 'change' the animal to benefit the relationship. But this may take considerable time and patience and there is no guarantee of success in changing the 'personality' of an animal.

The cat's personality is the second factor affecting the human–cat relationship that we want to consider. This aspect of cat behaviour is best appreciated by cat owners, and scientists are now trying to distinguish and understand the causes of personality differences.

One important finding for practical purposes is that a kitten's socialisation to people is partly dependent on the kitten's own temperament, as measured by activity level and vocalisation frequency (Karsh, 1984; Moelk, 1979). Under the same (good)

conditions for cat-to-human socialisation, about 15 per cent of the kittens seem to resist socialisation; these kittens have an extreme (slow/quiet) temperament, which can already be observed shortly after birth and may be inherited.

Some behavioural patterns or characteristics may be especially important to the owner and represent 'key-attributes' for a good human–cat relationship, at least from the viewpoint of the owner. These might include: socialisation towards people; playfulness or tolerance of close physical contact (Mertens & Turner, in press); excitability; aggressiveness, and sociability towards other cats. According to Mendl & Harcourt (Chapter 4) some personality traits are stable over time or across situations, while others are less so. The critical attributes of the cat will be the stable ones, since owners probably can't modify them very much and have to accept these.

Usually potential owners choose their pet based on its physical appearance. Since the human–cat relationship depends greatly on the cat's ability to satisfy the owner's expectations, we should pay more attention to personality traits before adopting a kitten. We can make fairly good predictions of the cat's future behaviour by looking precisely at its socialisation conditions, temperament and perhaps other stable factors. This means that one should observe the kitten and its breeder, perhaps visit the place several times, before making a decision. Since adult cats often express their personality traits more readily, one might also consider adopting an older animal, e.g. from an animal shelter.

Human expectations probably differ between cat owners; we know that cats differ greatly from individual to individual. We suspect that the quality of a human–cat relationship increases, the more cat owners are aware of these differences, and the more effort they make to match the cat to themselves. To date it is unknown whether the sex of a cat and its reproductive status (intact or neutered) are important for optimal matching. Since neutering is a very common practice, we need to consider next the ramifications of this surgical procedure.

The significance of castrating a cat

There are some good reasons for neutering a cat, whether male or female, indoor or outdoor cat. Unrestricted females are often spayed because it is difficult to find a good home for every kitten born (about eight to ten per year) and most people are unwilling to put down surplus kittens. Indoor females, which can easily be prevented from breeding, are very often a nuisance to the owner when 'singing' during oestrus. And some intact or sterilised females are in oestrus most of the year, if they are not mated. Males are castrated to prevent or reduce spraying in the house and because of their corporal odour when intact.

For the purpose of population regulation, castration of males and females is certainly the only effective method. The opinion that the cat population has to be controlled is growing with increasing numbers of feral and stray cats. But apart from this important reason, castration has long been practised upon the owner's request, without considering the consequences the operation may have for the cat's later life. What is the influence of castration on spatial and social behaviour? What is the influence on the human–cat relationship?

Scientific studies examining the effects of castration aim almost exclusively at the owner's interests or problems arising for the owners. Hart & Barrett (1973) found that 87 per cent of the castrated males reduce their spraying frequency drastically after the operation. Jemmett & Skerritt (1979) observed a correlation between the number of cats per household and the probability of spraying by at least one of the cats. This probability is 100 per cent in households with more than ten cats. This supports our earlier recommendation, not to keep too many cats in restricted environments (see p. 185). According to Borchelt & Voith (1982), some cats *start* spraying after castration. The proximity of conspecifics can provoke a neutered cat to spray, and the odours, sights and/or sounds of strange cats may have the same effect.

Hart & Barrett (1973) report that most adult male cats drastically change (reduce) their roaming and fighting behaviour after castration. The influence of the age at which a cat is castrated was studied by Hart & Cooper (1984): the likelihood of spraying and fighting in adult male and females is the same, regardless of whether the cat is castrated at six or ten months of age. As far as spraying and fighting is concerned, it is therefore not so important that the cat be castrated before puberty; about ten per cent of all animals still spray in adulthood, regardless of the treatment they received. However, castrated males live longer than their intact counterparts and prepubertal castration

promises a longer life than post-pubertal operation, even though deaths from leukemias are more frequent in the former cats (Hamilton, Hamilton & Mestler, 1969).

Rees (1981) and Neville & Remfry (1984) comment on more general changes in free-roaming cat behaviour after castration. But lack of quantitative data requires caution, and more work needs to be done to clarify whether social organisation, social bonds between cats, and fear of persons change after castration, as they suggest.

Our overall impression on castration from the available information is positive in the sense that it often (though not always) reduces so-called 'behavioural problems' allowing a better fulfilment of human expectations from the relationship. In the following section we will, however, see that urine spraying is only one of the problems frequently encountered and that many 'problems' involve quite natural behaviour of the cat.

Some frequent problems with cats

It is rarely easy to determine the cause of a problem in a given owner–cat pair. Not all problem situations with cats are due to the cat or its housing conditions; they are often related to the owner's lack of knowledge about normal cat behaviour or to his/her attitude and (false) expectations towards the cat. An anthropomorphic view of the cat is very common among owners, but this fosters misunderstanding. A cat should always be seen as a cat, not as a human being, and a better understanding of 'how the cat functions' will eliminate some of the 'problems'.

The following discussion of classical problems with cats is included to show the spectrum one is dealing with. It is impossible to treat each point in detail here; additional information on causes and treatment possibilities from the veterinarian's point of view is given in Voith (1980b, 1983) and Hart & Hart (1985). Generally, there are three main methods of influencing undesired behaviour, irrespective of whether the behaviour is normal or abnormal from the standpoint of the cat:

manipulating the environment;
changing the owners' behaviour (including counter-
    conditioning procedures) or their attitude towards
    the cat;
medicinal or surgical treatment of the animal.

Inappropriate defecation, urination and urine spraying

This is the most common complex of problems owners are confronted with. The list of potential reasons for such inappropriate behaviour is long: although defecation and urination in unacceptable places may be caused by disease, they are often an expression of problems the cat has with the litter box. A toilet alongside the food is unnatural for the cat. Some cats insist upon a perfectly clean litter box, some won't share it with other cats and still others don't accept the quality or quantity of the litter material. Many cats react with inappropriate defecation and urination when something suddenly changes in their life. This may be the addition of a new cat, the arrival of a new family member (e.g. a baby), or a change of daily routine. Depending on the severity of the change and on the cat's general ability to adapt, inappropriate defecation and urination can disappear quickly or remain a problem.

Since free-ranging cats preferably defecate and urinate outside the proper core area and have a tendency not to cover their faeces there (Liberg, 1980; Schär & Tschanz, 1982) this may also stress relations with human neighbours. Unfortunately, outdoor cats are less controllable and some are forced to become indoor cats only because of this problem.

Many cat owners are unaware that urine spraying is a *normal* cat behaviour. Its frequency differs with sex, the individual and the social status of the cat (Liberg, 1981; Panaman, 1981). That females also spray is unknown to many cat owners; and although they spray generally less often than males (e.g. Hart & Hart, 1985), some individual females do this as often as an intact, active male (Panaman, 1981). Relative to the amount of interest cat owners have in this potential problem, there are few studies investigating the social function of spraying (Matter, personal communication; Natoli, 1985b). A better knowledge of this might also increase our chances of influencing the behavioural pattern, without disrupting the cat's social life.

Scratching and climbing

Scratching and climbing (furniture) are, again, not problems for the cat, but rather for the owner. When cats scratch in inappropriate places, they endanger a good human–cat relationship. Feral and outdoor cats

normally scratch trees and other wooden surfaces (see e.g. Schär & Tschanz, 1982). They do this partly to condition their claws; by scratching (sometimes by biting), they remove a frayed and worn outer claw, exposing a new and sharp claw which has been growing underneath (Hart & Hart, 1985). This must be done by every cat and is part of its comfort behaviour (normal body care). When an indoor cat cannot find a suitable surface for this purpose, such as a scratching post, it will turn to the furniture, which is perfectly acceptable for the cat but not the owner.

There is general agreement among scientists that scratching also has a social function. It may serve as a visual and chemical mark (a geographical signpost [Leyhausen, 1979; Hart & Hart, 1985]), as threat or display behaviour when done in the presence of conspecifics (Leyhausen, 1979), and during interactions with humans, as a general indication of excitement (Schär, 1986).

Climbing is another part of the cat's normal behaviour repertoire. Some cats climb up the curtains, e.g. to reach an elevated resting place, to escape, or in the course of hunting insects and playing. The operative removal of the claws, as is sometimes practised to protect the furniture and curtains, is an act of abuse and should be forbidden by law in all, not just a few countries.

Predation

While the two former 'problems' are more frequently encountered in indoor cats, predation is usually only a problem for owners of outdoor cats. Some owners are pleased when their cat brings prey home and have a cat *because* of its prey-catching abilities. Other owners are horrified by the sight of a (perhaps half-dead) mouse or bird and would prefer their cat to stop hunting, or at least not bring the prey animals home.

The domestic cat will always remain a predator (even though some individuals don't hunt) and part of its prey-catching and prey-handling behaviour is innate (Leyhausen, 1979). There is no evidence that a cat hunts less when well-fed by the owner, nor more, when it isn't fed (Kuo, 1930). The tendency to catch prey and the skill at doing it is partly influenced by the mother, the siblings, early and adult experience and heredity (see Martin & Bateson, chapter 2). Play with live and dead prey is common in the domestic cat, but also occurs in wild adult felids (Leyhausen, 1979). Cat owners, who do not tolerate play with live prey, can take the prey item away from the cat and replace it with a substitute play object; of course, they will then have to dispose of the prey animal themselves.

We are asked by cat owners why some cats (including castrated males) bring home their prey and present it to the owner. Although no study has yet concentrated on this behaviour, Turner & Meister (Chapter 9) summarise the proposed explanations available.

Cats which hunt birds instead of mice pose another problem to some owners (though rarely to the bird populations, according to Fitzgerald, Chapter 10). Many owners accept mouse hunting, but not bird hunting, and ask how to influence their bird-catching cat. Apart from the usually successful trick of placing a collar with a small bell around the cat's neck, we can offer no further advice, since basic information on how and why a cat becomes a bird-specialist is missing.

Social problems with conspecifics

Some people do not appreciate their cat fighting with other animals, partly because of the injuries they cause and receive, partly for humane reasons. Others complain of their cat 'not accepting' a new cat in the same household, being 'jealous' of group members, being 'too timid' with strange cats and so on. Once again, these 'problems' do not represent behavioural disorders in the cat, and are often a species-specific way of dealing with different situations. Other problems are related to the cat's age (e.g. flexibility in new situations) or to its life history and personality. An indoor cat that has lived as the only pet in a household for years may have difficulties in dealing with a newcomer. A cat that was not socialised during its ontogeny will probably never be interested in social contacts with conspecifics. Such situations can often be avoided, however, by more thoughtfulness on the part of the owner.

We are often asked if there is an ideal way to combine cats within the same household. From practical experience we can make some suggestions: it is always better to place two young animals together (if possible, litter mates), which are still flexible and easily adjust to each other. But quite often only one of the two cats has to be replaced and the remaining cat will be older. Here we also advise the owner to choose a young cat, since it is probable that older cats show the 'cute response' (Serpell, 1986) to the kitten, and that dominance is clear from the start (the resident cat

having higher status and being less upset by the intruder). As for the sex combination, we can only say that males with housemates of the same sex fight and spray less than those with housemates of the opposite sex (Hart & Cooper, 1984). But we should not forget the distinction between sociable and solitary cats (see above)! Owners wanting more than one cat should make sure they procure sociable cats, and owners who prefer having only one cat should make sure it is of the solitary type.

Finally we must caution that every rule has its exceptions, which are probably largely due to personality; and this makes it very difficult to offer general solutions for such problems without knowing the specific situation.

Social problems with humans (owners)

Often the personality of the pet and the owner don't match well, which invariably leads to problems within their mutual relationship (see Karsh & Turner, Chapter 12). A cat may be too shy, too attached, too independent, too lively, and in rare cases even too aggressive towards humans. Often the real problem is that the cat does not satisfy the owner's (false) expectations.

Some undesired properties of the cat can be modified by changing one's own behaviour. E.g. a shy cat may become quite confident, if the owner gives the animal enough time and doesn't force it into close contact. Cats which are too aggressive in their play behaviour with the owner may become more quiet if the owner spends generally more time interacting with the cat or changes his/her own style of play.

As the studies on socialisation to people (Karsh & Turner, Chapter 12) and on personality or individuality (Mendl & Harcourt, Chapter 4) demonstrate, some traits are difficult to change in an adult cat. It is especially important that people, who adopt an adult cat of unknown parentage and life history, realise this. The older the cat, the lower the chance of changing its relationship towards people through learning. Instead, owners should learn to accept the cat's characteristics as they are, and pay more attention to them when selecting a cat. For example Mertens & Turner (in press) found that within equally well socialised cats, there are some which clearly prefer playing with persons and others which clearly prefer being petted. These two aspects of the human–cat relationship (the cat's readiness to interact playfully or allow prolonged body-contact) are usually important to the owner, and can be checked before adopting either a kitten or an adult.

Concluding remarks

Since the proportion of strictly indoor cats is growing and represents that part of the cat population which lives in closest contact with man, our closing comments particularly concern these individuals.

Pet cats not only enrich our lives, entertain us and reduce loneliness, they themselves have species-specific needs and behaviour, which we must know, accept and take into consideration. To accomplish this each cat owner should have a general knowledge about cats and that has to be determined and made available by scientists studying cats.

The fact that most practical (i.e. behavioural) problems arise with indoor cats probably has two main reasons: living conditions for many indoor cats are unnatural to the point where the cat can no longer adapt successfully; and/or many owners of indoor cats (mostly inhabitants of cities) have such a poor knowledge of the cat's natural behaviour, that it is impossible for the cat to satisfy the owner's false expectations.

We are convinced that three parameters strongly influence the cat's behaviour and the human–cat relationship: housing conditions, characteristics of the owner and characteristics of the cat itself. The important aspects under housing conditions are the amount and quality of space we offer our cat, the presence or absence of conspecifics, and the number and age of human partners for the cat. Important characteristics of the owner are a series of demographic variables, but also attitude and expectations towards the cat. And finally, we know of seven, partly interdependent variables, which affect the cat's behaviour: age, sex, breed, personality, early experience, learning and castration.

The scientific data on unrestricted farm, feral and stray cats show an enormous variability with respect to home range size, space utilisation and social organisation, due to ecological factors, but also to characteristics of the individual cat. This variability and adaptability makes the cat an ideal pet, predisposed to live under a variety of conditions with humans. The apparent disposition of many cats to sociality is of great practical value, since a social partner for a strictly indoor cat can help compensate for the lack of space, hunting opportunities, exploration, etc. and reduce boredom.

The cohabitation of man and cat, two highly developed species, is very complex and influenced by so many variables that each constellation is in some way unique. This not only renders the treatment of behavioural problems and disharmony in the human–cat relationship difficult; this uniqueness also provides a powerful stimulus for cat ownership when the relationship is harmonious.

Acknowledgements

Our experience with cats was gained partly during research projects supported by the Swiss National Science Foundation (Grants 3.338.82 and 3.247.85 to Turner [and Mertens]) and consultations with cat owners through an office for feline behavioural problems in Berne, Switzerland (Schär).

VI

Postscript

14

Questions about cats

Patrick Bateson and Dennis C. Turner

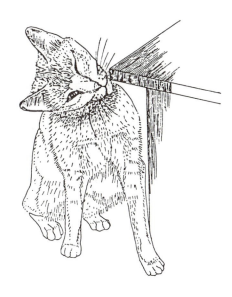

Introduction

Anybody who has kept cats as pets will have seen them behave in ways which have no obvious explanation. Why do they rub their heads against us, for instance? Those of us who study the behaviour of cats scientifically are often asked to provide the *real* answers. Unfortunately, many aspects of cat behaviour that most interest the lay public have not been the subject of extensive investigation. In part this is because the implied question, 'Why does the animal *need* to behave in this way?', is not an easy one to answer. To understand the functional value to the animal of behaving in a particular fashion, we must know how it behaves in the environment to which it is adapted. How does each aspect of its behaviour help it to survive and breed? If some patterns of behaviour have worked better than others in the past and they were inherited, they would eventually tend to be shared by most members of the cat population. The presumption is that by the process of Darwinian evolution, cats behave in a way that is well adapted to the type of

social and physical environment in which their ancestors lived.

Understandably, much of what is commonly known about cats is based on what people see them do in their own homes. Furthermore, when scientific studies are carried out, such work is usually done in the artificial environment of a laboratory. Studies of free-living cats in natural conditions are still in their infancy. This means that when asked, say, why cats rub against us, in all honesty we usually have to reply that we don't really know. However, some speculative answers will be given here, since most non-scientists like to be offered an informed guess and the scientists may want to be guided to the new areas of research.

The behaviour patterns considered here are described in *Cat Behavior* by Paul Leyhausen (1979). While he wrote his book before field studies of feral cats had been carried out, he was able to compare his house cats with other members of the cat family which he had kept in his laboratory. Also, the results of field studies on the big cats, particularly lions, were becoming available at the time, so he was able to make some reasonable suggestions for the functions of the behaviour patterns which seem so puzzling when seen in the home. Unless we give other references, authority for many of the statements we make can be found in Leyhausen's book. More recently in *Catwatching*, Desmond Morris (1986) has ventured answers to most, if not all, the questions that cat owners are likely to ask about their pets. He was clearly not writing a scholarly work and none of his claims are supported by references to original sources. In many cases the evidence simply does not exist. On the other hand, Morris is characteristically perceptive and in what follows, we shall often base our own speculations on his, although we do not always agree with him.

This chapter is primarily concerned with what the cat's patterns of behaviour mean in terms of its own survival and reproduction. When a cat behaves socially towards a human, the person has been treated as though he or she were a cat, although very possibly a particular *type* of cat. So an understanding of why cats behave as they do in their own interests is important in understanding the cat–human relationship. But there is more to it than that, since anybody who loves cats is irresistibly drawn to treat them as though they had some of the characteristics of humans. We project ourselves inside the heads of cats and, in so doing, empathise with them. The chapter will therefore also briefly consider that side of the relationship.

What is the environment to which cats are adapted?

What *is* the natural world of a cat? Have some populations of cats been in contact with humans long enough for the artificially created environment of humans to have become the one to which cats are now best adapted? Has the cat itself been subject to artificial selection by humans so that characteristics have been picked out that would never have been maintained under harsh, competitive conditions? Some of the characters which humans have selected would surely be disastrous for a cat in an unsupported environment. Take, for example, the long coat of the Persian breeds, the virtually non-existent coat of the Rex breeds, or the limp response of the Ragdoll when handled. Cats that maintain kittenish behaviour are especially attractive to people. As a consequence, some of the things that cats do as adults, such as kneading and mouthing soft tissues as if they were suckling like a kitten, may also have been the unwitting consequence of artificial selection for other aspects of the behaviour of young cats. How domesticated is the cat? The best answer would come from comparing the domestic cat with what is thought to be its wild ancestor, the African wild cat (*Felis silvestris libyca*). Unfortunately, little is as yet known about the behaviour of the African wild cat under either free-living or captive conditions.

Domestic cats resemble other domesticated mammals in that they probably produce more variable offspring than non-domesticated forms, other things being equal. Studies of the frequency with which chromosomes cross over suggest that domestic cats (like dogs, sheep and goats) have higher rates than would be expected for a wild-living animal which reaches sexual maturity at the same age (Burt & Bell, 1987). This indicates that the cats commonly found in homes and laboratories have probably been under intense artificial selection for producing novelties among their offspring or have been released from the pressure to keep variability in check. However, many feral cats live under conditions that are quite as harsh and as competitive as any endured by non-domesticated species. In the case of the feral cat, then, products of artificial selection are likely to be stripped away very quickly. Furthermore, many other members of the cat family behave in ways that are almost identical to the domestic cat. Biologists recognise that some useless characters are maintained in the repertoire of an animal because they are by-products linked to the expression of other beneficial traits (pleiotropy and allometry), because they do no harm, or because insufficient time has elapsed for them to have been purged after a change in the environment to which they had been adapted. The line taken here is that, if behaviour patterns are found in breeding populations of feral cats and better still in other members of the cat family, we are probably not wasting our time in supposing that the behaviour patterns represent adaptations to a natural environment. As will be seen in some cases, though, behaviour patterns that originally evolved because they were useful in one context might then have been coopted and modified for another use.

Why do cats purr?

Domestic cats resemble many other species of cat in their ability to purr, although it is often claimed that the large roaring cats (genus *Panthera*) do not do it. The precise way in which purring is accomplished is not known, but the purr can be produced with the mouth closed and continued for long periods of time. Purring almost certainly is a form of communication inasmuch as it indicates to other individuals that the purring animal is in a particular state (presumably relaxed and contented). Kittens first purr while suckling when they are a few days old. Their purring might signal to the mother that all is well, acting like the smile of a baby. If so, the purr helps to establish and maintain a close relationship. Probably for similar reasons, the purr is used by adults in social and sexual contexts. For instance, an adult female will purr while suckling her kittens and when she courts a male. Again like the human smile, purring can be used in appeasement by a subordinate animal towards a dominant one. The implication is that purring reduces the likelihood of attack. Whether or not relationships are impaired when purring does not occur has never been investigated as far as we know. It would be possible as a first stab in such a study to exploit the considerable natural variation that is found in the amounts that cats purr. As things stand this most familiar and distinctive feature of the cat remains largely uninvestigated.

Why do cats scratch with their fore-claws?

House cats often stretch themselves upwards, extend their forelegs and scratch furniture, sofa, and curtains. Feral cats do the same on trees and other rough surfaces. Less frequently scratching is done with the back legs accompanied by treading movements. Since claw sheaths are sometimes found where cats have been scratching, people usually suppose that the cats are sharpening their claws. Indeed, this may have been its original function. However, dominant cats will sometimes ostentatiously scratch their claws in front of subordinate ones. In such cases it looks like a display of confidence. Claw-scratching may also occur in bouts of oestrous rolling. If during the rolling the cat's forepaws come into contact with a rough surface, she may briefly scratch. Similarly, claw-scratching sometimes occurs in bouts of play as do other displays, such as arching. Finally, claw-scratching might involve some scent-marking (see below) by smearing secretions of glands on the feet onto the scratching posts.

Why do cats spray?

When cats spray urine, they behave differently from when they are simply emptying their bladders. When merely excreting, cats dig a hole, urinate in to it without tail movements, turn, sniff, and then cover the hole, often sniffing again and covering some more. Spraying is characterised by tail-quivering, and by the cat rarely sniffing the sprayed surface afterwards. Spraying is most commonly done onto a vertical surface (erect-spraying) but sometimes onto the ground (squat-spraying). In erect spraying the tail is held at 45–90° and quivered during spraying. The cat's hindquarters are held high, and one or both hind feet may leave the ground briefly during spraying. In squat-spraying the cat makes several abrupt treading movements with its hind feet, lowers its hind-quarters and the tail quivers as it sprays. Here again it walks away without sniffing the marked surface. All reproductive adult males and most females will spray urine onto trees, fence poles, shrubs, walls and so forth. The male's sprayed urine has a particularly pungent and characteristic odour.

While the usual interpretation of spraying is that it scares away intruders, cats have rarely been observed to approach an object marked by another cat, sniff it *and withdraw*. Cats periodically remark the same object. The scents left after spraying are likely to indicate that another animal of the same or a different sex has recently passed by. So it may act either as an advertisement, indicating that a female is in oestrus or an adult male is in the area, or serve a similar function as a visual threat, reducing the likelihood that the marker and the sniffer will come into physical contact. It is not yet known whether a cat that sprays or marks in other ways receives any benefit from doing so. But spraying, like front claw-scratching, is performed by confident cats and, as such, could play an important role in the assessments that cats, like other animals, continually make of each other.

Why do cats bury their faeces?

The belief that cats invariably bury their faeces is incorrect. In feral cats most scats are not buried and many are left elevated on grass tussocks (Corbett, 1979; Fitzgerald & Karl, 1979). Domestic cats close to home do tend to bury their scats, but when further afield often leave them exposed (Liberg, 1980). Panaman (1981) following female domestic cats, observed them defecate 58 times, but only on two occasions were brief attempts made to dig a hole before defecating. The substrate was scraped over more than half the holes, though most faeces were not completely covered. Significantly more scats were left exposed outside the home area. This picture was confirmed by Macdonald *et al.* (1987). The evidence suggests, then, that faeces are by no means always buried even by house cats. Near the main living area, burying is commonplace and may be done for hygienic reasons. It may also be the case that the habit has been encouraged by humans selecting those animals that were 'clean'. Further away from home, scats are much less likely to be buried and may be used as another form of marking in free-ranging cats.

Why do cats rub?

Cats frequently rub parts of their body against objects and other animals. Robert Prescott, working at Cambridge in the early 1970s, was the first to suggest that such familiar patterns of behaviour involve scent-marking; work by others followed in due course (e.g. Verberne & De Boer, 1976; Macdonald *et al.*, 1987). The patches between the eyes and the ears (which are only lightly covered with fur), the lips, the chin and the tail are all richly supplied with glands producing fatty secretions. The lips, chin and tail are primarily used in marking objects and the head patches and also the tail are used in marking other cats. Paul Leyhausen (1979) noted that his cats rubbed people much more actively than they did each other. He suggested that the relaxed, uncompetitive relationship that people have with their pet cats allows the expression of behaviour that would normally only be seen in young cats with their mother. However, relaxed, uncompetitive relationships are not simply limited to humans. Studies of feral cats have shown that rubbing by one friendly adult against another is commonplace in well established groups, but is particularly likely to be expressed by a subordinate individual towards a dominant one (see Chapter 6; Macdonald *et al.*, 1987). David Macdonald (personal communication) suggests that a pet cat rubbing on its owner behaves as it would towards a dominant cat and is, therefore, like a pet dog fawning and tail wagging to a human.

The result of marking with the head patch may sometimes be seen if a friendly cat on the other side of a window can be persuaded to approach and rub. If the light is right, a broad smear, which quickly dries, may be seen where the cat has pushed its head against the glass. Given that other cats are marked with the patch and the rubbing is reciprocated, it would seem that all the cats in a social group end up smelling alike. If that is so then the common odour would be an olfactory badge which might denote common kinship (see Chapter 6). Head-rubbing is frequent in the early stages of courtship and commonly the male comes from outside the female's own social group. However, study is needed of whether or not such rubbing involves assessment of how closely related the other animal might be. Verberne & De Boer (1976) found that a wooden peg which had been lip-rubbed by a female cat was sniffed significantly longer than an unmarked peg. The duration of sniffing by males probably varies with the state of oestrus of the female.

Rubbing with the tail by females occurs intensively in the early stages of oestrus. This could indicate to passing males that a female in heat is nearby. Tail-rubbing of objects (and humans) also occurs when cats are not sexually motivated. So does rubbing with the upper lip and chin. Pet owners can readily see their cat rub its lip along the corners of new cardboard boxes. Outside the house, cats also do it on head-height branches and twigs on plants. As with claw-scratching and spraying, such rubbing is sometimes performed vigorously by a confident animal after aggressive encounters with other animals. When no other cats are present, rubbing with the tail, chin and upper lip may simply give notice to other cats that an individual has recently been in the area. If this interpretation is correct, the behaviour may be very similar in function to spraying. A question remains about why so many different forms of scent-marking are used. Is it possible that some more patterned form of information is provided by combinations of scents?

Why do cats grimace after sniffing?

Apart from the tongue and the nose, the cat has a third organ for sensing chemical stimuli. This is the vomero-nasal organ found throughout the cat family and some other mammalian groups such as the horses. The entrance to this organ is in the roof of the mouth. When cats use it, they first locate the source which is to be investigated, approach it closely and then hold their heads still with partially retracted lips. This grimace, known by the German word *flehmen*, may be held for a second or more and is often misinterpreted as a threat. After sampling in this fashion, the cat usually licks its nose. Cats use the vomero-nasal organ when they are analysing urine sprayed by other cats, faeces, gland secretions and also many other non-biological odours.

What indicates that a cat is friendly?

Apart from purring and rubbing, which have already been discussed, one of the most characteristic signals of a cat entering a social group is the raising of its tail. Extending the tail upwards like this may facilitate inspection of the rear-end, as Morris (1986) suggests. However, the tail is also raised when cats leave their social group. It seems more likely, then, that the raised tail is a visual signal to the others (as it is to humans) that the individual is relaxed and friendly. Such signals may be performed regularly because, like a human hand-shake, the cat maintains stable social relationships in this way and reduces the chances that it will be disrupted in its daily round by the other individuals with which it lives. If so, do naturally tail-less cats such as the Manx experience any difficulties in their social relationships with other cats because they are unable to give the tail-up signal?

Another friendly gesture is the blink. A prolonged stare is intimidating and may cause a subordinate cat to withdraw. Perhaps for this reason, non-aggressive cats when staring at other cats or at humans will blink, thereby signalling that the scrutiny is not hostile. In Darwinian terms, once again, cats that did this were more likely to maintain their social relationships and thereby derive the benefits that such relationships provide.

Although many of the friendly interactions between pet cats and their human owners can be related to identical interactions seen between one cat and another, the meaning may change as the kitten grows up within a human household. Such special significance attached to certain types of behaviour could develop because the human–cat relationship is generally relaxed and rarely competitive. Some of the friendly behaviour directed at a person may be strengthened by the human reciprocating particularly strongly when a cat behaves in a certain way, such as rubbing. So what starts as perfectly natural piece of marking a dominant group member may be reinforced by stroking. Eventually, the behaviour pattern is expressed by cats in search of human attention.

Do cats cooperate?

The house cat's independence has encouraged a widespread view that it is unsocial and uncooperative. However, the studies of feral cats have revealed that, apart from an intense early family life, the females in particular may stay in groups as adults (see Chapters 6 and 7). While living together, cats may help each other in terms of mutual defence against intruders and caring for each other's offspring.

It is a myth that, because wild animals are the products of an intense struggle for existence, they always are in a state of social conflict. Two evolutionary explanations for cooperation are now widely accepted. The first is that, at least in the past, the aided individuals were relatives. Cooperation is like parental care and has evolved for similar reasons; by successfully helping close kin, the patterns of behaviour involved in such care become common in the population. The second evolutionary explanation is that cooperating individuals jointly benefited, even though they were not related; the cooperative behaviour has evolved because those that did it were more likely to survive and reproduce than those that did not. In keeping with these ideas, modern work strongly suggests that the cooperative behaviour of animals is exquisitely tuned to current conditions. The benefits to the individual of cooperation change as conditions change and, in really difficult circumstances, previously existing mutualistic arrangements may break down. Or if members of a group are not familiar with each other, no mutual aid may occur until they have been together for some time. As familiarity grows, individuals come to sense the reliability of each other. Furthermore, expectation of an indefinite number of future meetings means that deception or conflict are much less attractive options. Once evolutionary stability of cooperative behaviour under some conditions was reached in a social animal, features that maintained and enhanced the coherence of the behaviour would then have tended to evolve. Signals that predicted what one individual was about to do, and mechanisms for responding appropriately to them, would have become mutually beneficial. Furthermore, the maintenance of social systems that promoted quick interpretation of the actions of familiar individuals would have become important. Finally, when the quality or quantity of cooperation depended on social conditions, increasing sensitivity and self-awareness would have become advantageous. All these evolutionary changes probably occurred in the cat.

As discussed in Chapters 3 and 6, the most striking form of cooperation in feral female cats is in suckling young. Another more subtle example could be the nipple preferences formed by kittens. In the early stages after birth, kittens compete vigorously for access to nipples. With powerful sideways and backward thrusts with their front legs they can easily displace a sibling from a nipple. The claws are sharp and it is sometimes possible to see scratches on the heads of the kittens. Over the first week after birth, the scrabbling subsides and kittens will feed peacefully, often showing a strong preference for a particular nipple (Ewer, 1959). Some nipples produce more milk of better quality than others and the reduction in overt competition may simply reflect the establishment of a dominance hierarchy, with the most powerful kittens 'owning' the best nipples. However, a different interpretation, which needs to be investigated, is that the stability that is achieved represents peaceful coexistence. The benefits of having a preferred nipple in terms of reduced conflict outweigh any marginal improvement in food intake by keeping up the struggle.

How does weaning occur in the cat?

Weaning in the domestic cat is characterised by a gradual reduction in the ease with which kittens can obtain maternal care, rather than by overt maternal rejection. Weaning may be described as the period during which the rate of parental investment drops most sharply (see Chapter 2). Starting at about four weeks after birth, mothers make suckling more and more difficult for their kittens, both by avoiding them and by progressively adopting body postures in which their nipples are less accessible. By about seven weeks after birth, suckling frequencies have generally dropped to a low level, kittens are usually obtaining most of their nutrition in the form of solid food, and weaning may be considered to have finished.

Weaning in the domestic cat is not usually accompanied by aggressiveness on the part of the mother. None the less, the normally tranquil weaning process may sometimes be markedly disrupted if conditions are adverse – for example if the mother's food supply is inadequate (see Martin, 1986).

A number of questions concerning weaning – none of which has yet been fully answered for any species, let alone the domestic cat – therefore arise. What environmental factors affect the timing and nature of the weaning process? Is it the case, for example, that

mothers whose food supply is limited, or who are nursing many kittens, wean their kittens earlier than normal? Under adverse conditions, mothers might curtail investment in current offspring, by weaning them early, in order to preserve themselves for future reproduction (Bateson, 1981b). However, the opposite prediction is equally plausible: mothers with large litters or poor food supplies may have to nurse their kittens longer in order to get them to the minimum size and weight at which they can become independent. Or possibly, as conditions become more adverse mothers wean their offspring later, but at a certain point food is so restricted that they abruptly cease caring for their offspring and abandon them, so that they themselves can survive and reproduce later when conditions may have improved. At present, though, all this remains conjecture and badly needs investigation in free-living conditions.

Whatever the precise nature of their effects, naturally varying factors such as the mother's nutrition and the number of kittens she is nursing are likely to have systematic effects on the timing of weaning and its abruptness. The weaning period is a time of major changes for the developing kitten, during which it must make the transition from complete dependence on maternal care to partial or complete independence. If weaning occurs much earlier than normal, how does the kitten adapt, both in behavioural and physiological terms, and what are the long-term consequences? Is it the case that kittens which are forced to grow up more rapidly than normal, perhaps because their mother's food supply was poor, pay a cost in terms of later behavioural abilities? Here again much remains to be discovered.

Why do cats scratch the floor near food?

Cats sometimes cover up left-overs or food items that they have rejected in the same way that they cover up urine and faeces. This looks especially bizarre on a hard floor on which they may sometimes scratch without effect for minutes on end. Sometimes, these actions may be purely for sanitary reasons, since they are typically performed beside food for which they do not have much liking. However, they could represent attempts by the cat to cache left-over food. Occasionally feral cats have been observed to retrieve uneaten food that has been cached in this way (B. M. Fitzgerald, personal communication).

How do cats hunt?

Cats become specialists in hunting for particular types of prey. That much is clear to many pet-owners and from some laboratory studies (see Chapters 2 and 9). However, a host of questions remain to be answered by fieldwork. Is it the case that a cat specialising on birds will turn its attention to voles if there should be a vole plague? Will an individual employ different hunting strategies such as roaming and stalking as well as sitting and waiting? If so, under what conditions do they change from one to the other? At present we know little about the conditions in which a cat will switch the mode of hunting which it normally uses. The change ought to be easy for such clever animals, but maybe the change in habits is more difficult and costly in time than we suppose.

As with the issues of prey preferences and hunting style, little is known about what influences a cat as to when it should start to hunt, where it should hunt, when it should change hunting places and when it should give up hunting. For instance, how do local differences in prey availability within the home range affect where cats hunt? What do cats do when faced with a conflict between hunting and performing other activities? What do mothers do, for example, when hunting means they must leave their offspring? Do mothers faced with the heavy load of providing milk for their offspring have different nutritional requirements from males and non-lactating females? Do they take different prey? Many of these questions could be answered in part by field experiments in which the diet of feral cats is supplemented at the home area.

Why are cats so different from each other?

For those who know cats well, they seem as different from each other as do humans. Why should this be? If they were adapted in the past to a common set of conditions, should they not all be alike? The answer may be 'no' for several reasons. First, if one member of a social group behaves in a particular way it may be advantageous to other individuals to behave differently. An obvious case would be when a dominant animal is monopolising a limited source of food. Second, climate and habitat are not uniform and specialisations for one set of environmental conditions might be quite inappropriate in another. The same applies to social conditions. Finally, some of the variation seen in

cats may be the product of artificial selection. We have already mentioned the evidence of Burt & Bell (1987) that domestication of animals seems to have led to higher levels of variability than is found in comparable undomesticated forms.

As far as scientific investigation is concerned the extent to which individual differences can be induced by the conditions of early life is an active area of research at the moment (see Chapter 2). A fruitful area that is ripe for exploration is the study of behavioural genetics in the domestic cat. Much, of course, is known about genetic influences on morphological characters of the cat, such as the length and coloration of the coat. However, remarkably little attention has been paid to the role of genetic factors in the development of individual differences in behaviour (see Chapter 4). This stands in stark contrast to the extensive body of research on the genetics of breed differences in behaviour in dogs (e.g. Scott & Fuller, 1965). Cats are particularly suitable subjects for such analysis because kittens are easily cross-fostered to another mother. So, it would not be difficult to investigate the extent to which differences in kittens' friendliness to humans are affected by the genes they inherit from their true mothers and how much their personalities were affected by the temperaments of their foster mothers. In practice, of course, such questions rarely reduce to simple answers and what happens to an individual depends on an interplay between its own behaviour and that of its caregiver. None the less, such matters should not be prejudged and some personality characteristics may be expressed in a very wide variety of care-giving conditions.

Do cats think?

Most people, who watch their pets closely and form strong attachments to them, attribute intentions to their pets. Cats give the strong impression that they think like humans. How much of this is real? Humans have a well-known tendency to attribute to animals emotions and conscious experience that they feel themselves. If we are imaginative we can project ourselves inside plants and inanimate objects as well as other animals. We wonder what it would be like to be an oak tree, a house, a mountain, possibly even the Andromeda galaxy. Given this propensity, two issues need to be distinguished. First, we should be clear about the ways in which we create our perception of the world by projecting ourselves onto it. Second, we should specify the criteria that lead us to suppose that the parts of the non-human world operate as we do ourselves.

The urge to empathise is strong, but is often rewarded by understanding. Good welfare often depends on identification with the animals in question. So, often, does some good science. When an animal is thought of as a piece of clockwork machinery, then some of its most interesting attributes are almost certainly overlooked. For a different reason, biologists commonly attribute purpose to the things they study. When pressed, they claim to use a shorthand, but their stance is one that often helps to clarify and focus problems. The value of teleology as a heuristic device is also well known in the physical sciences, bringing order to human minds wrestling with systems that have complex dynamic properties. Therefore, attributing intention to an animal, so that we can better understand it, does not mean that, when our efforts are crowned with success, we have proved that the animal has intentions. Even if we find it helpful to suppose that animals have intentions, the way that we think about them is not evidence that they think.

What objective evidence may be obtained for thought in a cat? Currently a great deal of argument ranges around what sorts of criteria should be used in order to attribute intention, planning abilities and consciousness to an animal (see Dennett, 1983). Speech is not required, since most people would attribute thought to mute humans. What then about the ability to learn? Certainly, in the early days of experimental psychology cats were popular (and successful) subjects in studies of learning. They are excellent escape artists and would quickly learn to get out of puzzle boxes with novel types of catches on the lids and doors (Thorndike, 1911). Later, when apparatus was developed in which the animal had to press a lever in order to obtain food on a regular schedule, cats performed disappointingly, doing much less well than pigeons. This should not be taken as evidence that cats are stupid, however. Cats eat intelligent prey such as mice, under natural conditions rather than immobile objects, such as seeds. The cat must not only discover the places where prey are most commonly found, it must also avoid becoming too regular itself, lest its own movements are predicted by its potential prey. That is a complex job and may explain why cats are not well adapted to learning a monotonous task that involves repeated pressing of a lever in order to obtain food, even though they are very good at mastering other problems. While we have every reason to believe that cats are clever, so too are computers to which we do not attribute forethought or consciousness. So where does that leave us in trying to answer whether cats think as we do ourselves?

Many anecdotes suggest that cats perform acts while having some foreknowledge of the consequences. One of us had a cat called Polly that had a tense but dominant relationship with Olga, the other cat in the household. One day Polly was sitting on her owner's lap in a back-room of the house. Olga, who had been outside, had to pass in front of a long window in the room to reach a cat-door. She was seen by Polly, who jumped off the lap and crouched by the cat-door. As soon as Olga started to push the door flap open, Polly beat down on the other side with her forepaws. Poor, startled Olga fled back into the garden, while Polly confidently scratched her claws on the door mat inside the cat-door. Most owners will recount similar stories. A recurring one is the frustrated or ignored cat urinating in a place, such as a bed, that causes maximum inconvenience to its owner. In one case, the owner was preoccupied in a game of chess and the cat urinated in the middle of the chess board. What we make of such stories depends on how difficult it would be to explain them without invoking conscious thought. At present there is little agreement. Even so, it could be profitable to build up a collection of accounts of seemingly planned activity in order to discover whether systematic patterns can be detected. By degrees it should be possible to uncover the conditions that are required for these aspects of the cat's behaviour to be acquired and expressed.

Concluding remarks

We do not think that cats become less interesting as some of their enigmatic qualities yield to scientific research. As so often happens, new questions are posed by the answering of old ones. We hope, though, that interested cat owners and professional scientists alike will have gained pleasure from the increased understanding. The cat is much more social than popular myth would suggest. It is exquisitely sensitive to the behaviour of other individuals and, when it is kept as a pet, to the actions and moods of its human owner. A great deal of its own behaviour is devoted to maintaining its social relationships. That much is clear, but many of the influences on its behaviour remain uncertain. As yet the astonishing differences between individual cats are largely unexplained in terms of both how they are generated and why they might exist. We hope that this book will have served to stimulate the lay-reader and the professional scientist to view the cat with even greater sympathy and also to whet their appetites for what remains to be discovered.

Acknowledgements

We are grateful to Michael Fitzgerald, David Macdonald, Michael Mendl, Eugenia Natoli and James Serpell for their help in preparing this chapter.

References

Aberconway, C. (1949). *A Dictionary of Cat-Lovers: XV Century BC–XX Century AD*. London: Michael Joseph.

Achterberg, H. & Metzger, R. (1978). Untersuchungen zur Ernährungsbiologie von Hauskatzen aus dem Kreis Haldensleben und dem Stadtkreis Magdeburg. *Jahresschrift des Kreismuseums Haldensleben*, **19**, 69–78.

Achterberg, H. & Metzger, R. (1980). Neue Untersuchungen und Erkenntnisse zur Bedeutung der Hauskatze (*Felis silvestris f. catus*) für die Niederwildhege. *Jahresschrift des Kreismuseums Haldensleben*, **21**, 74–83.

Adamec, R. E., Stark-Adamec, C. & Livingston, K. E. (1980a). The development of predatory aggression and defense in the domestic cat (*Felis catus*). II. The development of aggression and defense in the first 164 days of life. *Behavioural and Neural Biology*, **30**, 410–34.

Adamec, R. E., Stark-Adamec, C. & Livingston, K. E. (1980b). The development of predatory aggression and defense in the domestic cat (*Felis catus*). III. Effects on development of hunger between 180 and 365 days of age. *Behavioural and Neural Biology*, **30**, 435–47.

Adamec, R. E., Stark-Adamec, C. & Livingston, K. E. (1983). The expression of an early developmentally emergent defensive bias in the adult domestic cat (*Felis catus*) in non-predatory situations. *Applied Animal Ethology*, **10**, 89–108.

Adler, H. E. (1955). Some factors of observation learning in cats. *Journal of Genetic Psychology*, **86**, 159–77.

Alderton, D. (1983). *The Cat: the most complete illustrated practical guide to cats and their world*. London: MacDonald.

Andersson, M. & Erlinge, S. (1977). Influence of predation on rodent populations. *Oikos*, **29**, 591–7.

Apps, P. J. (1981). Behavioural ecology of the feral house cat (*Felis catus* L.) on Dassen Island. M.Sc. thesis, University of Pretoria.

Apps, P. J. (1983). Aspects of the ecology of feral cats on Dassen Island, South Africa. *South African Journal of Zoology*, **18**, 393–9.

Apps, P. J. (1986). Home ranges of feral cats on Dassen Island. *Journal of Mammalogy*, **67**, 199–200.

Arkow, P. (1985). The human society and the human-companion animal bond: reflections on the broken bond. *Veterinary Clinics of North America*, **15**, 455–66.

Arkow, P. & Dow, S. (1983). The ties that do not bind. In *The Pet Connection: its influence on our health and quality of life*, ed. R. K. Anderson, B. L. Hart & L. A. Hart. Minneapolis: University of Minnesota Press.

Baerends, G. P. (1941). Fortpflanzungsverhalten und Orientierung des Grabwespe Ammophila campestris Jur. *Tijdschrift voor Entomologie*, **84**, 68–275.

Baerends-van Roon, J. M. & Baerends, G. P. (1979). *The Morphogenesis of the Behaviour of the Domestic Cat*. Amsterdam: North-Holland Publishing Co.

Bailey, T. N. (1974). Social organization in a bobcat population.

Journal of Wildlife Management, **38**, 435–46.

Bailey, T. N. (1981). Factors of bobcat social organization and some management implications. In *Proc. Worldwide Fur-bearer Conference, Vol. II*, ed. J. A. Chapman & D. Pursley. College Park:University of Maryland Press.

Bailey, T. N., Bangs, E. E., Portner, M. F., Malloy, J. C. & McAvinchey, R. J. (1986). An apparent overexploited lynx population on the Kenai Peninsula, Alaska. *Journal of Wildlife Management*, **50**, 279–90.

Baron, A., Stewart, C. N. & Warren, J. M. (1957). Patterns of social interaction in cats (*Felis domesticus*). *Behaviour*, **11**, 56–66.

Barrett, P. & Bateson, P. (1978). The development of play in cats. *Behaviour*, **66**, 106–20.

Bateson, P. (1976). Rules and reciprocity in behavioural development. In *Growing Points in Ethology*, ed. P. P. G. Bateson & R. A. Hinde. Cambridge: Cambridge University Press.

Bateson, P. (1979). How do sensitive periods arise and what are they for? *Animal Behaviour*, **27**, 470–86.

Bateson, P. (1981a). Control of sensitivity to the environment during development. In *Behavioral Development*, ed. K. Immelmann, G. W. Barlow, L. Petrinovich & M. Main. Cambridge: Cambridge University Press.

Bateson, P. (1981b). Discontinuities in development and changes in the organisation of play in cats. In *Behavioral Development*, ed. K. Immelmann, G. W. Barlow, L. Petrinovich & M. Main. Cambridge: Cambridge University Press.

Bateson, P. (1983). The interpretation of sensitive periods. In *The Behavior of Human Infants*, ed. A. Oliverio & M. Zappella. New York: Plenum.

Bateson, P. (1987a). Imprinting as a process of competitive exclusion. In *Imprinting and Cortical Plasticity*, ed. R. Rauschecker & P. Marler. New York: Wiley.

Bateson, P. (1987b). Biological approaches to the study of behavioural development. *International Journal of Behavioral Development*, **10**, 1–22.

Bateson, P., Martin, P. & Young, M. (1981). Effects of inter-rupting cat mothers' lactation with bromocriptine on the subsequent play of their kittens. *Physiology and Behaviour*, **27**, 841–5.

Bateson, P. & Young, M. (1979). The influence of male kittens on the object play of their female siblings. *Behavioural and Neural Biology*, **27**, 374–8.

Bateson, P. & Young, M. (1981). Separation from the mother and the development of play in cats. *Animal Behaviour*, **29**, 173–80.

Bayly, C. P. (1976). Observations on the food of the feral cat (*Felis catus*) in an arid environment. *South Australian Naturalist*, **51**, 22–4.

Bayly, C. P. (1978). A comparison of the diets of the red fox and the feral cat in an arid environment. *South Australian Naturalist*, **53**, 20–8.

Beadle, M. (1977). *The Cat: History, Biology and Behaviour*. London: Collins & Harvill Press.

Beaver, B. V. (1976). Feline behavioral problems. *Veterinary Clinics of North America*, **6**, 333–40.

Beaver, B. V. (1977). Mating behaviour in the cat. *Veterinary Clinics of North America*, **7**, 729–33.

Beaver, B. V. (1980). *Veterinary Aspects of Feline Behavior*. St Louis: C. V. Mosby Co.

Beck, A. M. (1983). Animals in the city. In *New Perspectives on our Lives with Companion Animals*, ed. A. H. Katcher & A. M. Beck. Philadelphia: University of Pennsylvania Press.

Beck, A. M. & Katcher, A. H. (1984). A new look at pet-facilitated therapy. *Journal of the American Veterinary Medical Association*, **184**, 414–21.

Berg, W. E. (1979). Ecology of bobcats in northern Minnesota. *National Wildlife Federation Sci. Tech. Series*, **6**, 55–61.

Bertram, B. C. R. (1975). The social system of lions. *Scientific American*, **232** (5), 54–65.

Bertram, B. C. R. (1978). *Pride of Lions*. New York: Charles Scribner's Sons.

Biben, M. (1979). Predation and predatory play behaviour of domestic cats. *Animal Behaviour*, **27**, 81–94.

Bloch, S. A. & Martinoya, C. (1981). Reactivity to light and development of classical cardiac conditioning in the kitten. *Developmental Psychobiology*, **14**, 83–92.

Block, J. (1977). Advancing the psychology of personality: Paradigmatic shift or improving the quality of research? In *Personality at the Crossroads*, ed. N. S. Endler & D. Magnusson. New York: John Wiley & Sons.

Bond, S. (1981). *A Hundred and One Uses of a Dead Cat*. London: Methuen.

Borchelt, P. L. & Voith, V. L. (1982). Diagnosis and treatment of elimination behavior problems in cats. *Veterinary Clinics North America. Small Animal Practice*, **12**, 673–81.

Borkenhagen, P. (1978). Von Hauskatzen (*Felis sylvestris f. catus* L., 1758) eingetragene Beute. *Zeitschrift für Jagdwissenschaft*, **24**, 27–33.

Borkenhagen, P. (1979). Zur Nahrungsökologie streunender Hauskatzen (*Felis sylvestris f. catus* Linné, 1758) aus dem Stadtbereich Kiel. *Zeitschrift für Säugetierkunde*, **44**, 375–83.

Braastad, B. O. & Heggelund, P. (1984). Eye-opening in kittens: effects of light and some biological factors. *Developmental Psychobiology*, **17**, 675–81.

Bradt, G. W. (1949). Farm cat as predator. *Michigan Conservation*, **18**, 23–5.

Brambell, F. W. R. (1970). *The Transmission of Passive Immunity from Mother to Young*. Amsterdam: North-Holland.

Brand, C. J., Keith, L. B. & Fischer, C. A. (1976). Lynx responses to changing showshoe hare densities in central Alberta. *Journal of Wildlife Management*, **40**, 416–28.

Brooker, M. G. (1977). Some notes on the mammalian fauna of the western Nullarbor Plain, Western Australia. *Western Australian Naturalist*, **14**, 2–15.

Brothers, N. P. (1984). Breeding, distribution and status of burrow-nesting petrels at Macquarie Island. *Australian Wildlife Research*, **11**, 113–31.

Brown, D. (1984). Personality and gender influences on human relationships with horses and dogs. In *The Pet Connection: its influence on our health and quality of life*, ed. R. K. Anderson, B. L. Hart & L. A. Hart. Minneapolis: University of Minnesota Press.

Brown, R. E. & Macdonald, D. W. (1985). *Social Odours in Mammals*. London: Oxford University Press.

Brown, K. A., Buchwald, J. S., Johnson, J. R. & Mikolich, D. J. (1978). Vocalization in the cat and kitten. *Developmental Psychobiology*, **11**, 559–70.

Burt, A. & Bell, G. (1987). Mammalian chiasma frequencies as a test of two theories of recombination. *Nature*, **326**, 803–5.

Buss, A. H. & Plomin, R. (1986). The EAS approach to temperament. In *The Study of Temperament: changes, continuities and challenges*, ed. R. Plomin & J. Dunn. Hillsdale, New Jersey: Lawrence Erlbaum.

Bygott, J. D., Bertram, B. C. R. & Handy, J. P. (1979). Male lions in large coalitions gain reproductive advantages. *Nature*, **282**, 840–1.

Caro, T. M. (1979a). Relations between kitten behaviour and adult predation. *Zeitschrift für Tierpsychologie*, **51**, 158–68.

Caro, T. M. (1979b). The development of predation in cats. Ph.D. thesis, University of St Andrews, Scotland.

Caro, T. M. (1980a). The effects of experience on the predatory patterns of cats. *Behavioural and Neural Biology*, **29**, 1–28.

Caro, T. M. (1980b). Effects of the mother, object play and adult experience on predation in cats. *Behavioural and Neural Biology*, **29**, 29–51.

Caro, T. M. (1980c). Predatory behaviour in domestic cat mothers. *Behaviour*, **74**, 128–48.

Caro, T. M. (1981a). Sex differences in the termination of social play in cats. *Animal Behaviour*, **29**, 271–9.

Caro, T. M. (1981b). Predatory behaviour and social play in kittens. *Behaviour*, **76**, 1–24.

Caro, T. M., Roper, R., Young, M. & Dank, G. R. (1979). Inter-observer reliability. *Behaviour*, **69**, 303–15.

Carr, G. M. & Macdonald, D. W. (1986). The sociality of solitary foragers: A model based on resource dispersion. *Animal Behaviour*, **34**, 1540–9.

Catling, P. C. (1988). Similarities and contrasts in the diet of foxes (*Vulpes vulpes*) and cats (*Felis catus*) relative to fluctuating prey populations and drought. *Australian Wildlife Research*, in press.

Chamove, A. S., Eysenck, H. J. & Harlow, H. F. (1972). Personality in monkeys: Factor analysis of rhesus social behaviour. *Quarterly Journal of Experimental Psychology*, **24**, 496–504.

Chazeau, E. de (1965). *Of Houses and Cats*. New York: Random House.

Cheke, A. S. (1984). Lizards of the Seychelles. In *Biogeography and Ecology of the Seychelles Islands*, ed. D. R. Stoddart. *Monographiae Biologicae 55*. The Hague: Dr W. Junk, Publishers.

Chesler, P. (1969). Maternal influence in learning by observation in kittens. *Science*, **166**, 901–3.

Childs, J. E. (1986). Size-dependent predation on rats (*Rattus norvegicus*) by house cats (*Felis catus*) in an urban setting. *Journal of Mammalogy*, **67**, 196–9.

Christian, D. P. (1975). Vulnerability of meadow voles, *Microtus pennsylvanicus*, to predation by domestic cats. *American Midland Naturalist*, **93**, 498–502.

Clough, G. C. (1976). Current status of two endangered Caribbean rodents. *Biological Conservation*, **10**, 43–7.

Clutton-Brock, J. (1969). Carnivore remains from the excavations of the Jericho tell. In *The Domestication and Exploitation of Plants and Animals*, ed. P. J. Ucko & G. W. Dimbleby. London: Duckworth.

Clutton-Brock, J. (1981). *Domesticated Animals from Early Times*. London: Heinemann and British Museum of Natural History.

Clutton-Brock, T. H. & Harvey, P. H. (1978). Mammals, resources and reproductive strategies. *Nature*, **273**, 191–5.

Cogger, H. G. (1983). *Reptiles and Amphibians of Australia*, revised edition. Sydney: Reed.

Cole, D. D. & Shafer, J. B. (1966). A study of social dominance in cats. *Behaviour*, **27**, 39–53.

Collard, R. R. (1967). Fear of strangers and play behavior in kittens with varied social experience. *Child Development*, **38**, 877–91.

Coman, B. J. & Brunner, H. (1972). Food habits of the feral house cat in Victoria. *Journal of Wildlife Management*, **36**, 848–53.

Connelley, M. E. & Todd, N. B. (1972). Age at first parity, litter size and survival in cats. *Carnivore Genetics Newsletter*, **2**, 50–2.

Cook, L. M. & Yalden, D. W. (1980). A note on the diet of feral cats on Deserta Grande. *Bocagiana*, **52**, 1–4.

Corbett, L. K. (1979). Feeding ecology and social organisation of wild cats (*Felis silvestris*) and domestic cats (*Felis catus*) in Scotland. PhD thesis, University of Aberdeen, Scotland.

Corbett, L. K. (1983). Feeding ecology and social organization of wildcats (*Felis silvestris*) and domestic cats (*Felis catus*) in Scotland. Poster, 18th International Ethological Conference, Brisbane, 1983.

Corionos, J. D. (1933). Development of behavior in the fetal cat. *Genetics Psychology Monographs*, **14**, 283–383.

Csiza, C. K., Scott, F. W., De Lahunta, A. & Gillespie, J. H. (1971). Immune carrier state of feline panleucopaenia virus-infected cats. *American Journal of Veterinary Research*, **32**, 419–26.

Dale-Green, P. (1963). *Cult of the Cat*. London: Heinemann.

Dards, J. L. (1978). Home ranges of feral cats in Portsmouth dockyard. *Carnivore Genetics Newsletter*, **3**, 242–55.

Dards, J. L. (1979). The population ecology of feral cats (*Felis catus* L.) in Portsmouth dockyard. Ph.D. thesis, University of Southampton.

Dards, J. L. (1981). Habitat utilisation by feral cats in Portsmouth dockyard. In *The Ecology and Control of Feral Cats*, ed. Universities Federation for Animal Welfare. Potters Bar: UFAW.

Dards, J. L. (1983). The behaviour of dockyard cats: interactions of adult males. *Applied Animal Ethology*, **10**, 133–53.

Darnton, R. (1984). *The Great Cat Massacre and Other Episodes in French Cultural History*. London: Allen Lane.

Darwin, C. (1872). *The Origin of Species by Means of Natural Selection*. 6th edition. London: John Murray.

Davies, E. M. & Boersma, P. D. (1984). Why lionesses copulate with more than one male. *American Naturalist*, **123**, 594–611.

Davies, N. B. (1982). Behaviour and competition for scarce resources. In *Current Problems in Sociobiology*, ed. King's College Sociobiology Group. Cambridge: Cambridge University Press.

Davies, N. B. & Houston, H. I. (1984). Territory economics. In *Behavioural Ecology: an evolutionary approach*, ed. J. R. Krebs & N. B. Davies. Oxford: Blackwells.

Davis, D. E. (1957). The use of food as a buffer in a predatory-prey system. *Journal of Mammalogy*, 38, 466–72.

Davis, J. L. & Jensen, R. A. (1976). The development of passive and active avoidance learning in the cat. *Developmental Psychobiology*, 9, 175–9.

Deag, J. M., Lawrence, C. E. & Manning, A. (1987). The consequences of differences in litter size for the nursing cat and her kittens. *Journal of Zoology (London)*, 213, 153–79.

De Boer, J. B. (1977). Dominance relations in pairs of domestic cats. *Behaviour Processes*, 2, 227–42.

Denenberg, V. H. (1970). Experimental programming of life histories and the creation of individual differences. In *Effects of early Experience*, ed. M. R. Jones. Coral Gables: University of Miami Press.

Dennett, D. C. (1983). Intentional systems in cognitive ethology: The 'Panglossian paradigm' defended. *Behavioral and Brain Sciences*, 6, 343–90.

Derenne, P. (1976). Note sur la biologie du chat haret de Kerguelen. *Mammalia*, 40, 531–5.

Derenne, P. & Mougin, J. L. (1976). Données écologiques sur les mammifères introduits de l'île aux Cochons, Archipel Crozet (:46°06′S, 50°14′E). *Mammalia*, 40, 21–53.

Dewsbury, D. A. (1972). Patterns of copulatory behavior in male mammals. *The Quarterly Review of Biology*, 47, 1–32.

Dilks, P. J. (1979). Observations on the food of feral cats on Campbell Island. *New Zealand Journal of Ecology*, 2, 64–6.

Dominey, W. J. (1984). Alternative mating tactics and evolutionary stable strategies. *American Zoologist*, 24, 385–96.

Dunbar, R. I. M. (1982). Intraspecific variations in mating strategy. In *Perspectives in Ethology, Vol. 5*, ed. P. P. G. Bateson & R. A. Hinde. New York: Plenum Press.

Eaton, R. L. (1970). Group interactions, spacing and territoriality in cheetahs. *Zeitschrift für Tierpsychologie*, 27, 481–91.

Eaton, R. L. (1973). *The World's Cats*. Portland, Oregon: World Wildlife Safari Publications.

Eaton, R. L. (1978). Why some felids copulate so much: a model for the evolution of copulation frequency. *Carnivore*, 1, 42–51.

Eberhard, T. (1954). Food habits of Pennsylvania house cats. *Journal of Wildlife Management*, 19, 284–6.

EFFEMS (1984). *Heimtierhaltung in der Schweiz: Wichtigste Daten aus einer Studie der Scope AG Luzern*, durchgeführt 1984 im Auftrag der Effems AG. Zürich: Trimedia Public Relations.

Ehret, G. & Romand, R. (1981). Postnatal development of absolute auditory thresholds in kittens. *Journal of Comparative Physiology and Psychology*, 95, 304–11.

Eloff, F. C. (1973). Ecology and behaviour of the Kalahari lion. In *The World's Cats, Vol. I*. Portland, Oregon: World Wildlife Safari Publications.

Elton, C. S. (1927). *Animal Ecology*. London: Sidgwick & Jackson.

Elton, C. S. (1953). The use of cats in farm rat control. *British Journal of Animal Behaviour*, 1, 151–5.

Erlinge, S., Göransson, G., Hansson, L., Högstedt, G., Liberg, O., Nilsson, N., Nilsson, T., von Schantz, T. & Sylvén, M. (1983). Predation as a regulating factor on small rodent populations in southern Sweden. *Oikos*, 40, 36–52.

Erlinge, W., Göransson, G., Högstedt, G., Jansson, G., Liberg, O., Loman, J., Nilsson, I. N., von Schantz, T. & Sylvén, M. (1984a). Can vertebrate predators regulate their prey? *American Naturalist*, 123, 125–33.

Erlinge, S., Frylestam, B., Göransson, G., Högstedt, G., Liberg, O., Loman, J., Nilsson, I. N., von Schantz, T. & Sylvén, M. (1984b). Predation on brown hare and ring-necked pheasant populations in southern Sweden. *Holarctic Ecology*, 7, 300–4.

Erlinge, S. & Sandell, M. (1986). Seasonal changes in the social organization of male stoats, *Mustela erminea*: an effect of shifts between two decisive resources. *Oikos*, 47, 57–62.

Errington, P. L. (1936). Notes on food habits of southern Wisconsin house cats. *Journal of Mammalogy*, 17, 64–5.

Errington, P. L. (1967). *Of Predation and Life*. Ames: Iowa State University Press.

Ewer, R. F. (1959). Suckling behaviour in kittens. *Behaviour*, 15, 146–62.

Ewer, R. F. (1961). Further observations on suckling behaviour in kittens, together with some general considerations of the interrelations of innate and acquired responses. *Behaviour*, 17, 247–60.

Ewer, R. F. (1969). The instinct to teach. *Nature*, 222, 698.

Ewer, R. F. (1973). *The Carnivores*. London: Weidenfeld & Nicholson.

Fagen, R. (1978). Population structure and social behavior in the domestic cat (*Felis catus*). *Carnivore Genetics Newsletter*, 3, 276–80.

Farsky, O. (1944). Potrava toulavých kocek. *Moravské Prirodovedecké Spolecnosti*, 16, 1–28.

Feaver, J. M., Mendl, M. T. & Bateson, P. (1986). A method for rating the individual distinctiveness of domestic cats. *Animal Behaviour*, 34, 1016–25.

FEDIAF (1982). *The European Pet Food Industry*. Brussels: European Pet Food Industry Federations.

Fennell, C. (1975). Some demographic characteristics of the domestic cat population in Great Britain with particular reference to feeding habits and the incidence of the feline urological syndrome. *Journal of Small Animal Practice*, 16, 775–83.

Fitzgerald, B. M. (1988). Cats. In *Handbook of New Zealand Mammals*, ed. C. M. King. Oxford: Oxford University Press.

Fitzgerald, B. M. & Karl, B. J. (1979). Food of feral house cats (*Felis catus* L.) in forests of the Orongorongo Valley, Wellington. *New Zealand Journal of Zoology*, 6, 107–26.

Fitzgerald, B. M. & Karl, B. J. (1986). Home range of feral house cats (*Felis catus* L.) in forests of the Orongorongo Valley, Wellington, New Zealand. *New Zealand Journal of Ecology*, 9, 71–81.

Fitzgerald, B. M. & Veitch, C. R. (1985). The cats of Hereko-pare Island, New Zealand: their history, ecology and effects on birdlife. *New Zealand Journal of Zoology*, **12**, 319–30.

Fogle, B. (ed.) (1981). *Interrelations Between People and Pets*. Springfield, Illinois: Charles C. Thomas.

Fogle, B. (1983). *Pets and Their People*. London: Collins Harvill.

Folk, G. E., Fox, M. W. & Folk, M. A. (1970). Physiological differences between alpha and subordinate wolves in a captive sibling pack. *American Zoologist*, **10**, 487.

Fox, M. W. (1969). Behavioral effects of rearing dogs with cats during the 'critical period of socialization'. *Behaviour*, **35**, 273–80.

Fox, M. W. (1970). Reflex development and behavioral organization. In *Developmental Neurobiology*, ed. W. A. Himwich. Springfield, Illinois: Charles C. Thomas.

Fox, M. W. (1972). Socio-ecological implications of individual differences in wold litters: a developmental and evolutionary perspective. *Behaviour*, **41**, 298–313.

Fox, M. W. (1974). *Understanding Your Cat*. New York: Coward, McCann & Geoghegan.

Fox, M. W. (1975). The behaviour of cats. In *The Behaviour of Domestic Animals, IIIrd edition*, ed. E. S. E. Hafez. Baltimore: Williams & Wilkins.

Fox, M. W. & Andrews, R. V. (1973). Physiological and biochemical correlates of individual differences in behaviour of wolf cubs. *Behaviour*, **46**, 129–40.

Frederickson, C. J. & Frederickson, M. H. (1979). Emergence of spontaneous alternation in the kitten. *Developmental Psychobiology*, **12**, 615–21.

Freed, E. X. (1965). Normative data on a self-administered projective question for children. *Journal of Projective Technique and Personal Assessment*, **29**, 3–6.

Freedmann, D. G., King, J. A. & Elliot, O. (1961). Critical period in the social development of dogs. *Science*, **133**, 1016–17.

Freye, H. A. (1985). Urban-ökologische Bemerkungen zum Heimtier. In *Die Mensch-Tier-Beziehung*, ed. Institut für interdisziplinäre Erforschung der Mensch-Tier-Beziehung. Wien: Selbstverlag.

Friedmann, E., Katcher, A. H. & Meislich, D. (1983). When pet owners are hospitalized: Significance of companion animals during hospitalization. In *New Perspectives on our Lives with Companion Animals*, ed. A. H. Katcher & A. M. Beck. Philadelphia: University of Pennsylvania Press.

Friedmann, E., Katcher, A. H., Eaton, M. & Berger, B. (1984). Pet ownership and psychological status. In *The Pet Connection: its influence on our health and quality of life*, ed. R. K. Anderson, B. L. Hart & L. A. Hart. Minneapolis: University of Minnesota Press.

Galef, B. G. Jr (1981). The ecology of weaning: parasitism and the achievement of independence by altricial mammals. In *Parental Care in Mammals*, ed. D. J. Gubernick & P. H. Klopfer. New York: Plenum Press.

Gallo, P. V., Werboff, J. & Knox, K. (1980). Protein restriction during gestation and lactation: development of attachment behaviour in cats. *Behavioural Neural Biology*, **29**, 216–23.

Gallo, P. V., Werboff, J. & Knox, R. (1984). Development of home orientation in offspring of protein-restricted cats. *Developmental Psychobiology*, **17**, 437–49.

Geering, K. (1986). Der Einfluss der Fütterung auf die Katze-Mensch-Beziehung. Thesis, Zoology Institute, University of Zürich-Irchel, Switzerland.

George, W. G. (1974). Domestic cats as predators and factors in winter shortages of raptor prey. *Wilson Bulletin*, **86**, 384–96.

George, W. G. (1978). Domestic cats as density independent hunters and 'surplus killers'. *Carnivore Genetics Newsletter*, **3**, 282–7.

Gibb, J. A., Ward, G. D. & Ward, C. P. (1969). An experiment in the control of a sparse population of wild rabbits (*Oryctolagus c. cuniculus* L.) in New Zealand. *New Zealand Journal of Science*, **12**, 509–34.

Gibb, J. A., Ward, G. D. & Ward, C. P. (1978). Natural control of a population of rabbits, *Oryctolagus cuniculus* (L.), for ten years in the Kourarau enclosure. DSIR Bulletin 223. New Zealand.

Gibbons, J. (1984). Iguanas of the South Pacific. *Oryx*, **18**, 82–91.

Goldschmidt-Rothschild, B. & Lüps, P. (1976). Untersuchungen zur Nahrungsökologie 'verwilderter' Hauskatzen (*Felis sylvestris f. catus* L.) im Kanton Bern (Schweiz). *Revue Suisse de Zoologie*, **83**, 723–35.

Goldsmith, H. H., Buss, A. H., Plomin, R., Rothbart, M. K., Thomas, A., Chess, C., Hinde, R. A. & McCall, R. B. (1987). What is temperament? Four approaches. *Child Development*, **58**, 505–29.

Goszczynski, J. (1977). Connections between predatory birds and mammals and their prey. *Acta Theriologica*, **22**, 399–430.

Gottlieb, G. (1971). Ontogenesis of sensory function in birds and mammals. In *The Biopsychology of Development*, ed. E. Tobach, L. R. Aronson & E. Shaw. New York: Academic Press.

Guggisberg, C. A. W. (1975). *Wild Cats of the World*. London: David & Charles.

Guyot, G. W., Cross, H. A. & Bennett, T. L. (1983). Early social isolation of the domestic cat: Responses during mechanical toy testing. *Applied Animal Ethology*, **10**, 109–16.

Haas, A. (1962). Phylogenetisch bedeutungsvolle Verhaltensänderungen bei Hummeln. *Zeitschrift für Tierpsychologie*, **19**, 356–70.

Haas, A. (1965). Weitere Beobachtungen zum 'Generischen Verhalten' bei Hummeln. *Zeitschrift für Tierpsychologie*, **22**, 305–20.

Haltenorth, T. & Diller, H. (1980). *A Field Guide to the Mammals of Africa including Madagascar*. London: Collins.

Hamilton, J. B., Hamilton, R. S. & Mestler, G. E. (1969). Duration of life and causes of death in domestic cats: influence of sex, gonadectomy, and inbreeding. *Journal of Gerontology*, **24**, 427–37.

Hamilton, P. H. (1976). The movements of leopards in Tsavo National Park, Kenya, as determined by radio-tracking. M.Sc. thesis, Nairobi University.

Hamilton, W. D. (1964). The genetical evolution of social behaviour. *Journal of Theoretical Biology*, 7, 1–52.

Harlow, H. F. & Harlow, M. K. (1962). Social deprivation in

monkeys. *Scientific American*, **207** (5), 136–44.

Harrington, F. H. (1987). Aggressive howling in wolves. *Animal Behaviour*, **35**, 7–12.

Hart, B. L. & Barrett, R. E. (1973). Effects of castration on fighting, roaming, and urine spraying in adult male cats. *Journal of the American Veterinary Medical Association*, **163**, 290–2.

Hart, B. L. & Cooper, L. (1984). Factors related to urine spraying and fighting in prepubertally gonadectomized male and female cats. *Journal of the American Veterinary Medical Association*, **184**, 1255–8.

Hart, B. L. & Hart, L. A. (1984). Selecting the best companion animal: breed and gender specific behavioral profiles. In *The Pet Connection: its influence on our health and quality of life*, ed. R. K. Anderson, B. L. Hart & L. A. Hart. Minneapolis: University of Minnesota Press.

Hart, B. L. & Hart, L. A. (1985). *Canine and Feline Behavioral Therapy*. Philadelphia: Lea & Febiger.

Hartel, R. (1972). Frequenzspektrum und akustische Kommunikation der Hauskatze. *Wiss. Zeitschrift Universität Berlin, Math-Nat. R.*, **21**, 371–4.

Hartel, R. (1975). Zur Struktur und Funktion akustischer Signale im Pflegesystem der Hauskatze (*Felis catus* L.). *Biologisches Zentralblatt*, **94**, 187–204.

Haskins, R. (1977). Effect of kitten vocalizations on maternal behavior. *Journal of Comparative Physiology and Psychology*, **91**, 930–8.

Haskins, R. (1979). A causal analysis of kitten vocalization: an observational and experimental study. *Animal Behaviour*, **27**, 726–36.

Heidemann, G. (1973). Weitere Untersuchungen zur Nahrungsökologie 'wildernder' Hauskatzen (*Felis sylvestris* f. catus Linné, 1758). *Zeitschrift für Säugetierkunde*, **3**, 216–24.

Heidemann, G. & Vauk, G. (1970). Zur Nahrungsökologie 'wildernder' Hauskatzen (*Felis sylvestris* f. catus Linné, 1758). *Zeitschrift für Säugetierkunde*, **35**, 185–90.

Hemker, T. P., Lindzey, F. G. & Ackerman, B. B. (1984). Population characteristics and movement patterns of cougars in southern Utah. *Journal of Wildlife Management*, **48**, 1275–84.

Hemmer, H. (1979). Gestation period and postnatal development in felids. *Carnivore*, **2**, 90–100.

Herbert, M. J. & Harsh, C. M. (1944). Observational learning by cats. *Journal of Comparative Psychology*, **37**, 81–95.

Hess, E. H. (1959). Imprinting. *Science*, **130**, 133–41.

Hinde, R. A. & Atkinson, S. (1970). Assessing the roles of social partners in maintaining mutual proximity, as exemplified by mother–infant relations in rhesus monkeys. *Animal Behaviour*, **18**, 169–76.

Hinde, R. A. & Bateson, P. (1984). Discontinuities versus continuities in behavioural development and the neglect of process. *International Journal of Behavioural Development*, **7**, 129–43.

Hochstrasser, G. (1970). Hauskatze frisst Heuschrecken zur Sättigung. *Säugetierkundliche Mitteilungen*, **18**, 278.

Holmes, W. G. & Sherman, P. W. (1983). Kin recognition in animals. *American Scientist*, **71**, 46–75.

Hornocker, M. (1969). Winter territoriality in mountain lions. *Journal of Wildlife Management*, **33**, 457–64.

Howard, R. D. (1978). The evolution of mating strategies in bullfrogs, *Rana catesbiana*. *Evolution*, **32**, 850–71.

Howe, C. (1982). 'Yorkshire kittens rule O.K.!' *Mammal Society Youth News, Number 17*.

Howey, M. O. (1930). *The Cat in the Mysteries of Religion and Magic*. London: Rider & Co.

Hrdy, S. B. (1977). *The Langurs of Abu*. Cambridge, Mass: Harvard University Press.

Hubbs, E. L. (1951). Food habits of feral house cats in the Sacramento Valley. *California Fish and Game*, **37**, 177–89.

Ikeda, H. (1979). Physiological basis of visual acuity and its development in kittens. *Child Care and Health Dev*, **5**, 375–83.

Imaizumi, Y. (1976, 1977). *Report on the Iriomote cat project, Part I & II*. Tokyo: Environmental Agency, Government of Japan. (In Japanese.)

Immelmann, K. & Suomi, S. J. (1981). Sensitive phases in development. in *Behavioral Development*, ed. K. Immelmann, G. W. Barlow, L. Petrinovich & M. Main. Cambridge: Cambridge University Press.

Inselman, B. R. & Flynn, J. P. (1973). Sex-dependent effects of gonadal and gonadotrophic hormones on centrally-elicited attack in cats. *Brain Research*, **60**, 1–19.

Iverson, J. B. (1978). The impact of feral cats and dogs on populations of the west Indian rock iguana, *Cyclura carinata*. *Biological Conservation*, **14**, 63–73.

Izawa, M. (1984). Ecology and social systems of the feral cats (*Felis catus* Linn.). Ph.D. thesis, Kuyshu University, Japan.

Izawa, M., Doi, T. & Ono, Y. (1982). Grouping patterns of feral cats (*Felis catus*) living on a small island in Japan. *Japan Journal of Ecology*, **32**, 373–82.

Jackson, W. B. (1951). Food habits of Baltimore, Maryland, cats in relation to rat populations. *Journal of Mammalogy*, **32**, 458–61.

Janetos, A. C. (1980). Strategies of female mate choice: a theoretical analysis. *Behavioral Ecology and Sociobiology*, **7**, 107–12.

Jehl, J. R. Jr & Parkes, K. C. (1983). 'Replacements' of landbird species on Socorro Island, Mexico. *Auk*, **100**, 551–9.

Jemmett, J. E. & Skerritt, G. (1979). Poster display, Annual Meeting of the American Veterinary Medical Association, 1979.

Jensen, R. A., Davis, J. L. & Shnerson, A. (1980). Early experience facilitates the development of temperature regulation in the cat. *Developmental Psychobiology*, **13**, 1–6.

John, E. R., Chesler, P., Bareltt, F. & Victor, I. (1968). Observation learning in cats. *Science*, **159**, 1489–91.

Johnson, N. H. & Galin, S. (1979). *The Complete Kitten and Cat Book*. London: Hale.

Johnson, R. H., Margolis, G. & Kilham, L. (1967). Microbiology: identity of feline ataxia virus with feline panleucopaenia virus. *Nature*, **214**, 175–7.

Jones, E. (1977). Ecology of the feral cat, *Felis catus* (L.) (Carnivora: Felidae) on Macquarie Island. *Australian Wildlife Research*, **4**, 249–62.

Jones, E. & Coman, B. J. (1981). Ecology of the feral cat, *Felis catus* (L.), in south-eastern Australia. I. Diet. *Australian Wildlife Research*, **8**, 537–47.

Jones, E. & Coman, B. J. (1982). Ecology of the feral cat, *Felis catus* (L.) in South Eastern Australia. III. Home ranges and population ecology in semi-arid North West Victoria. *Australian Wildlife Research*, **9**, 409–20.

Jung, C. G. (1959). *The Archetypes and the Collective Unconscious*. New York: Pantheon.

Kagan, J. (1984). *The Nature of the Child*. New York: Basic Books.

Karl, B. J. & Best, H. A. (1982). Feral cats on Stewart Island: their foods and their effects on kakapo. *New Zealand Journal of Zoology*, **9**, 287–94.

Karsh, E. B. (1983a). The effects of early handling on the development of social bonds between cats and people. In *New Perspectives on Our Lives with Companion Animals*, ed. A. H. Katcher & A. M. Beck. Philadelphia: University of Pennsylvania Press.

Karsh, E. B. (1983b). The effects of early and late handling on the attachment of cats to people. In *The Pet Connection, Conference Proceedings*, ed. R. K. Anderson, B. L. Hart & L. A. Hart, St Paul: Globe Press.

Karsh, E. B. (1984). Factors influencing the socialization of cats to people. In *The Pet Connection: its influence on our health and quality of life*, ed. R. K. Anderson, B. L. Hart & L. A. Hart. Minneapolis: University of Minnesota Press.

Kellert, S. R. (1984). Attitudes towards animals: age-related development among children. In *The Pet Connection: its influence on our health and quality of life*, ed. R. K. Anderson, B. L. Hart & L. A. Hart. Minneapolis: University of Minnesota Press.

Kerby, G. (1984). Small cats. In *The Encyclopaedia of Mammals, Vol. I*, ed. D. Macdonald. London: George Allen & Unwin.

Kerby, G. (1987). The social organisation of farm cats (*Felis catus* L.). D.Phil. thesis, University of Oxford.

Kidd, A. H., Kelley, H. T. & Kidd, R. M. (1984). Personality characteristics of horse, turtle, snake, and bird owners. In *The Pet Connection: its influence on our health and quality of life*, ed. R. K. Anderson, B. L. Hart & L. A. Hart. Minneapolis: University of Minnesota Press.

Kirk, G. (1967). Werden Spitzmäuse (Soricidae) von der Hauskatze (*Felis catus*) erbeutet und gefressen? *Säugetierkundliche Mitteilungen*, **15**, 169–70.

Kirkpatrick, R. B. & Rauzon, M. J. (1986). Foods of feral cats *Felis catus* on Jarvis and Howland Islands, central Pacific Ocean. *Biotropica*, **18**, 72–5.

Kitchings, J. T. & Story, J. D. (1984). Movements and dispersal of bobcats in East Tennessee. *Journal of Wildlife Management*, **48**, 957–61.

Klamming, B. (1983). Scandinavian pet environment. In *Nutrition and Behavior in Dogs and Cats: Proceedings of the First Nordic Symposium on Small Animal Veterinary Medicine, Oslo, 1982*, ed. R. S. Anderson. Oxford: Pergamon Press.

Kleimann, D. G. & Eisenberg, J. F. (1973). Comparisons of canid and felid social systems from an evolutionary perspective. *Animal Behaviour*, **21**, 637–59.

Koepke, J. E. & Pribram, K. H. (1971). Effect of milk on the maintenance of suckling behavior in kittens from birth to six months. *Journal of Comparative Physiology and Psychology*, **75**, 363–77.

Kolb, B. & Nonneman, A. J. (1975). The development of social responsiveness in kittens. *Animal Behaviour*, **23**, 368–74.

Konecny, M. J. (1983). Behavioural ecology of feral house cats in the Galapagos Islands, Ecuador. Ph.D. thesis, University of Florida, Gainsville.

Konrad, K. W. & Bagshaw, M. (1970). Effects of novel stimuli on cats reared in a restricted environment. *Journal of Comparative Physiology and Psychology*, **70**, 157–64.

Krutch, J. W. (1961). *The World of Animals*. New York: Simon & Schuster.

Kruuk, H. (1972). Surplus killing by carnivores. *Journal of Zoology (London)*, **166**, 233–44.

Kruuk, H. (1976). Functional aspects of social hunting in carnivores. In *Function and Evolution in Behaviour*, ed. G. Baerends, A. Manning & C. Beer. London: Oxford University Press.

Kruuk, H. (1978). Spatial organisation and territorial behaviour of the European badger, *Meles meles*. *Journal of Zoology (London)*, **184**, 1–19.

Kuo, Z. Y. (1930). The genesis of the cat's response to the rat. *Journal of Comparative Psychology*, **11**, 1–35.

Kuo, Z. Y. (1938). Further study on the behavior of the cat toward the rat. *Journal of Comparative Psychology*, **25**, 1–8.

Kuo, Z. Y. (1960). Studies on the basic factors in animal fighting. VII. Interspecies coexistence in mammals. *Journal of Genetic Psychology*, **97**, 211–25.

Kuo, Z. Y. (1967). *The Dynamics of Behavior Development: an epigenetic view*. New York: Random House.

Langeveld, M. & Niewold, F. (1985). Aspects of a feral cat (*Felis catus* L.) population on a Dutch island. In *Proc. XVIIth Congress International Union of Game Biologists*.

Larson, M. A. & Stein, B. E. (1984). The use of tactile and olfactory cues in neonatal orientation and localization of the nipple. *Developmental Psychobiology*, **17**, 423–36.

Latimer, H. B. & Ibsen, H. L. (1932). The postnatal growth in body weight of the cat. *Anatomical Record*, **52**, 1–5.

Laundré, J. (1977). The daytime behaviour of domestic cats in a free-roaming population. *Animal Behaviour*, **25**, 990–8.

Laurie, A. (1983). Marine iguanas in Galapagos. *Oryx*, **17**, 18–25.

Lawrence, C. W. (1981). Individual differences in the mother–kitten relationship in the domestic cat, *Felis catus*. Ph.D. thesis, University of Edinburgh.

Leitch, I., Hytten, F. E. & Billewicz, W. Z. (1959). The maternal and neonatal weights of some mammalia. *Proceedings of the Zoological Society, London*, **133**, 11–28.

Lehner, P. (1979). *Handbook of Ethological Methods*. Holland: Van Nostrand-Rheinohold.

Levinson, B. M. (1961). The dog as co-therapist. *Mental Hygiene*, **46**, 59–65.

Levinson, B. M. (1983). The future of research into relationships between people and their animal companions. In *New Perspectives on Our Lives with Companion Animals*, ed. A. H. Katcher & A. M. Beck. Philadelphia: University of

Pennsylvania Press.

Leyhausen, P. (1954). Die Entdeckung der relativen Koordination: Ein Beitrag zur Annäherung von Physiologie und Psychologie. *Studium Generale*, 7, 45–60.

Leyhausen, P. (1956a). Verhaltensstudien an Katzen. *Zeitschrift für Tierpsychologie Beiheft*, 2, 1–120.

Leyhausen, P. (1956b). *Verhaltensstudien an Katzen*. Berlin: Paul Parey.

Leyhausen, P. (1956c). Das Verhalten der Katzen (Felidae). *Handbuch der Zoologie* VIII (10), 1.34.

Leyhausen, P. (1965a). Ueber die Funktion der relativen Stimmungshierarchie (dargestellt am Biespiel der phylogenetischen und ontogenetischen Entwicklung des Beutefangs von Raubtieren). *Zeitschrift für Tierpsychologie*, 22, 412–94.

Leyhausen, P. (1965b). The communal organization of solitary mammals. *Symposia of the Zoological Society of London*, 14, 249–63.

Leyhausen, P. (1979). *Cat Behavior: The Predatory and Social Behavior of Domestic and Wild Cats*. New York: Garland STPM Press.

Leyhausen, P. (1985a). The cat who walks by himself. In *Leaders in the Study of Animal Behavior: Autobiographical Perspectives*, ed. D. A. Dewsbury. Lewisburg, PA: Bucknell University Press.

Leyhausen, P. (1985b). The image of the cat: mirror of people. In *The Human–Pet Relationshio: Proceedings of the International Symposium*. Vienna: Austrian Academy of Sciences/IEMT.

Leyhausen, P. & Wolff, R. (1959). Das Revier einer Hauskatze. *Zeitschrift für Tierpsychologie*, 16, 666–70.

Liberg, O. (1980). Spacing patterns in a population of rural free roaming domestic cats. *Oikos*, 35, 336–49.

Liberg, O. (1981). Predation and social behaviour in a population of domestic cats: an evolutionary perspective. Ph.D. thesis, University of Lund, Sweden.

Liberg, O. (1982a). Hunting efficiency and prey impact by a free-roaming house cat population. *Transactions of the International Congress of Game Biology*, 14, 269–75.

Liberg, O. (1982b). Home range and territoriality in free ranging house cats. *Third International Theriological Congress, Helsinki, 1982*.

Liberg, O. (1983). Courtship behaviour and sexual selection in the domestic cat. *Applied Animal Ethology*, 10, 117–32.

Liberg, O. (1984). Home range and territoriality in free ranging house cats. *Acta Zoologica Fennica*, 171, 283–5.

Liche, H. (1939). Oestrous cycle in the cat. *Nature*, 143, 900.

Litvaitis, J. A., Sherburne, J. A. & Bissonette, J. A. (1986). Bobcat habitat use and home range size in relation to prey density. *Journal of Wildlife Management*, 50, 110–17.

Llewellyn, L. M. & Uhler, F. M. (1952). The foods of fur animals of the Patuxent Research Refuge, Maryland. *American Midland Naturalist*, 48, 193–203.

Lorenz, K. (1935). Der Kumpan in der Umwelt des Vogels. *Zeitschrift für Ornithologie*, 83, 137–213, 289–413.

Lorenz, K. (1937). The companion in the bird's world. *Auk*, 54, 245–73.

Lorenz, K. (1940). Durch Domestikation verursachte Störungen des arteigenen Verhaltens. *Zeitschrift für angewandte Psychologie und Charakterkunde*, 59, 1–81.

Lorenz, K. (1954). *Man Meets Dog*. London: Methuen.

Loxton, H. (1981). *Cats*. London: Kingfisher.

Loxton, H. (1983). *Cats*. London: Granada.

Lüps, P. (1972). Untersuchungen an streunenden Hauskatzen im Kanton Bern. *Naturhistorisches Museum Bern, Kleine Mitteilungen*, 4, 1–8.

Lüps, P. (1976). Hauskatzen in Feld und Wald: Ihre rechtliche Stellung und Rolle als Beutemacher. *Natur und Mensch*, 18, 172–5.

Lüps, P. (1984). Beobachtungen zur Fellfärbung bei erlegten freilaufenden Hauskatzen, *Felis sylvestris f. catus*, aus dem schweizerischen Mittelland. *Säugetierkundliche Mitteilungen*, 31, 271–3.

Lundberg, U. (1980). Experimentelle Ergebnisse zu Normen und Leistungsprinzipien des Beutesuchverhaltens von Hauskatzen. *Zeitschrift für Psychologie*, 188, 430–49.

Macbeth, G. & Booth, M. (1979). *The Book of Cats*. London: Penguin.

Macdonald, D. W. (1981). The behavioural ecology of farm cats. In *The Ecology and Control of Feral Cats*, ed. Universities Federation for Animal Welfare. Potters Bar: Universities Federation for Animal Welfare.

Macdonald, D. W. (1983). The ecology of carnivore social behaviour. *Nature*, 301, 379–89.

Macdonald, D. W. (1985). The carnivores: Order Carnivora. In *Mammalian Social Odours*, ed. R. E. Brown & D. W. Macdonald. Oxford: Oxford University Press.

Macdonald, D. W. & Apps, P. J. (1978). The social behaviour of a group of semi-dependent farm cats, *Felis catus*: a progress report. *Carnivore Genetics Newsletter*, 3, 256–68.

Macdonald, D. W., Apps, P. J., Carr, G. M. & Kerby, G. (1987). Social dynamics, nursing coalitions and infanticide among farm cats, *Felis catus*. *Advances in Ethology* (suppl. to *Ethology*), 28, 1–64.

Macdonald, D. W. & Moehlman, P. D. (1982). Cooperation, altruism, and restraint in the reproduction of carnivores. In *Perspectives in Ethology*, ed. P. P. G. Bateson & P. Klopfer. London: Plenum Press.

Mackenzie, D. A. (1913). *Egyptian Myth and Legend*. London: Gresham Publishing.

Maddock, I. T. (1983). Lesser long-eared bat *Nyctophilus geoffroyi*. In *The Australia Museum Complete Book of Mammals*, ed. R. Strahan. Sydney: Angus & Robertson.

Maes, J. P. (1939). Neural mechanisms of sexual behaviour in the female cat. *Nature*, 144, 598–9.

Mahood, I. T. (1980). The feral cat. *Post-Graduate Committee in Veterinary Science, University of Sydney, Proceedings No. 53*, 447–56.

Marshall, W. H. (1961). A note on the food habits of feral cats on Little Barrier Island, New Zealand. *New Zealand Journal of Science*, 4, 822–4.

Martin, P. (1982). Weaning and behavioural development in the cat. Ph.D. thesis, University of Cambridge, UK.

Martin, P. (1984a). The (four) whys and wherefores of play in cats: a review of functional, evolutionary, developmental and causal issues. In *Play in Animals and Humans*, ed. P. K. Smith. Oxford: Basil Blackwell.

Martin, P. (1984b). The meaning of weaning. *Animal Behaviour*, 32, 1257–9.

Martin, P. (1985). Weaning: A Reply to Counsilman and Lim. *Animal Behaviour*, 33, 1024–6.

Martin, P. (1986). An experimental study of weaning in the domestic cat. *Behaviour*, 99, 221–49.

Martin, P. & Bateson, P. (1985a). The ontogeny of locomotor play in the domestic cat. *Animal Behaviour*, 33, 502–10.

Martin, P. & Bateson P. (1985b). The influence of experimentally manipulating a component of weaning on the development of play in domestic cats. *Animal Behaviour*, 33, 511–18.

Martin, P. & Caro, T. M. (1985). On the function of play and its role in behavioral development. *Advances in the Study of Behaviour*, 15, 59–103.

Martin, P. & Kraemer, H. C. (1987). Individual differences in behaviour and their statistical consequences. *Animal Behaviour*, 35, 1366–75.

McCord, C. M. & Cardoza, J. E. (1982). Bobcat and lynx. In *Wild Mammals of North America: biology, management, and economics*, ed. J. A. Chapman & G. A. Fieldhamer. Baltimore: Johns Hopkins University Press.

McDougall, Ch. (1981, 1982, 1983). Long Term Tiger Monitoring Project, Royal Chitwan National Park. Reports 1–3, unpublished.

McGinty, D. J., Stevenson, M., Hoppenbrouwers, T., Harper, R. M., Sterman, M. B. & Hodgman, J. (1977). Polygraphic studies of kitten development: sleep state patterns. *Developmental Psychobiology*, 10, 455–69.

McMurray, F. B. & Sperry, C. C. (1941). Food of feral house cats in Oklahoma, a progress report. *Journal of Mammalogy*, 22, 185–90.

Mead, C. J. (1982). Ringed birds killed by cats. *Mammals Review*, 12, 183–6.

Mech, L. D. (1970). *The Wolf: the ecology and behavior of an endangered species*. New York: Natural History Press.

Mech, L. D. (1980). Age, sex, reproduction, and spatial organization of lynxes colonizing Northeastern Minnesota. *Journal of Mammalogy*, 61, 261–7.

Meier, G. W. (1961). Infantile handling and development in Siamese kittens. *Journal of Comparative Physiology and Psychology*, 54, 284–6.

Meier, M. & Turner, D. C. (1985). Reactions of home cats during encounters with a strange person: evidence for two personality types. *Journal of the Delta Society*, 2, 45–53.

Mendl, M. T. (1986). Effects of litter size and sex of young on behavioural development in domestic cats. Ph.D. thesis, University of Cambridge.

Mertens, C. & Turner, D. C. (1988). Experimental analysis of human-cat interactions: factors influencing the behavior of both partners during first encounters. *Anthrozoös*, in press.

Merton, D. V. (1970). Kermadec Islands expedition reports: a general account of birdlife. *Notornis*, 17, 147–99.

Mery, F. (1967). *The Life, History and Magic of the Cat*. Transl. by E. Street. London: Hamlyn.

Mery, F. (1968). *The Life, History, and Magic of the Cat*. New York: Grosset & Dunlap, Inc.

Messent, P. R. & Horsfield, S. (1985). Pet population and the pet–owner bond. In *The Human–Pet Relationship. Proceedings of the International Symposium*. Vienna: Austrian Academy of Sciences/ IEMT. Oest. Akad. Wissenschaft/ IEMT.

Messent, P. R. & Serpell, J. A. (1981). A historical and biological view of the pet–owner bond. In *Interrelations between People and Pets*, ed. B. Fogle. Springfield, Illinois: Charles C. Thomas.

Metcalfe, C. (1980). *Cats*. London: Hamlyn.

Michael, R. P. (1958). Sexual behaviour and the vaginal cycle in the cat. *Nature*, 181, 567–8.

Michael, R. P. (1961). Observations upon the sexual behaviour of the domestic cat (*Felis catus* L.) under laboratory conditions. *Behaviour*, 18, 1–24.

Miller, B. & Mullette, K. J. (1985). Rehabilitation of an endangered Australian bird: the Lord Howe Island woodhen *Tricholimnas sylvestris* (Sclater). *Biological Conservation*, 34, 55–95.

Miller, S. D. & Speake, D. W. (1979). Progress report: Demography and home range of the bobcat in South Alabama. *National Wildlife Federation Science Technology Series*, 6, 123–4.

Mills, M. G. L. (1982). The mating system of the brown hyaena, *Hyaena brunnea*, in the Southern Kalahari. *Behavioral Ecology and Sociobiology*, 10, 131–6.

Moelk, M. (1979). The development of friendly approach behavior in the cat: a study of kitten–mother relations and the cognitive development of the kitten from birth to eight weeks. In *Advances in the Study of Behaviour, Vol. 10*, ed. J. S. Rosenblatt, R. A. Hinde, C. Beer & M. Busnel. New York: Academic Press.

Mohr, C. O. & Stumpf, W. A. (1966). Comparison of methods for calculating areas on animal activity. *Journal of Wildlife Management*, 30, 293–304.

Morris, D. (1986). *Catwatching*. London: Cape.

Muckenhirn, N. & Eisenberg, J. R. (1973). Home ranges and predation of the Ceylon leopard (*Panthera pardus fusca*). In *The World's Cats, Vol. I*. Portland, Oregon: World Wildlife Safari Publications.

Mugford, R. A. & Thorne, C. (1980). Comparative studies of meal patterns in pet and laboratory housed dogs and cats. In *Nutrition of Dog and Cat*, ed. R. S. Anderson. Oxford: Pergamon Press.

Nader, I. A. & Martin, R. L. (1962). The shrew as prey of the domestic cat. *Journal of Mammalogy*, 43, 417.

Natoli, E. (1983). Behavioural evolution in the feral cat (*Felis catus* L.) as a response to urban ecological conditions. *Monitore Zool. Italiana (N.S.)*, 17, 200–1.

Natoli, E. (1985a). Spacing patterns in a colony of urban stray cats (*Felis catus*, L.) in the historic centre of Rome. *Applied Animal Ethology*, 14, 289–304.

Natoli, E. (1985b). Behavioural responses of urban feral cats to different types of urine marks. *Behaviour*, 94, 234–43.

Necker, C. (1970). *The Natural History of Cats*. New Jersey: Random House.

Nelson, N. S., Berman, E. & Stara, J. F. (1969). Litter size and sex distribution in an outdoor feline colony. *Carnivore Genetics Newsletter*, 1, 181–91.

Neugarten, B. L., Havinghurst, R. J. & Tobin, S. S. (1961). The measurement of life satisfaction. *Journal of Gerontology*, 16, 134–43.

Neville, P. F. & Remfry, J. (1984). Effect of neutering on two groups of feral cats. *Behaviour*, 94, 234–43.

Niewold, F. J. J. (1986). Voedselkeuze, terreingebruik en aantalsregulatie van in het veld oplrerende Huiskatten *Felis catus* L., 1758. *Lutra*, 29, 145–87.

Nilsson, N. N. (1940). The role of the domestic cat in relation to game birds in the Willamette Valley, Oregon. M.Sc. thesis, Oregon State College.

Norton, T. T. (1974). Receptive-field properties of superior colliculus cells and development of visual behavior in kittens. *Journal of Neurophysiology*, 37, 674–90.

Nussbaum, R. A. (1984a). Snakes of the Seychelles. In *Biogeography and Ecology of the Seychelles Islands*, ed. D. R. Stoddard. *Monographiae Biologicae 55*. The Hague: Dr W. Junk, Publishers.

Nussbaum, R. A. (1984b). Amphibians of the Seychelles. In *Biogeography and Ecology of the Seychelles Islands*, ed. D. R. Stoddard. *Monographiae Biologicae 55*. The Hague: Dr W. Junk, Publishers.

O'Brien, S. J. (1980). The extent and character of biochemical genetic variation in the domestic cat. *Journal of Heredity*, 71, 2–8.

Oliver, W. R. B. (1955). *New Zealand Birds*, 2nd edition. Wellington: A. H. & A. W. Reed.

Olmstead, C. E. & Villablanca, J. R. (1980). Development of behavioral audition in the kitten. *Physiology and Behaviour*, 24, 705–12.

Olmstead, C. E., Villablanca, J. R., Torbiner, M. & Rhodes, D. (1979). Development of thermoregulation in the kitten. *Physiology and Behaviour*, 23, 489–95.

Oppenheimer, E. C. (1980). *Felis catus* population densities in an urban area. *Carnivore Genetics Newsletter*, 4, 72–80.

Ory, M. G. & Goldberg, E. L. (1984). An epidemiological study of pet ownership in the community. In *The Pet Connection: its influence on our health and quality of life*, ed. R. K. Anderson, B. L. Hart & L. A. Hart. Minneapolis: University of Minnesota Press.

Owens, M. & Owens, D. (1985). *Cry of the Kalahari*. London: William Collins Sons & Co.

Packer, C. (1986). The ecology of sociality in felids. In *Ecological Aspects of Social Evolution*, ed. D. I. Rubenstein & R. W. Wrangham. Princeton: Princeton University Press.

Packer, C. & Pusey, A. E. (1983). Cooperation and competition in lions. *Nature*, 302, 356.

Pallaud, B. (1984). Hypotheses on mechanisms underlying observational learning in animals. *Behavioural Processes*, 9, 381–94.

Palmer, J. (1983). *Cats*. Poole: Blandford.

Panaman, R. (1981). Behaviour and ecology of free-ranging female farm cats (*Felis catus* L.). *Zeitschrift für Tierpsychologie*, 56, 59–73.

Panwar, H. S. (1979). Population dynamics and land tenures of tiger in Kanha National Park. International Symposium on Tiger, New Delhi, 1979.

Parker, G. A. (1970). Sperm competition and its evolutionary consequences in the insects. *Biological Review*, 45, 525–67.

Parmalee, P. W. (1953). Food habits of the feral house cat in east-central Texas. *Journal of Wildlife Management*, 17, 375–6.

Partridge, L. (1983). Genetics and behaviour. In *Animal Behaviour, Vol. 3, Genes, Development and Learning*, ed. T. R. Halliday & P. J. B. Slater. Oxford: Blackwell Scientific Publications.

Pascal, M. (1980). Structure et dynamique de la population du chat haret de l'archipel des Kerguelen. *Mammalia*, 44, 161–82.

Pavlov, I. P. (1927). *Conditioned Reflexes*. Transl. by G. V. Anrep. London: Oxford University Press.

Pearson, O. P. (1964). Carnivore-mouse predation: an example of its intensity and bioenergetics. *Journal of Mammalogy*, 45, 177–88.

Pearson, O. P. (1966). The prey of carnivores during one cycle of mouse abundance. *Journal of Animal Ecology*, 35, 217–33.

Pearson, O. P. (1971). Additional measurements of the impact of carnivores on California voles (*Microtus californicus*). *Journal of Mammalogy*, 52, 41–9.

Pearson, O. P. (1985). Predation. In *Biology of New World Microtus*, ed. R. H. Tamarin. Special Publication of the American Society of Mammalogists, 8, 535–66.

Pericard, J.-M. (1986). Le rôle du chat dans l'épidemiologie de la rage sylvatique. Importance de la sensibilité au virus et de l'etho-ecologie des chats errants. Vet.D. thesis, Université Paul Sabatier, Toulouse, France.

Pervin, L. A. (1980). *Personality: Theory Assessment and Research*. New York: John Wiley & Sons.

Peters, S. E. (1983). Postnatal development of gait behaviour and functional allometry in the domestic cat (*Felis catus*). *Journal of Zoology (London)*, 199, 461–86.

Peters, R. P. & Mech, L. D. (1975). Scent-marking in wolves. *American Scientist*, 63, 628–37.

Pettersson, R. (1968). Mejtodik vid studier av näringsval hos katter. *Särtryck ur Zoologisk Revy*, 29, 1–9.

Pielowski, Z. (1976). Cats and dogs in the European hare hunting ground. In *Ecology and Management of European Hare Populations*, ed. Z. Pielowski & Z. Pucek. Warsaw: Polish Hunting Association.

Pielowski, Z. & Raczyński, J. (1976). Ecological conditions and rational management of hare populations. In *Ecology and Management of European Hare Populations*, ed. Z. Pielowski & Z. Pucek. Warsaw: Polish Hunting Association.

Pitt, F. (1944). *Wild Animals in Britain*, 2nd edition. London: Batsford.

Plomin, R. (1981). Ethological behavioral genetics and development. In *Behavioral Development*, ed. K. Immelmann, G. W. Barlow, L. Petrinovich & M. Mann. Cambridge: Cambridge University Press.

Plomin, R., DeFries, J. C. & McClearn, G. E. (1980). *Behavioral Genetics: a primer*. San Francisco: W. H. Freeman & Co.

Pond, G. & Raleigh, I. (eds) (1979). *A Standard Guide to Cat Breeds*. London: MacMillan.

Prescott, C. W. (1973). Reproduction patterns in the domestic cat. *Australian Veterinary Journal*, 49, 126–9.

Quigley, J. S., Vogel, L. E. & Anderson, R. K. (1983). A study of perceptions and attitudes toward pet ownership. In *New Perspectives on our Lives with Companion Animals*, ed. A. H. Katcher & A. M. Beck. Philadelphia: University of Pennsylvania Press.

Rasa, O. A. E. (1975). Mongoose sociology and behaviour as related to zoo exhibition. *International Zoo Yearbook*, 1975, 65–73.

Rauschecker, J. & Marler, P. (eds.) (1987). *Imprinting and Cortical Plasticity*. New York: Wiley.

Rees, P. (1981). The ecological distribution of feral cats and the effects of neutering on a hospital colony. In *The Ecology and Control of Feral Cats*, ed. Universities Federation for Animal Welfare. Potters Bar: UFAW.

Rheingold, H. & Eckermann, C. (1971). Familiar social and nonsocial stimuli and the kitten's response to a strange environment. *Developmental Psychobiology*, 4, 71–89.

Rieger, I. & Walzthoeny, D. (1979). Markieren Katzen beim Wangenreiben? *Zeitschrift für Tierpsychologie*, 44, 319–20.

Ritvo, H. (1985). Animal pleasures: popular zoology in eighteenth and nineteenth century England. *Harvard Library Bulletin*, 33, 239–79.

Robinson, R. (1977). *Genetics for Cat Breeders*, 2nd edition. London: Pergamon Press.

Robinson, R. (1984). Cat. In *Evolution of Domesticated Animals*, ed. I. L. Mason. London: Longman.

Robinson, R. & Cox, H. W. (1970). Reproductive performance in a cat colony over a 10-year period. *Laboratory Animals*, 4, 99–112.

Rockwell, J. (1978). *Cats and Kittens*. New York: F. Watts.

Rodel, H. (1986). Faktoren, die den Aufbau einer Mensch-Katze-Beziehung beeinflussen. Thesis, Zoology Institute, University of Zürich-Irchel, Switzerland.

Rose, A. B. (1975). Domestic cats that kill wildlife. *Australian Birds*, 10, 12–13.

Rosenblatt, J. S. (1971). Suckling and home orientation in the kitten: A comparative developmental study. In *The Biopsychology of Development*, ed. E. Tobach, L. R. Aronson & E. Shaw. New York: Academic Press.

Rosenblatt, J. S. (1972). Learning in newborn kittens. *Scientific American*, 227 (6), 18–25.

Rosenblatt, J. S. (1976). Stages in the early behavioural development of altricial young of selected species of non-primate animals. In *Growing Points in Ethology*, ed. P. P. G. Bateson & R. A. Hinde. Cambridge: Cambridge University Press.

Rosenblatt, J. S. & Aronson, L. R. (1958). The decline of sexual behaviour in male cats after castration with special reference to the role of prior sexual experience. *Behaviour*, 12, 285–338.

Rosenblatt, J. S. & Schneirla, T. C. (1962). The behaviour of cats. In *The Behaviour of Domestic Animals*, ed. E. S. E. Hafez. London: Ballière, Tindall & Co.

Rosenblatt, J. S., Turkewitz, G. & Schneirla, T. C. (1961). Early socialization in the domestic cat as based on feeding and other relationships between female and young. In *Determinants of Infant Behaviour*, ed. B. M. Foss. London: Methuen.

Rosenblatt, J. S., Turkewitz, G. & Schneirla, T. C. (1962). Development of suckling and related behaviour in neonate kittens. In *Roots of Behaviour*, ed. E. L. Bliss. New York: Harper & Brothers.

Rosenblatt, J. S., Turkewitz, G. & Schneirla, T. C. (1969). Development of home orientation in newly born kittens. *Transactions of the New York Academy of Science*, 31, 231–50.

Rowe-Rowe, D. T. (1978). The small carnivores of Natal. *Lammergeyer*, 25, 1–48.

Ryszkowski, L., Goszczynski, J. & Truszkowski, J. (1973). Trophic relationships of the common vole in cultivated fields. *Acta Theriologica*, 18, 125–65.

Sandell, M. (1969). Development of home orientation in newly born kittens. *Transactions of the New York Academy of Science*, 31, 231–50.

Sandell, M. (1986). Movement patterns of male stoats *Mustela erminea* during the mating season: differences in relation to social status. *Oikos*, 47, 63–70.

Santana, F., Martin, A. & Nogales, M. (1986). Datos sobre la alimentacion del gato cirmarron (*Felis catus* Linnaeus, 1758) en los montes de Pajonales, Ojeda e Inagua (Gran Canaria). *Vieraea*, 16, 113–337.

Schaller, G. B. (1967). *The Deer and the Tiger*. Chicago: University of Chicago Press.

Schaller, G. B. (1972). *The Serengeti Lion: a study of predator–prey relations*. Chicago: University of Chicago Press.

Schaller, G. B. & Crawshaw, P. G. (1980). Movement patterns of jaguar. *Biotropica*, 12, 161–8.

Schär, R. (1983). Influence of man on life and social behaviour of farm cats. Poster, International Symposium on the Human–Pet Relationship, Vienna, 1983.

Schär, R. (1986). Einfluss von Artgenossen und Umgebung auf die Sozialstruktur von fünf Bauernkatzengruppen. Lizentiatsarbeit. Bern: Druckerei der Universität Bern.

Schär, R. & Tschanz, B. (1982). Social behaviour and space utilization of farm cats using biotelemetry. In *Proceedings of the 7th International Symposium on Biotelemetry*, ed. J. D. Meindl & P. Kimmich. Stanford.

Schneirla, T. C. & Rosenblatt, J. S. (1961). Behavioural organization and genesis of the social bond in insects and mammals. *American Journal of Orthopsychiatry*, 31, 223–53.

Schneirla, T. C., Rosenblatt, J. S. & Tobach, E. (1963). Maternal behavior in the cat. In *Maternal Behavior in Mammals*, ed. H. R. Rheingold. New York: John Wiley.

Scott, J. P. (1962). Critical periods in behavioral development. *Science*, 138, 949–57.

Scott, J. P. (1970). Critical periods in the development of social behavior in dogs. In *The Postnatal Development of the Phenotype*, ed. S. Kazda & V. Denenberg. Prague: Academia.

Scott, J. P. (1980). The domestic dog: a case of multiple identities. In *Species Identity and Attachment*, ed. M. A. Roy. New York: Garland STPM Press.

Scott, J. P. & Fuller, J. L. (1965). *Genetics and the Social Behavior of the Dog*. Chicago: University of Chicago Press.

Scott, J. P. & Marston, M. V. (1950). Critical periods affecting the development of normal and maladjustive social behavior in puppies. *Journal of Genetic Psychology*, 77, 25–60.

Scott, J. P., Stewart, J. & DeGhett, V. J. (1974). Critical periods in the organization of systems. *Developmental Psychobiology*, 7, 489–513.

Scott, P. P. (1970). Cats. In *Reproduction and Breeding Techniques for Laboratory Animals*, ed. E. S. E. Hafez. Philadelphia: Lea & Febiger.

Seidensticker, J. C., Hornocker, M. G., Wiles, W. V. & Messick, J. P. (1973). Mountain lion social organization in the Idaho Primitive Area. *Wildlife Monographs*, 35, 1–60.

Seitz, P. F. D. (1959). Infantile experience and adult behavior in animal subjects. II. Age of separation from the mother and adult behavior in the cat. *Psychosomatic Medicine*, 21, 353–78.

Serpell, J. A. (1983). The personality of the dog and its influence on the pet–owner bond. In *New Perspectives on Our Lives with Companion Animals*, ed. A. H. Katcher & A. M. Beck. Philadelphia: University of Pennsylvania Press.

Serpell, J. A. (1986). *In the Company of Animals: a study of human–animal relationships*. Oxford: Basil Blackwell.

Simonson, M. (1979). Effects of maternal malnourishment, development and behavior in successive generations in the rat and cat. In *Malnutrition, Environment and Behavior*, ed. D. A. Levitsky. Ithaca: Cornell University Press.

Simpson, M. J. A. (1985). Effects of early experience on the behaviour of yearling rhesus monkeys (*Macaca mulatta*) in the presence of a strange object: classification and correlational approaches. *Primates*, 26, 57–72.

Sireteanu, R. (1985). Forced-choice preferential looking acuity in very young kittens: a model for human development. *Journal of the American Optometrics Association*, 56, 644–8.

Sitton, L. W., Wallen, S., Weaver, R. A., & MacGregor, W. G. (1976). *California Mountain Lion Study*. Sacramento: California Dept. of Fish and Game.

Slater, P. J. B. (1981). Individual differences in animal behaviour. In *Perspectives in Ethology, Vol. 4, Advantages of Diversity*, ed. P. P. G. Bateson & P. H. Klopfer. New York: Plenum Press.

Smith, B. A. & Jansen, G. R. (1977a). Brain development in the feline. *Nutrition Reports International*, 16, 487–95.

Smith, B. A. & Jansen, G. R. (1977b). Maternal undernutrition in the feline: brain composition of offspring. *Nutrition Reports International*, 16, 497–512.

Smith, B. A. & Jansen, G. R. (1977c). Maternal undernutrition in the feline: behavioral sequelae. *Nutrition Reports International*, 16, 513–26.

Smith, H. S. (1969). Animal domestication and animal cult in dynastic Egypt. In *The Domestication and Exploitation of Plants and Animals*, ed. P. J. Ucko and G. W. Dimbleby. London: Duckworth.

Smithers, R. H. N. (1968). Cat of the pharaohs. *Animal Kingdom*, 61, 16–23.

Spencer-Booth, Y. & Hinde, R. A. (1969). Tests of behavioural characteristics for rhesus monkeys. *Behaviour*, 33, 179–211.

Spittler, H. (1978). Untersuchungen zur Nahrungsbiologie streunender Hauskatzen (*Felis sylvestris f. catus* L.). *Zeitschrift für Jagdwissenschaft*, 24, 34–44.

Sterman, M. B., Knauss, T., Lehmann, D. & Clemente, C. D. (1965). Circadian sleep and waking patterns in the laboratory cat. *Electroencephalography and Clinical Neurophysiology*, 19, 509–17.

Stevenson-Hinde, J. (1983). Individual characteristics: a statement of the problem. In *Primate Social Relationships*, ed. R. A. Hinde. Oxford: Blackwell.

Stevenson-Hinde, J. (1986). Towards a more open construct. In *Temperament Discussed*, ed. D. Kohnstamm, pp. 97–106. Holland: Swets & Zeitlinger.

Stevenson-Hinde, J., Stillwell-Barnes, R. & Zunz, M. (1980a). Individual differences in young rhesus monkeys: consistency and change. *Primates*, 21, 498–509.

Stevenson-Hinde, J., Stillwell-Barnes, R. & Zunz, M. (1980b). Subjective assessment of rhesus monkeys over four successive years. *Primates*, 21, 66–82.

Stevenson-Hinde, J. & Zunz, M. (1978). Subjective assessment of individual rhesus monkeys. *Primates*, 19, 473–82.

Stonehouse, B. (1962). Ascension Island and the British Ornithologists' Union Centenary Expedition 1957–59. *Ibis*, 103, 107–23.

Strong, B. W. & Low, W. A. (1983). Some observations of feral cats *Felis catus* in the southern Northern Territory. Conservation Commission of the Northern Territory, Technical Report No. 9.

Sunquist, M. E. (1981). The social organization of tigers (*Panthera tigris*) in Royal Chitawan National Park, Nepal. *Smithsonian Contributions to Zoology*, 336, 1–98.

Suomi, S. J. (1983). Social development in rhesus monkeys: a consideration of individual differences. In *The Behavior of Human Infants*, ed. A. Oliverio & M. Zapella. New York: Plenum Press.

Tabor, R. (1981). General biology of feral cats. In *The Ecology and Control of Feral Cats*, ed. Universities Federation for Animal Welfare. Potters Bar: UFAW.

Tabor, R. (1983). *The Wildlife of the Domestic Cat*. London: Arrow Books.

Tan, P. L. & Counsilman, J. J. (1985). The influence of weaning on prey-catching behaviour in kittens. *Zeitschrift für Tierpsychologie*, 70, 148–64.

Taylor, R. H. (1979). Predation on sooty terns at Raoul Island by rats and cats. *Notornis*, 26, 199–202.

Thoman, E. B. & Levine, S. (1970). Hormonal and behavioral changes in the rat mother as a function of early experience treatments of the offspring. *Physiological Behavior*, 5, 1417–27.

Thomas, E. & Schaller, F. (1954). Das Spiel der optisch isolierten Kaspar-Hauser-Katze. *Naturwissenschaften*, 41, 557–8.

Thomas, K. (1983). *Man and the Natural World: changing attitudes in England 1500–1800*. London: Allen Lane.

Thompson, W. R. & Melzack, R. (1956). Early environment. *Scientific American*, 194, 30–42.

Thorn, F., Gollender, M. & Erickson, P. (1976). The development of the kitten's visual optics. *Vision Research*, 16, 1145–9.

Thorndike, E. L. (1911). *Animal Intelligence*. New York: Macmillan.

Thorne, C. (1985). Cat feeding behaviour. *Pedigree Digest*, 12, 4–6.

Tinbergen, N. (1951). *The Study of Instinct*. London: Oxford University Press.

Todd, N. B. (1977). Cats and commerce. *Scientific American*, **237**, 100–7.

Todd, N. B. (1978). An ecological, behavioural genetic model for the domestication of the cat. *Carnivore*, **1**, 52–60.

Toner, G. C. (1956). House cat predation on small animals. *Journal of Mammalogy*, **37**, 119.

Triggs, B., Brunner, H. & Cullen, J. M. (1984). The food of fox, dog and cat in Croajingalong National Park, south-eastern Victoria. *Australian Wildlife Research*, **11**, 491–9.

Trivers, R. L. (1972). Parental investment and sexual selection. In *Sexual Selection and the Descent of Man*, ed. B. Campbell. Chicago: Aldine Press.

Turner, D. C. (1985a). Reactions of domestic cats to an unfamiliar person: comparison of mothers and juveniles. *Experimentia*, **41**, 1227.

Turner, D. C. (1985b). The human/cat relationship: methods of analysis. In *The Human–Pet Relationship: Proceedings of the International Symposium*. Vienna: Austrian Academy of Sciences/IEMT.

Turner, D. C. (1988). Cat behaviour and the human/cat relationship. *Animalis Familiaris*, in press.

Turner, D. C., Feaver, J., Mendl, M. & Bateson, P. (1986). Variations in domestic cat behaviour towards humans: a paternal effect. *Animal Behaviour*, **34**, 1890–2.

Turner, D. C. & Mertens, C. (1986). Home range size, overlap and exploitation in domestic farm cats (*Felis catus*). *Behaviour*, **99**, 22–45.

Universities Federation for Animal Welfare (ed.) (1981). *The Ecology and Control of Feral Cats*. Potters Bar: Universities Federation for Animal Welfare.

van Aarde, R. J. (1978). Reproduction and population ecology in the feral house cats, *Felis catus*, at Marion Island. *Carnivore Genetics Newsletter*, **3**, 288–316.

van Aarde, R. J. (1979). Distribution and density of the feral house cat *Felis catus* on Marion Island. *South African Journal of Antarctic Research*, **9**, 14–19.

van Aarde, R. J. (1980). The diet and feeding behaviour of feral cats, *Felis catus*, at Marion Island. *South African Journal of Wildlife Research*, **10**, 123–8.

Van de Castle, R. L. (1983). Animal figures in fantasy and dreams. In *New Perspectives on Our Lives with Companion Animals*, ed. A. H. Katcher & A. M. Beck. Philadelphia: University of Pennsylvania Press.

Van Orsdol, K. (1982). Feeding behaviour of lions. International Cat Symposium, 1982. Kingsville, Texas.

Van Orsdol, K., Hanby, J.-P. & Bygott, J. D. (1985). Ecological correlates of lion social organization (*Panthera leo*). *Journal of Zoology (London)*, **206**, 97–112.

Van Rensburg, P. J. J. (1985). The feeding ecology of a decreasing feral house cat, *Felis catus*, population at Marion Island. In *Antarctic Nutrient Cycles and Food Webs*, ed. W. R. Siegfried, P. R. Condy & R. M. Laws. Berlin: Springer Verlag.

Veitch, C. R. (1985). Methods of eradicating feral cats from offshore islands in New Zealand. In *Conservation of Island Birds*, ed. P. J. Moors. International Council for Bird Preservation, Technical Publication No. 3.

Verberne, G. & De Boer, J. N. (1976). Chemocommunication among domestic cats mediated by the olfactory and vomeronasal senses. *Zeitschrift für Tierpsychologie*, **42**, 86–109.

Verberne, G. & Leyhausen, P. (1976). Marking behaviour of some Viverridae and Felidae: time-interval analysis of the marking pattern. *Behaviour*, **58**, 192–253.

Villablanca, J. R. & Olmstead, C. E. (1979). Neurological development in kittens. *Developmental Psychobiology*, **12**, 101–27.

Voith, V. L. (1980a). Play behavior interpreted as aggression or hyperactivity: case histories. *Modern Veterinary Practice*, **61**, 707–9.

Voith, V. L. (1980b). Therapeutic approaches to feline urinary behavior problems. *Modern Veterinary Practice*, **61**, 539–42.

Voith, V. L. (1983). Animal behavior problems: an overview. In *New Perspectives on our Lives with Companion Animals*, ed. A. H. Katcher & A. M. Beck. Philadelphia: University of Pennsylvania Press.

Voith, V. L. (1985). Attachment of people to companion animals. *Veterinary Clinics of North America*, **15**, 289–95.

Von Uexküll, J. (1921). *Umwelt und Innenwelt der Tiere*. 2nd edition. Berlin.

Ward, R. M. P. & Krebs, C. J. (1985). Behavioural responses of lynx to declining snowshoe hare abundance. *Canadian Journal of Zoology*, **63**, 2817–24.

Warner, R. E. (1985). Demography and movements of free-ranging domestic cats in rural Illinois. *Journal of Wildlife Management*, **49**, 340–6.

Waser, P. M. & Wiley, R. H. (1979). Mechanisms and evolution of spacing in animals. In *Handbook of Behavioral Neurobiology, Vol. 3*, ed. P. Marler & J. G. Vandenbergh. New York: Plenum Press.

Watson, D. L. (1980). Immunological functions of the mammary gland and its secretions – comparative review. *Australian Journal of Biological Science*, **33**, 403–22.

West, M. J. (1974). Social play in the domestic cat. *American Zoologist*, **14**, 427–36.

West, M. J. (1979). Play in domestic kittens. In *The Analysis of Social Interactions*, ed. R. B. Cairns. Hillsdale, New Jersey: Lawrence Erlbaum.

Whalen, R. E. (1963). Sexual behaviour of cats. *Behaviour*, **20**, 321–42.

Wildt, D. E., Guthrie, S. & Seager, S. W. (1978). Ovarian and behavioural cyclicity of the laboratory maintained cat. *Hormones and Behaviour*, **10**, 251–7.

Wilkinson, F. & Dodwell, P. C. (1980). Young kittens can learn complex visual pattern discriminations. *Nature*, **284**, 258–9.

Williams, G. C. (1975). *Sex and Evolution*. Princeton: Princeton University Press.

Wilson, C. & Weston, E. (1947). *The Cats of Wildcat Hill*. New York: Duell, Sloan & Pearce.

Wilson, E. O. (1975). *Sociobiology*. Cambridge, Mass.: Belknap, Harvard University Press.

Wilson, M., Warren, J. M. & Abbott, L. (1965). Infantile stimulation, activity, and learning by cats. *Child Development*, **36**, 843–53.

Windle, W. F. & Fish, M. W. (1932). The development of the vestibular righting reflex in the cat. *Journal of Comparative Neurology*, **54**, 85–96.

Winegarner, M. S. (1985). Pugmarks and the biology of the bobcat, *Lynx rufus*. *Zeitschrift für Saugetierkunde*, **50**, 166–74.

Winer, B. (1962). Statistical principles in experimental design. *Development*, **36**, 843–53.

Winslow, C. (1938). Observations of dominance-subordination in cats. *Journal of Genetic Psychology*, **52**, 425–8.

Wright, M. & Walters, S. (1980). *The Book of the Cat*. New York: Summit Books.

Wyrwicka, W. (1978). Imitation of mother's inappropriate food preference in weanling kittens. *Pavlovian Journal of Biological Science*, **13**, 55–72.

Wyrwicka, W. & Long, A. M. (1980). Observations on the initiation of eating of new food by weanling kittens. *Pavlovian Journal of Biological Science*, **15**, 115–22.

Yasuma, Sh. (1981). Feeding behaviour of Iriomote cat (*Prionailurus iriomotensis* Imaizumi 1967). *Bull. Tokyo Univ. Forests*, **70**, 81–140. (In Japanese.)

Zeuner, F. E. (1963). *A History of Domesticated Animals*. London: Hutchinson. New York: Harper & Row.

Zezulak, D. S. & Schwab, R. G. (1979). A comparison of density, home range and habitat utilization of bobcat at Lava Beds and Joshua Tree National Monuments, California. *National Wildlife Federation Sci. Tech. Series*, **6**, 74–9.

Index

Page numbers in italics refer to illustrations, figures and tables

Abyssinian cat, 169
acoustic cues in hunting, 113
acquired behaviour, 22
active avoidance, 12
    sociability, 73–4
activity level, 170
    of kittens, 186
    in placing cats with owners, 174
adaptation, behavioural, 58
African wild cat, 194
age–sex class distinctions, 75–8
aggression,
    at cat shows, 51
    between social partners, 185
    and context of behavioural style, 51
    during weaning, 28, 35
    of females during mating, 101
    interaction rate, 76
    in isolated cats, 163
    male, 52
    of mother cats, 25, 35
    in play, 189
    reduction of male to kittens, 108
    in social groups, 70, 71, 184
    social interaction, 75
air-righting reaction, 11
allomarking, 71
allomaternal behaviour, 80
alternative tactics of behaviour, 52

ambushing, 115
angling behaviour, 59
animal-facilitated therapy, 171
anthropomorphism, 187
anxiety, 50
appearance of cat, 173–4
archaeological remains, 151, 152
artificial
    brooder, 18
    separation of kittens from mother, 18
attitudes to cats, 155–7, 180–1
auditory system of kitten, 9
autonomic response in isolated cats, 49
autonomy of behaviour, 58
avoidance behaviour, 12, 69, 71

Baerends, G. P., 58
Bastet, 153, 154
Bay lynx, 62
behavioural
    changes during development, 10
    profile, 78
    recording, 44–5, 46
binary discrimination, 115
bird
    hunting, 112, 113, 189
    population and effect of predation, 131,
        141–3
birth weight, 9, 32

bob-tailed cat, 156
bob-cat, 62, 68
    range size, 96
body posture, 38
    direct behavioural recording, 46
    in hunting, 112
    of mother cat, 26, 27
body-righting reaction, 11
bodyweight,
    of kittens, 33, 34
    of males, 25, 32–3
    of mothers, 34
boredom, 183, 185
brain,
    growth deficit and malnutrition, 20
    weight, 11
breed characteristics, 48
breeders and effect on socialisation, 186
breeding,
    experience, 4
    season, 88
burrows and hunting techniques, 112, 113

call,
    of kittens, 26
    of mother cats, 27
    ultrasonic, 28
carrion, 126–7

217

castration, 116–17
  age at, 187
  effects on cat personality, 181
  significance, 186–7
Cat Behaviour, 3, 193
Cat Watching, 194
cat-to-person attachment, 166–8; *see also*
    human– cat relationship
  feeding behaviour, 168
  later experiences, 168
characteristics of behaviour, 46, 47
cheetahs, 61
chemical stimuli sensing, 196
choice of cat, 173–4
classification, 151
claw removal, 188
climbing, 188
coat colour, 20, 173, 174
  and deafness, 48
colonies,
  of farm cats, 4
  on oceanic islands, 4, 130–2, 141–3
  size, 72
colostrum, 37–8
communal
  denning, 80
  nursing, 24, 37–8, 197
communication,
  in lions, 68
  purring, 26, 194–5
Companion cats, 172–3, 174
  social type, 185
context, effect on behaviour, 51
cooperative behaviour, 197
copulation, 78–9
  behaviour, 102, 106, 107
  females' acceptance, 101
cortisol level, 51
courting behaviour of males, 101, 102,
    104, 106, 107
critical period, 161, 162
cross-situational temperament character-
    istics, 51

deafness, 48
defaecation, 27, 188, 195–6
density of females, 4
desert cat, 62
diet, 123–36
  age of cat, 132–3
  availability, 133, 135–6
  country cats, 125–6
  effect of latitude, 127, *128*
  faecal analysis, 123
  frequency of prey species, 128–30
  gut samples, 123
  island cats, 130
  of kittens, 21
  palatability of prey, 128–30
  prey records, 123, 124
  quantitative studies, 125
  seasonal variation, 133, *134, 135*
  size of cat, 132–3
  studies of food types, *146–7*

town cats, 125–6
direct behavioural recording, 46
disease transmission, 80
diurnal activity, 117
domestication, 4, 152–3
  constraints on behaviour, 44, 181–5,
    187–90
dominance,
  categories of male cats, 88
  hierarchy, 71–2
  introduction of new cat, 189
  and restricted environments, 184–5
  riding up, 185
  scratching behaviour, 195
drive, 60

early influences on behaviour, 14
ears, 113
eating,
  patterns, 117
  prey, 119
Egyptians, 152, 153–4, 159
elimination, voluntary in kittens, 12
embryo, tactile sensitivity, 9
encounters in social groups, 70
energy source, 57
environment,
  adaptation to, 194
  influence on behaviour, 49
equifinality, system theory concept, 13
etymology, 152
European wild cat, 62, 63, 68, 151
  population density, 84
  taming, 151
executive system, 162
experience,
  and adult behaviour patterns, 13–14
  and learning, 60, 61
exploration behaviour of kittens, 28
eye–paw coordination, 12
eye,
  development in kittens, 10–11
  kitten, 9, 10
  shape, 153
  time of opening, 21

faecal analysis, *see* scat analysis
faeces and social odour, 69
farm cats,
  colony size, 72–3
  control of rabbits, 137–8
  effect on rat population, 137, 140
  female social groups, 71
  male social groups, 70
  social interaction, 74–5
  society, 72–80
fearfulness, 50
feeding,
  ecology, 67
  human–cat relationship, 168
feet and social odour, 69
Felis chaus, 151
F. libyca, 62
F. manul, 151

F. margarita, 62
F. nigripes, 62
F. silvestris, 62, 63, 68, 84
F. silvestris catus, 67, 151
F. silvestris libyca, 9, 117, 194
F. silvestris silvestris, 151
feral cats, 4
  caching food, 198
  colony in Rome, 100–1
  conditions for, 194
  diet, 125–6
  diet and prey population, 136
  food sources, 101
  group living, 91
  habits, 83
  hunting efficiency, 115
  infanticide, 108
  population density, 84
  social groups, 68
  social organisation, 23, 24, 64
  spatial requirements, 182
  suckling, 16
  and trapping index of rats, *140*
fighting, 61, 62, 187, 189
Fishing cat, 62, 63
folliculin, 116
food,
  abundance, 84, *85*
  acceptance by kittens, 17
  availability, 4, 68, 69, 133, 135–6
  distribution, 85, 93
  hunting behaviour and availability of,
    116, 117
  preference by kittens and imitation of
    mother, 17
  resources, 90–1
  sources for feral cats, 101
  studies, *146–7*
  supply and social groups, 69, 70
forest hunting grounds, 119
friendliness,
  characteristics of, 185–6
  and early handling, 176
  and handling, 186
  indications, 197
  to humans, 171, *172*

gait of kittens, 11
Garfield, 159
gene expression, 4, 20, 22
genetic
  constitution, 67
  differences between populations, 62
  diversity, 108
  factors in individuality, 199
  influence on behaviour, 20, 21–2, 48, 49
  paternal contribution, 108
  variation, 48, 49
gestation, 9
grass eating, 127
gregariousness, 4
group, 67–8
  living, 69, 90–2
  range, 69, 70

size, 69–70
stability, 91
structure, 69–70
growth,
  and malnutrition, 20
  period, 4
  rate of kittens, 32, 36
  sex differences in kittens, 33

Haas, A., 64
habitats, 67
handling, 49
  in cat-to-person relationship, 166–7
  early and effect on behaviour of kittens, 20
  and friendliness, 176, 186
  kittens, 49, 161, 164–5
  and mother's presence, 167–8
  number of people, 167
  puppies, 163
head-rubbing, 196
hearing, 10
heart-rate, 51
  conditioning in kittens, 12
hierarchies of moods and instincts, 58, 59
historical aspects, 153–7
Historie of Foure-Footed Beastes, 153
home range, 68, 70, 72
  artificial restriction, 181
  characteristics, 89
  dominant males, 95
  food abundance and size, 85
  and hunting patterns, 118–19
  overlap, 92–5, 97–8
  and population density, 89
  seasonal variation in size, 88, 96–7
  size, 85, 88–90
  of unrestricted cats, 180
  of wild felids, 96
hooking behaviour, 59
hormones, 116
house cat, habits, 83
housing conditions for cats, 180
Huc, P. E., 153
human–animal interactions, 171
human–cat relationship, 159–61
  cat's personality, 186
  changes in older cats, 189
  effect of spaying, 187
  problems in, 179, 187–90
  scientific basis, 179–80
humans,
  association with, 4–5
  attachment to cats, 171
  attitudes to pets, 155–7, 180–1
  cat personality and attachment to, 168–71
  choice of cat, 173–4
  cohabitation with cats, 185–6
  expectations of pet, 186, 187, 189
  feeding and cat relationship, 168
  matching cats to, 174
  physical effects of cat ownership, 173
  psychological effects of cat ownership,

173
  quality of life, 173
  relationship of cat with, 185–6
  response of cats to, 46, 47
  social problems of cats with, 189
hunter,
  and predatory behaviour, 117
  and prey catching, 58
hunting, 111–20
  activity patterns, 117–18
  for birds, 112, 113
  by mother and time spent with litter, 24
  contact with other cats, 119
  definition, 111–12
  direct behavioural recording, 46
  distance travelled, 118
  duration of excursions, 116
  effect of castration, 116–17
  and food availability, 116, 117
  individual differences, 115–16
  influence of hunger, 117
  locality, 118–19
  methods, 4, 112–13
  mobile strategy, 115
  opportunist strategy, 113–14
  prey preference, 199
  for rodents, 112
  and sex hormones, 116
  simulation in artificially restricted home range, 183
  and social organisation, 115
  stationary strategy, 115
  strategies, 113–14
  style, 199
  success rate, 4, 114–17
  time for capture, 115, 116
hybridisation, 151

immunity transmission from mother to kitten, 37–8
immunoglobulins, 37–8
imprinting, 161–2
inbreeding, 95
individual behavioural differences, 4, 46
individuality,
  causes, 44, 199
  consequences, 44
  differences between individuals, 42
  in domestication, 156
  evolutionary based approach, 52
  in hunting behaviour, 115–16
  meaning, 42
  measurement, 44–6, 46–8
  methods of study, 42–3
  origins, 48
  perceived, 42–3
  and pet qualities, 181
  physiological basis, 51
  research model, 44
  stability across situations, 51
  sum total of animal's behaviour, 42
infanticide, 80
  in feral cats, 108
information, adaptations for acquiring, 4

initiators of relationships, 75–6, 77
injury and effect on behaviour patterns, 14
innate behaviour, 22
insect hunting, 112
instinct order, 58–9, 60
interactions,
  between farm cats, 74–5
  in colonies, 76, 77, 78
interest for a locus, 112
Iriomote cat, 62
isolation, 49, 163

Japan, 156
Jungle cat, 151
Just So Stories, 57, 152

Kipling, R., 57, 152
kitten,
  activity level, 170
  age and relationship with mother, 30–1
  approaches to mother, 28
  behaviour differences, 39
  dependence, 31
  displaced from nest, 25
  environmental influences on behaviour, 49
  frequency of approaching and leaving, 38
  friendliness, 49, 50
  growth rate, 36
  handling, 49, 161, 164–5, 167–8, 186
  handling prey, 120
  individual differences within litter, 25
  isolated, 163
  number to keep, 185
  predictability of adult behaviour, 169–70
  purring, 195
  rearing conditions, 166
  relationship with mother, 25
  removal from mother, 186
  sensitive period of socialisation, 163–6
  sex ratio, 33, *34*
  sex and size, 33
  social contact, 64
  social interaction, 184
  socialisation, 186
  survival and mother's behaviour, 26
  type of cry, 26

lactation,
  amount of milk produced, 34–5
  bodyweight of mother, 34
  stress on mother, 23, 24, 25
learned performance in kittens, 12
learning, 60, 61
  ability, 200
  in kittens, 12, 17
  modification of innate behaviour, 22
leopard, 63, 68
leukaemia, 187
Leyhausen, P., 3, 193–4
licking, 75
Life Satisfaction Index, 173

limb-placing, 11
lion, 61
  prides, 92
  range size, 96
  roaring, 68
  social structure, 63–4
  synchrony of oestrus, 107
lip-rubbing, 196
literature, anti-cat, 157
litter,
  culling, 35
  discontinuity in weight, 36, *38*
  individual differences between kittens, 25
  kitten size and sex, 33
  mates in social development, 18
  mixed, 24
  sex ratio, 33, *34*
  size, 4, 23, 25
  size and birth weight, 32
  size and mother–kitten relationship, 31, 35
  spontaneous movement, 25
  time with, by mother cat, 28, *29*
litter box, 183
locomotor play, 12
Lorenz, K., 57–8, 160, 161
Lynx rufus, 62, 68, 96

male cats,
  behaviour after castration, 187
  body size, 25, 32–3
  breeders and non-breeders, 79
  courting behaviour, 101, 102, *104*, 106, 107
  dispersion from natal groups, 92
  groups, 70
  home range, 182
  mating system, 24
  odour, 187, 195
  reproductive success, 78
  social organisation, 24
  urine spraying, 69
malnutrition, 20–1
mammal hunting, 112, 113
maternal
  behaviour recording, 46
  care benefits and costs, 25
  condition, 23
mating, 99, 101, 102, 106
  female behaviour, 106, 107, 108
  frequency, 78
  mounting frequency, 107
  number of males to each female, 102, *106*
  season, 88
  success of dominant males, 96
  system, 24, 71
  tactics, 95–6
matrilineal organisation, 80–1
metabolism, *57*
milk,
  reward, 18
  supply, 34
milk production, 4

and bodyweight, 34
and litter size, 32
mobility of kittens, 11
morphology, 151
Morris, D., 194
mother cat,
  approaches to kitten, 28
  hunting behaviour, 116
  parity, 33–4
  relationship with litter, 23
  stressed, 35
  time spent with litter, 28, *29*
mother–kitten relationship, 17–18, 25
mothering styles, 38–9
motor
  abilities, 11
  patterns of play, 14
mountain lion, 96
mounting, 185; *see also* mating behaviour
mouse trails, 112
mummification, 154, 159

natural selection, 52
neighbourhood system, 62
nest
  orientation, 18
  site, 25, 79–80
nipple,
  preference by kittens, 36, 198
  selection by kittens, 31
nocturnal behaviour, 117
noradrenalin, 163
nursing, 11–12
  initiated by kittens, 11–12
  period and presence of other adult females, 4
nutrition,
  of kittens, 11
  of mother, 4, 20
  rehabilitation and effect on behavioural development, 20

object play, 14
observational learning, 17
observer rating of behaviour, 45, 46
obstacle avoidance, 10
oceanic islands, 4, 130–2, 141–3
odour, 68, 69
  of male cats, 187, 195
  response of kittens, 28
  and social groups, 71
  urine, 195
oestrus,
  behavioural patterns, 95
  calling, 71
  claw scratching, 195
  distribution of periods, 102, *103*
  duration, 102
  occurrence and length, 101
  problems to owners, 187
  rubbing with the tail, 196
  synchrony, 37, 101–2, 107
  timing, 107

olfactory stimuli to kitten, 9
organisation of behaviour, 58
orientation,
  behaviour of kittens, 10, 25
  nest, 18
  suckling, 10
  visual, 10
ovulation, induced, 71
owners' reports of behaviour, 45–6

Pallas's cat, 151
Panthera leo, 68
P. pardus, 68
parental behaviour, 76
parity of mother, 33–4
parturition, 25, 26
passive avoidance, 12
paternal uncertainty, 108
patterns of behaviour, consistent times of development, 9
perioral region, 69, 71
persecution, 4, 155, 159
Persian cat,
  coat, 194
  temperament, 169
person–cat attachment, 171–6; *see also* human–cat relationship
  negative attitudes, 176
  problems in development of relationship, 175
  strong relationship, 175
  weak relationship, 175–6
personality,
  of cat, 41–2, 181
  of cat and relationship to humans, 186
  profiles, 174, 180
  rating, 169
pets, 152–3, 155–7
  number to keep, 185
  owners, 180–1
  population, 179
  spatial requirements, 181–2
physiological changes during development, *10*
planned activity, 200
play, 12, 28
  in artificially restricted home range, 183
  changes in, 14
  development and time of weaning, 19
  and handling of cats, 161
  motor patterns, 14, *15*
  and predatory skills, 14–15
  sex differences in kittens, 33
polygyny, 24
population
  density, 67, 69, 70, 72, 84–5
  density and human control, 84
  density of wild felids, 96
  structure, 67
pouncing, 112
  number for prey capture, 116
  and prey type, 115
predation, 188–9
  behavioural development, 13, 14
  on bird populations, 141–3

by kittens, 11
on continental bird populations, 141
correlation of behaviour at different ages, 15–16
equifinality and development of skills, 13
individual variation, 13
on islands, 130–2, 141–3
multiple influences, 21
on rabbits, 137–9
on rats, 137, 140
on rodents, 139–40
skills and experience, 21
on small game, 140–1
and social experience, 17
social influences, 16–17
and weaning time, 19
predator,
defence mechanisms, 114–15
effect on prey population, 137–43
protection from at parturition, 25
predatory behaviour, 4
development in kittens, 27–8, 58
development of skills, 50
direct recording, 46
hungry and satiated cats, 58
organisation of, 58
sex differences, 33
predatory skills,
adult, 13
development, 13
experience of prey, 13, 16
and play, 14–15
teaching by mother, 16–17
presence percentage, 101
prey,
availability, 115
birds, 189
carrying home, 119–20
defensive behaviour, 115
experience of, 115
frequency of species in diet, 128–30
handling, 119–20
identification in gut samples, 124
killing, 119, 120
for kittens, 11, 16–17, 120
location, 113
major groups, 126–7, 130–2
palatability, 128–30
piracy, 120
playing with, 120
populations, 4, 137–43
records in diet analysis, 123, 124
rodents, 188–9
searching for, 112, 115
sharing, 120
size, 114–15, 132
species, 50
types, 115, 116
Prionailurus, 62, 63
Profelis concolor, 63
protection, 154
proximity index, 28
puma, 63
purring, 26, 194–5

rabbits,
control by cats, 137–9
hunting, 113, 115–16
radio tracking, 85
Ragdoll cat, 48, 194
range size,
for females, 85, 90
for males, 85, 88–90
recognition system, 162
recording behaviour, 44–5
Red cat, 194
reflex republics, 60
relatedness of offspring, 108
relative
coordination mechanisms, 60
hierarchy of moods, 61
religious
aspects of persecution, 155, 159
significance, 153–4, 155, 156
reproductive
history, 23
lifetime output, 24, 25
pattern, 67
success, 23, 25, 52
success of females, 79
success of males, 78
respiratory disease, 101
riding up, 185
righting reflex, 9
roamers, 97
rodent hunting, 115–16
Romans, 155
Rome, feral cat colony, 100–1
rubbing, 28, 101, 193, 196
social interaction, 75
running, 11
Russian Blue cat, 48

scat,
analysis, 123, *125*
burying, 195–6
scavenging, 113–14
scent-marking, 69, 72
in mating behaviour, 95
rubbing, 196
scratching, 188, 195
spraying, 195
scratching, 188, 195
floor near food, 198
search strategies, 115
seasonal
activity, 118
variation in diet, 133, *134*, *135*
self-domestication, 65
sensitive period of
behavioural development, 16
socialisation, 161–6, 184
separation distress, 160
serval cat, 59
sex of kittens, 33
sexual
maturity, 11
significance, 156
shelves, 183
shy behaviour, 47

Siamese cat,
behavioural distinctions, 48
temperament, 169
visual system, 20
siblings in social development, 18
sit-and-wait hunting, 112, 115
skeleton, 151
skills, adaptations for acquiring, 4
sleep,
patterns, 11
in social groups, 73–4
social
attachments, 16
avoidance behaviour, 69, 71
behaviour, 4, 72
contact with conspecifics, 189
culture, 65
distance, 64
diversity in domestic cats, 65
dominance, 51, 52; *see also* dominance
experience, 17
gatherings, 62
groups, 68, 71, 72
influences on development, 16–18
interaction, 184
interspecific system, 180
odour, 68, 69, 71
partners, 183–5
play, 12, 14
profile, 78
relationships, 67, 70
stress, 184–5
threat stimuli, 12
social organisation,
of domestic cats, 61–2
effect on mother–kitten relationship, 23, 24–5
and hunting behaviour, 115
of wild felids, 62
socialisation, 160
cat-to-cat, 184
sensitive period, 161–6
to humans, 161, 186
to other cats, 185
to other species, 160–1
sociality, 68
in domestic cats, 108, 184
facultative, 119
solitary cats, 68–9
behaviour, 183, 185
territoriality, 93
sound,
conditioned response in kittens, 12
response to, 10
space for pet cats, 180
spacing,
patterns, 4
of solitary cats, 68–9
spatial distribution, 92–5
of male cats, 94
of males around females in oestrus, 101, 102, *105*, 107
wild felids, 96–8
spatial organisation, 67, 68, 72
effect of population density, 84

spatial organisation (*cont.*)
  and feeding, 168
  of females, 168
  of males, 168
  studies, *86–7*
  of wild felids, 96
spatial requirements, 181–3
  behavioural problems, 182, 183
  of feral cats, 182
  minimum, 182
sperm competition, 108
spraying, 69, 71, 187, 188, 195
stalking, 112
stress-induced attachment, 162–3
suckling, 26
  approaches by mother and kittens,
    28–30
  behaviour with age, 31
  behaviour amongst feral cats, 16
  by other mothers, 24, 37–8, 80, 197
  cooperative behaviour, 197
  direct behavioural recording, 46
  discomfort to mother, 35
  during weaning, 28, 35
  initiation, 18, *30*
  intermittent, 12
  litter-mate competition, 18
  mother–kitten relationship, 18
  orientation, 10
  reasons for, 36
  time spent, 15, 26, 32

tactile
  contact-placing, 11

sensitivity, 9
  stimuli to kitten, 9
tail-rubbing, 196
taming, 151–2
teeth,
  changing, 11
  eruption, 11
temperament, 168–71
  inherited, 171, 186
temperature regulation, 11, 14
territorial behaviour, 61, 62–4, 92, 93
territory, 61–2
  breeding, 72
  of solitary cats, 69
The Cat Who Walked by Himself, 57, 152
The Chinese Empire, 153
thermal
  gradient detection in kittens, 11
  stimuli to kitten, 9
thinking capacity, 199–200
tiger, 63, 96
timidity, 165
  rating, 170
Tinbergen, N., 58
Topsell, P., 153, 155–6
transient male cats, 97
trauma, 14
treading movement of kitten, 27
trusting behaviour, 47

urbanisation and pet keeping, 179
urination, 188, 195
  by kittens, 12, 27
urine, social odour, 69
  see also spraying

variability of habits, 9
variation in behaviour style, 52
vestibular system, 9
violence by humans, 101
vision in hunting, 113
visual
  acuity, 10–11
  cell development, 16
  cliff, 10
  cortex, 16
  social stimuli and response of kittens, 28
  system, 9, 20
visually guided
  behaviour, 10, 18
  paw-placing, 10, 11
vocalisation, 26, 48, 101
vomero-nasal organ, 196
Von Uexkull, J., 58, 60, 61

walking, 11
weaning, 11, 27, 28, 198
  body posture, 26, 35
  changes in mother–kitten relationship,
    28
  conditions for, 198
  direct behavioural recording, 46
  introduction of prey, 35
  time and litter size, 35
  time and prey availability, 35
  variations in age, 18–19
wild cat, *see* European wild cat
  felids' social life, 62–5
witchcraft, 155–6, 159
  and irrational fear of cats, 176
woodland hunting grounds, 119